The Effective Prevention and Control of Symptoms in Cancer

The Effective Prevention and Control of Symptoms in Cancer

Edited by

Andrew Hoy FRCP FRCR
Consultant in Palliative Medicine, Princess Alice Hospice, Surrey and
Chairman, Association for Palliative Medicine of Great Britain and Ireland

Ilora Finlay FRCGP FRCP
Professor of Palliative Medicine/Vice-Dean, University of Wales College of Medicine and
Past Chairman, Association for Palliative Medicine of Great Britain and Ireland

Andrew Miles MSc MPhil PhD
Professor of Public Health Sciences, and Editor-in-Chief,
Journal of Evaluation in Clinical Practice,
Barts and The London, Queen Mary's School of Medicine and Dentistry,
University of London, UK

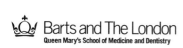

The Royal College
of
Radiologists

Association
of
Cancer Physicians

Association for Palliative
Medicine of Great Britain
and Ireland

AESCULAPIUS MEDICAL PRESS
LONDON SAN FRANCISCO SYDNEY

Published by

Aesculapius Medical Press (London, San Francisco, Sydney)
PO Box LB48, London EC1A 1LB, UK

© Aesculapius Medical Press 2004

First published 2004

British Library Cataloguing in Publication Data
A CIP catalogue record for this book is available from the British Library

ISBN: 1 903044 39 1

Further copies of this volume are available from:

Claudio Melchiorri
Aesculapius Medical Press
PO Box LB48, Mount Pleasant Mail Centre, Farringdon Road, London EC1A 1LB, UK

Fax: 020 8525 8661
Email: claudio@keyadvances4.demon.co.uk

Copy edited by The Clyvedon Press Ltd, Cardiff, UK

Typeset, printed and bound in Britain
Peter Powell Origination & Print Limited

Contents

Contributors

Paul L. R. Andrews BSc PhD, Professor of Comparative Physiology, St George's Hospital Medical School, London, UK

Richard Booton MB MRCP, Department of Medical Oncology, Christie Hospital, Manchester, UK

Shirley E. Crofts BSc SRN, Haematology Nurse Counsellor and Myeloma Nurse Specialist, Department of Haematology, Southampton University Hospitals NHS Trust, Southampton, UK

John Ellershaw MA FRCP, Medical Director, Marie Curie Centre Liverpool, UK

Marie T. Fallon MB ChB MD DCH DRCOG MRCGP FRCP, Senior Lecturer in Palliative Medicine, Edinburgh Cancer Centre, Western General Hospital, Edinburgh, UK

Jacqueline Filshie MB BS FRCA, Consultant in Anaesthesia and Pain Management, The Royal Marsden Hospital, London and Surrey, UK

Rob George MA MD FRCP, Consultant in Palliative Medicine, University College London Hospitals Trust, London, UK

Peter J. Hoskin BSc MD FRCP FRCR, Consultant Clinical Oncologist, Mount Vernon Hospital, London, UK

Samantha Jayasekera DCH MRCGP, Specialist Registrar in Palliative Medicine, St George's Hospital, London, UK

Robin L. Jones MB BS BSc MRCP, Specialist Registrar in Medical Oncology, Department of Medical Oncology, St George's Hospital, London, UK

Anne H. Kendall BM BS MRCP, Specialist Registrar in Medical Oncology, Department of Medical Oncology, St George's Hospital, London, UK

John Keown MA DPhil PhD, Rose F. Kennedy Professor of Christian Ethics, Georgetown University, USA

Albert Koomson MB ChB FRCA, Specialist Registrar in Anaesthesia, The Royal Marsden Hospital, London and Surrey, UK

Iain Lawrie BSc DipMedEd MB ChB MRCGP, Innovative Training Registrar, LOROS Hospice, Leicester, UK

Tim J. Littlewood MB BCh MD MRCP MRCPath, Consultant Haematologist, John Radcliffe Hospital, Oxford, UK

Mari Lloyd-Williams MD MRCGP MMedSci ILTM, Consultant in Palliative Medicine/Senior Lecturer/Director of Community Studies, Liverpool Marie Curie Centre and Royal Liverpool Hospital, University of Liverpool Medical School, Liverpool, UK

Jonathan Martin MMedSci MRCGP Macmillan GP, Facilitator in Palliative Medicine, Department of Primary Care, Royal Free & University College London Medical School, London, UK

Aleksandar Mijovic MBBS PhD MRCPath, Consultant Haematologist / Honorary Senior Lecturer, Department of Haematological Medicine, Kings College Hospital and the National Blood Service, London, UK

Rachel Newman MB ChB MRCP, Specialist Registrar in Palliative Medicine, Department of Palliative Care, Southampton University Hospitals NHS Trust, Southampton, UK

Nicholas Reed MB BS FRCR FRCP, Consultant Clinical Oncologist, Beatson Oncology Centre, Western Infirmary, Glasgow, UK

Jens Samol MD MRCP, Specialist Registrar in Haematology, John Radcliffe Hospital, Oxford, UK

Alastair G. Smith BSc MB ChB FRCP FRCPath, Consultant Haematologist and Honorary Clinical Senior Lecturer, Department of Haematology, Southampton University Hospitals NHS Trust, Southampton, UK

Patrick Stone, MA MD MRCP, Macmillan Senior Lecturer in Palliative Medicine, St George's Hospital Medical School, London, UK

Nicola S. Stoner BSc MRPharmS DipClinPharm PhD, Specialist Principal Pharmacist, The Churchill, Oxford Radcliffe Hospitals NHS Trust, Oxford, UK

Fiona Taylor BSc, Researcher, University of Leicester Medical School, Leicester, UK

Nicholas Thatcher PhD FRCP, Professor of Oncology, Christie Hospital, Manchester, UK

Catherine E. Urch BM BS BSc PhD MRCP, Consultant in Palliative Medicine, The Royal Marsden Hospital and Honarary Senior Lecturer in Neuropharmacology, University College, London, UK

John D. Walley MB ChB MRCP MRCGP, Specialist Registrar in Palliative Medicine, Edinburgh Cancer Centre, Western General Hospital, Edinburgh, UK

Preface

Cancer symptomatology arises from the local and systemic effects of the specific tumour, iatrogenic and personal factors. While these have both short and long term effects on quality of life and acknowledging that cancer is a chronic disease with survival often measured in years, it is now increasingly recognised that clinical care has too often focused preferentially on diagnosis, pathological features of disease, response to treatment and survival, and that the effective control of common symptoms during the course of the disease process is often neglected as a function of a failure to recognise the presence and severity of symptoms on the one hand and a failure to institute effective treatment strategies for the management of common symptoms on the other. Taking these observations into account we present in the current volume detailed, indeed state of the art, discussions of current scientific evidence and expert opinion for the management of some of the most common symptoms which occur during the course of advanced malignancy and which may benefit from direct clinical intervention in the ways described.

The past decade has seen a growing recognition that fatigue associated with cancer and its treatment is a major factor in reducing patient quality of life. A working definition of this type of fatigue would be a "subjective state of overwhelming, sustained exhaustion and decreased capacity for physical and mental work that is not relieved by rest". It is, we believe, true to say that fatigue has now become a major factor in patients' perception of the negative effects of chemotherapy, with a reported prevalence of 60–90% and representing the longest persisting symptom that patients will experience following the treatment of their cancer. In many ways, fatigue in cancer patients has increased in prominence because of the success we have achieved in treating the other, common side effects of therapy such as nausea and vomiting and the advancements made in increasing cancer cure rates and survival times.

Research on cancer-related fatigue has historically tended to focus on the characterisation of the phenomenon using survey techniques and the data that have been generated by drug trials focusing on the treatment of anaemia with recombinant erythropoietin. In contrast, research into the mechanisms of cancer-related fatigue has been limited, although this situation is now beginning to change as a consequence of the development and introduction of methods for the objective quantification of activity. In Chapter One, Kendall, Stone and Andrews provide a comprehensive account of our current knowledge of the physiological and pharmacological mechanisms of weakness and fatigue in cancer, identifying in addition the key questions for ongoing research which include the need to assess the relative contributions of the cancer and therapy (including surgery), the pathophysiological changes induced (e.g. elevation of TNF, anaemia) and the way in which these changes induce the sensation of fatigue and its associated symptoms such as depression and circadian rhythm disruption. The answers to these questions, the authors rightly contend, will allow the development of rational treatments for this and perhaps other protracted consequences of cancer and its treatment such as cognitive disorders and the so-called 'chemo-brain'.

In Chapter Two, Samol and Littlewood review our current knowledge of the management of weakness and fatigue in patients with haematological malignancies. As the authors discuss, a range of interventions may be employed with some efficacy in the amelioration of weakness and fatigue, including the treatment of anxiety and depression and an encouragement to exercise. As in haematological malignancy, weakness and fatigue presents a particular problem in the majority of patients with solid tumours, as Booton and Thatcher proceed to describe in Chapter Three. In lung cancer, for example, anaemia is a particularly common problem and complicated by the fact that patients with this disease often present with co-morbidities which of their nature cause greater sensitivity to the effects of anaemia. Here, as in haematological malignancy, modification of activity and rest patterns, stress management, attention to nutritional status and the use of antidepressants may all contribute to the management of fatigue but these particular interventions have not yet been systematically evaluated in order to allow clinical recommendations for treatment to be confidently made at the time of writing.

So what treatments may be considered particularly effective for the management of cancer-related fatigue? For decades, as Mijovic notes in Chapter Four, red cell transfusion has been the treatment of choice as an intervention designed for correcting cancer-related anaemia and has owed its appeal to a prompt and assured effect with few idiosyncratic reactions and, more recently, a lowered rate of infectious complications, although perhaps in contrast to HIV and HCV, the true risk of nvCJD transmission remains unknown. However, there are now real and increasing concerns in relation to the extent of blood usage within the British NHS in the face of a greatly reduced level of blood donation due to significantly narrowed donor selection and the refusal of appropriate donors to allow screening of donated blood. This is indeed worrying given the modern use of increasingly intensive chemotherapy, haemopoietic stem cell transplantation and the prolonged survival of patients with cancer, all of which contribute substantially to increased blood component usage. Haemato-oncology, for example, has been estimated to utilize 10–15% of donated red cells in developed countries and this may be set to increase.

Blood transfusions have always been viewed as a less expensive option and, currently, the NHS bears most of the cost of this acquiring, handling, processing, storing and administration of blood with the nominal cost to the hospital blood bank being in the region of £100 per unit. With a test for nvCJD likely to be introduced into the health service in due course there will, inevitably perhaps, be a further reduction in blood donation due to donors refusing to be tested and the cost of blood will therefore rise, probably to in excess of £200 per unit in the UK. This will double the cost of transfusions in 3 months of cancer treatment and a more serious problem may be represented by an acute shortage of blood which in any hospital is required for surgical as well as medical use.

So what alternatives are there to red cell transfusion in the face of such difficulties? Certainly, for both haematological malignancy and solid tumours, the use of erythropoietin for anaemia-related fatigue has a considerable evidence base. As the authors of chapters two, three and four discuss, randomized trials of erythropoietin in the treatment of anaemia in patients with a wide variety of cancers have demonstrated that most will benefit from treatment with an associated increase in haemoglobin concentration, a reduction in transfusion need and, perhaps most importantly, an improvement in quality of life. Economic studies comparing blood transfusion and erythropoietin in cancer patients are, however, still lacking, but new studies of the cost-effectiveness of this agent are underway and these, when available, together with the ongoing developments in the formulation of erythropoietin (including once weekly and even longer dosing) and better predictors of erythropoietin response, should translate into considerable improvements in fatigue management.

The use of red cell transfusion and erythropoietin administration to ameliorate cancer-related weakness and fatigue is certainly of considerable importance to effective symptom control but a further, and central issue for consideration, is the effect of prevailing anaemia on tumour biology, progression and the clinical outcome from disease and how these relate to the effectiveness and efficiency of current cancer treatments. In a fascinating contribution, Reed, writing in Chapter Five, describes how historical data have shown that anaemia appears to be an adverse risk factor for cancer outcome. As the author describes, tumours vary in the extent to which they are affected by lowered oxygen availability with squamous cancers, especially of cervix and of head and neck, together with sarcomas, being of particular interest. These tumours are commonly treated by irradiation with or without chemotherapy with good effect. Nevertheless, there are some patients who do not appear to respond to treatment and investigators are increasingly asking why this should be the case.

Anaemia is often associated with other adverse risk factors such as grade of tumour, size, nodal metastases and renal impairment. For over thirty years it has been recognised that the correction of anaemia apparently improves clinical outcome in cancer. Indeed, there is now evidence to suggest that the local microenvironment in the tumour cells is important. Hypoxia appears to exert effects at the molecular level with effects on both tumour suppressor and inducer genes, as well as local growth factors which promote metastasis and angioinvasion, now being documented. We are therefore entering an exciting new era in which validation of the hypotheses on the effects of tumour hypoxia on treatment efficacy and clinical outcome developed forty years ago may be confirmed, allowing us to overcome some aspects of tumour resistance to treatment and thus to maximise disease response to the treatments we use.

Since most cancers, by the time of diagnosis, remain incurable, establishing a reliable method for evaluating overall symptomatic improvement which complements survival data is, as Smith and colleagues point out in Chapter 6, the final chapter of Part 1 of this volume on the management of weakness and fatigue in cancer, an unfulfilled objective in clinical practice and research. These authors argue that quality of life assessment offers the most appropriate means to measure symptomatic improvement.

Comparatively little data are available in published randomised controlled cancer trials to date and a lack of standardization of the instruments which measure quality of life and a limited practicality of such methods in clinical settings are probably the main causal factors to which may be added the effect of the cultural 'gap' between biomedical and psychosocial research. Measurement of quality of life in trials needs to be focused on showing differences for groups of patients receiving different treatments whereas in clinical practice the emphasis is on individual patient quality of life. In the clinic there is potential utility in using quality of life data to improve communication and help decision making as well as enhancing the training of professionals in specialist teams. The authors' prominent experience in drawing up national guidelines for the management of malignant myeloma certainly supports the influence of quality of life in treatment recommendations and is now probably mirrored in the established or developing guidelines for other cancers. As they point out, further work is needed to standardize quality of life instruments and their utility and such developments will need to take place in parallel with the education of clinicians in the importance of quality of life data when making treatment decisions.

We move from Part One of the volume which has been dedicated to a thorough review of the management of cancer-related weakness and fatigue, to Part Two which we have dedicated to a description of recent advances in the understanding, prevention and control of pain in cancer. In the first chapter of this part, Chapter Seven, Hoskin provides a detailed review of the management of bone pain. As the author points out, the effective management of bone pain relies on the appropriate use of analgesics and adjuvant analgesic drugs supplemented by specific treatment to modify the underlying process in the bone with surgery, chemotherapy or hormone therapy, radiotherapy or bisphosphonates representing prominent interventions.

As Hoskin points out, there is a large literature on the use of chemotherapy and hormone therapy for the common cancers producing bone metastases. In breast cancer, for example, the complete response rate for bone pain may be as high as 84% but response times are relatively slow, many patients taking several months to achieve good pain control after chemotherapy or hormone therapy. In contrast, response to anti-androgen therapy in prostate cancer is rapid and typically seen within a few weeks and achieved by over 90% of patients in most studies independent of the specific anti-androgen therapy used with a median duration of 18 to 24 months. As he records, the use of local radiotherapy has relatively recently been subject to a Cochrane review reflecting the results of 13 randomised controlled trials and supporting its efficacy in metastatic bone pain. Wide field radiotherapy (hemibody radiotherapy) has, in contrast, less trial data to support its use. A further, and increasingly popular modality, is radioisotope therapy as part of nuclear medicine approaches to the management of bone pathology and this, as the author describes, has been subject to stringent evaluation with the classical pattern of Phase I, II & III trial data now being available. The most commonly used isotope in the UK, Strontium 89, has been evaluated in dose escalation studies with bone marrow toxicity being its limiting factor and randomised trials against both placebo and external beam radiotherapy showing it to be an effective means of pain control in metastatic bone pain with equivalent pain control to external beam or hemibody radiotherapy. Similar evidence for Samarium is also now available.

Of ongoing interest, as Hoskin discusses, is the use of bisphosphonate therapy in metastatic bone pain which, distinct from its adjuvant or prophylactic role, has also been evaluated in breast cancer in a recent Cochrane review. Four randomised controlled trials were identified which showed an improvement in bone pain with the use of bisphosphonates and two additional trials showed improvement in overall quality of life. One study, as the author describes, has randomised between the use of chemotherapy alone or chemotherapy with bisphosphonates in metastatic breast cancer and interestingly demonstrated an improved incidence of marked pain relief when the combination of pamidronate and chemotherapy was used. The relative role of ibandronate and radiotherapy is currently under evaluation in a multi-centred randomised trial. Optimal management for an individual patient will, of course, encompass the entire spectrum of treatment options that Hoskin has elegantly outlined.

Incident pain is usually understood to be a subtype of breakthrough pain, classically induced by movement or weight bearing. However, the term may also be used to encompass the triad of pain symptoms precipitated by invasion and destruction of bone by cancer: a background dull ache, acute severe pain on movement or weight bearing and spontaneous episodic pain. In addition, breakthrough pain is often used to cover all forms of acute, episodic pain, with no attempt to subdivide into different causes. In Chapter Eight, Urch reviews this confusion in classification and provides a characteristically detailed overview of the evaluation of therapeutics that has been enabled by recent animal models of disease. The difficulty in effectively reducing severe episodic (either movement induced or spontaneous) pain in cancer remains, as Urch points out, an elusive goal and with her we look forward to a foreseeable future where, as the unique nociceptive changes that occur in bone cancer pain are investigated, novel therapeutics will be developed.

In terms of available therapeutics, there is evidence that the opioids provide significant analgesia for neuropathic pain but the dosages required for adequate control are often associated with unacceptable side effects and it is to the formulation and use of clinical strategies for the effective management of this type of pain that Fallon and Walley turn in Chapter Nine. The use of an adjuvant analgesic from either the tricyclic antidepressant class or the anticonvulsant class will control neuropathic pain in one out of three patients (NNT = 3 from systematic reviews), providing direct evidence for their use in this context. Clearly, few pains in cancer are of just one mechanism and opioid/adjuvant combinations are, as the authors make clear, standard therapy unlike in non-malignant neuropathic pain where adjuvants are often used alone. However, despite our best efforts, some types of neuropathic pain remain very difficult to control, leading investigators to assess the merits of alternative approaches, for example, the use of NMDA antagonists. The authors, in addition, usefully discuss currently available evidence which suggests a clinical benefit in the use of topical agents such as capsaicin and lignocaine patches while they are less convinced, on the basis of recently published data and experience, about the usefulness of invasive anaesthetic techniques for resistant neuropathic pain.

While Hoskin in Chapter Seven, Urch in Chapter Eight and Fallon and Walley in Chapter Nine have been concerned to describe and evaluate the scientific evidence for management of pain in cancer deriving largely from quantitative biomedical studies such as randomised controlled trials, meta-analyses and systematic reviews, George and Martin, writing in Chapter 10, are preferentially concerned to discuss the integration of psychosocial and spiritual aspects of pain with medical ones, emphasising the need for an early, holistic, multi-disciplinary approach to the individual patient. The authors usefully enumerate ten distinct though related aspects which must be considered in this context and bring to an appropriate close Part Two of this volume.

Having examined in detail the evidence and opinion base for the prevention and amelioration of weakness and fatigue in cancer and also our current such knowledge for the control of malignant pain, Part Three of this text is devoted to a thorough review of current practice in the prophylaxis and control of therapy-related nausea and vomiting. In the opening chapter of this Section, Jones and Andrews contribute a particularly detailed exposition of the physiological mechanisms which appear to be involved.

Although nausea, the unpleasant sensation associated with the urge to vomit and capable of producing aversive responses, and vomiting, the forceful oral expulsion of gastric contents, are frequently encountered in a number of clinical contexts it is important to remember that they are components of the system which acts to protect the body against accidental ingestion of toxins. Nausea may be accompanied by indications of autonomic activation (tachycardia, cutaneous vasoconstriction, sweating, salivation) and it is certainly true that large increases in plasma vasopressin (ADH) and disturbed gastric motility are consistently associated with nausea, but a causal link has not been established. The precise brain pathways by which this sensation is generated are, as the authors discuss, not yet characterised but imaging studies have implicated the inferior frontal gyrus. In terms of vomiting, it is now recognised that, prior to its onset, the proximal stomach relaxes and a retrograde contraction of the small intestine occurs, both under vagal control. Vomiting then occurs as a result of the forceful compression of the stomach by the diaphragm and anterior abdominal muscles.

From a physiological point of view, the authors describe how the autonomic and somatic motor components are coordinated in the brainstem which receives inputs from four main sources capable of inducing retching and vomiting: the vestibular system, the 'higher' regions of the brain, the area postrema and the abdominal vagal afferents where the precise processes associated with each currently vary. Jones and Andrews are clear that the above emetic pathway(s) could be activated by the tumour and/or therapy, the latter including drugs such as morphine typically administered as part of palliative care. The physical presence of the tumour which may cause, for example, brainstem compression or gut obstruction, or the chemicals and the tumour-related factors released, could act on the above pathways to either induce emesis or to sensitise the pathway to other stimuli. The authors remind us that surgery is a common treatment for cancer and is itself associated with acute nausea and vomiting although radiotherapy and chemotherapy remain the best understood causes of acute emesis in the first 24 hours of treatment of cancer patients.

The authors provide particular insight into the physiological mechanisms of cancer-related nausea and vomiting by describing and considering the now substantial body of preclinical evidence that has implicated 5-hydroxytryptamine (5-HT) released from the enterochromaffin cells in the intestine in the activation of $5\text{-}HT_3$ receptors located on abdominal vagal afferents projecting to the brainstem. As the authors describe, some of the most recent data implicate the neurokinin1 receptor as part of the physiological response, and the development of NK-1 receptor antagonists which have demonstrated efficacy in the control of therapy-related nausea and vomiting show much promise as part of effective clinical strategies.

In the two chapters which follow, Chapters Twelve and Thirteen, Stoner provides a thorough overview of the assessment of severity of therapy-related nausea and vomiting and the indications for and evidentiary basis of current pharmacological approaches to management. Risk factors for chemotherapy-induced emesis include, as the author describes, exposure to previous chemotherapy, female gender, susceptibility to motion sickness, anxiety, sickness during pregnancy, underlying nausea and vomiting, young age and low alcohol intake and patients who experience acute emesis with chemotherapy are more likely to have delayed emesis.

The risk of emesis with radiotherapy varies with the treatment administered and the treatment field is one of the major determinants of emetic risk. Other considerations, as Stoner points out, include the dose of radiotherapy administered per fraction and the pattern of fractionation itself. In terms of classification for the purposes of the clinical assessment of severity, radiotherapy-induced emesis is classified as 'high risk', 'intermediate risk' and 'low risk'. The emetogenic potential of chemotherapy drugs differs slightly though significantly and is classified as 'high', 'moderate-high', 'low-moderate' and 'low' and it is recognised that drug combinations often have an additive emetogenic effect.

Having considered the factors influencing the risk of therapy-related nausea and vomiting, Stoner is subsequently concerned to examine anti-emetic therapy itself.

The immediate goal of anti-emetic therapy is, of course, to prevent emesis completely but despite improvements in the control of emesis over the last twenty years a significant number of patients continue to experience emesis. Factors that need to be considered when choosing an anti-emetic regimen, as she points out, include the emetogenicity of therapy, dose and schedule, the mechanism of action and routes of administration, the type of emesis being treated, that is, anticipatory, acute, delayed, the patient's risk of emesis and the adverse effects of the drugs. Overall, to achieve a significant degree of effectiveness, anti-emetics should be given regularly and prophylactically, remembering that, in general, combinations will prove significantly more effective than the use of single agents.

In terms of the precise pharmacological classes of drugs that have shown the highest degree of effectiveness in the prevention and control of cancer-related nausea and vomiting, Stoner is clear that the serotonin receptor antagonist anti-emetics (5-HT_3 antagonists) and corticosteroids are overwhelmingly two of the most effective classes of anti-emetics of proven use. Moreover, these agents have been observed to have the fewest side-effects and are convenient to use from a dosing perspective. They are recommended in combination for highly and moderately-highly emetogenic chemotherapy regimens and, where possible, should be given orally in single doses. Similar clinical experience has shown dexamethasone to be another agent with one of the most effective treatments for delayed emesis and many colleagues now recommend the dopamine antagonists as useful for maintenance therapy. Generally, if patients fail treatment with a 5-HT_3 antagonist (with or without dexamethasone), many clinical practice guidelines recommend that consideration should be given to the use of phenothiazines such as prochlorperazine or levomepromazine and to agents such as lorazepam or nabilone as part of a 'salvage' scenario. In terms of novel agents, Stoner touches upon the utility of the neurokinin-1 (substance P) antagonists which have been shown to be effective very recently in the management of acute and elayed emesis and it is interesting to note that other pharmacological strategies currently in development and under evaluation include CB_1 (cannabinoid) and 5-HT_{1A} receptor interacting drugs. We are left, after having considered her chapters, with much optimism for the future prevention and control of cancer-related nausea and vomiting.

Having considered, in no small detail, the physiological and pharmacological basis of the prophylaxis and management of therapy-induced nausea and vomiting, we now turn to the final chapter of Part Three of this volume. In Chapter Fourteen, Filshie and Koomson provide a stimulating and in-depth discussion of the role of so called 'non-pharmacological' approaches to treatment. As the impact of uncontrolled nausea and vomiting may be significant enough for patients to consider abandoning potentially curative or palliative anti-cancer treatment, non-pharmacological interventions are, as the authors argue, gaining increasing importance in the alleviation of symptoms such as pain, nausea and vomiting and dyspnoea, which are unrelieved by conventional medication.

Acupuncture is the first line treatment for many pain and non-pain conditions for therapeutic and preventive purposes and has been used in China for over 2000 years. As those colleagues familiar with this technique will already know, the procedure involves the insertion of fine needles at specific anatomical points to stimulate the 'flow of energy' (Traditional Chinese Acupuncture) and can also involve manipulation of segmental or extrasegmental nerves in order to stimulate 'the release of multiple endogenous substances to modulate neurophysiological changes' (Western Medical Acupuncture). Following pioneering work by the late Professor John Dundee using a single needle at the traditional acupuncture point PC6 on the forearm, numerous randomised controlled trials have been performed to assess the efficacy of the technique in reducing the extent of nausea and vomiting due to a variety of causes. While the traditional biomedical, and as some colleagues would argue 'reductionist', orientation of medical research in the current era of 'evidence-based medicine' holds much scepticism of the efficacy and place of acupuncture, several landmark reviews of its utility have, in fact, been conducted in recent times using the now established technique of systematic review. For example, in a systematic review in the mid 1990's, Vickers (1996) identified 27 out of 33 trials on acupuncture for nausea and vomiting as demonstrating a positive therapeutic response and highlighted 5 out of 5 studies on 151 subjects with chemotherapy-induced nausea and vomiting as demonstrating significant efficacy. Later, using the technique of meta-analysis, further efficacy of acupuncture was demonstrated in the context of management of post-operative nausea and vomiting. The phenomenon of nausea and vomiting in advanced terminal care is considerably more complex and often multifactorial and, like Filshie and Koomson, we await the accumulation of further evidence for the place of this particular intervention in that context.

In addition to acupuncture, Filshie and Koomson have also, in their review, considered the place of hypnosis as a 'non-pharmacological' intervention in the control of cancer-related nausea and vomiting. Hypnosis, as the authors define, is an altered state of consciousness that provides access to unconscious processes. Change in memory and perception and trance experiences have been used since the time of the ancient Greeks. Patients placed under hypnosis become absorbed in the hypnotic experience with distortion of time awareness and are curiously receptive to suggestions implanted at the time. In addition to the reduction of symptoms of procedure-related pain, hypnosis has been found helpful for alleviation of anticipatory chemotherapy-related nausea and vomiting as well as anxiety and stress. The authors conclude their contribution by examining the usefulness of this intervention and also others focused on herbal medicine, healing and therapeutic touch, massage, aromatherapy, reflexology and music therapy.

We have dedicated Part Four of the current volume, the penultimate Part, to the study of current clinical strategies for the management of depression and of anorexia in cancer. It can be difficult, as Lloyd-Williams and her colleagues discuss, to distinguish between what may be called 'appropriate' sadness at the end of life and a treatable depressive illness. As the authors outline in Chapter Fifteen, it is estimated that 20% of patients will have a formal psychiatric diagnosis, the most common being depression and, for a quarter of all patients admitted to a palliative care unit, depression will be a significant symptom. A survey of the literature suggests that up to 80% of the psychological and psychiatric morbidity which develops in cancer patients goes unrecognised and untreated. A reason for this low rate of detection is thought to be non-disclosure by patients who may either feel that they are 'wasting the doctor's time' or that they are in some way to blame for their distress and therefore choose to hide it. A further reason may well be represented by a lack of confidence in diagnosing this symptom by many medical and nursing staff. Screening tools can help in the assessment of depression but require prior validation. There are many effective antidepressants available, so patients identified within the last two to three months of life can still benefit from treatment. It is important that all professionals caring for palliative care patients have an understanding of the enormous impact that this symptom can have on the quality of life of patients and their families. We agree with Lloyd-Williams and her colleagues that much further work needs to be undertaken to explore why depression is still not recognised as often as it should be and that we also need to devote time to evaluate the relative clinical effectiveness of available therapeutic interventions.

Along with depression, anorexia is a common symptom in cancer patients. It can either exist alone or as part of cancer cachexia, a clinical syndrome characterized by anorexia, involuntary weight loss, tissue wasting, poor performance status and protein calorie malnutrition. In Chapter Sixteen, Jayasekera and Stone outline the aetiological basis of anorexia and proceed to discuss clinical approaches to effective management. The first step in managing this symtom will be, of course, the identification and treatment of reversible causes. For example, anorexia may improve with adequate attention to mouth care, suitable treatment of nausea and vomiting as outlined in earlier sections of this volume, and the resolution of any constipation. For many patients, however, no underlying treatable cause for the anorexia will be identified. For these patients, anorexia may be improved with sensible nutritional advice or the provision of nutritional supplements but while this approach has been shown to increase protein and colorie intake, little effect has been documented in relation to survival or quality of life. The authors usefully consider physical exercise as having been shown to have a role in the management of anorexia as have corticosteroids which can stimulate appetite in cancer patients, although these particular effects are short lived and there are numerous side effects to be considered. Progestational steroids, on the other hand, have proven efficacy in treating anorexia with a better side-effect profile and recent studies suggest that nutritional supplements enriched with fish oil may have beneficial effects on weight loss in cancer patients. Several other pharmacological approaches are currently under investigation, as Jayasekera and Stone discuss, and the results of these are awaited with much interest.

We turn now to Part Five of the current volume and to particularly difficult and often highly contentious areas of clinical practice in the care of the patient with highly advanced disease. In Chapter Seventeen, Keown considers the issues of withholding versus withdrawing treatment, Do Not Attempt Resuscitation (DNAR) orders and Advance Directives. His chapter falls into three parts, beginning with an outline of the Law as it relates to the withholding/withdrawing of treatment and to DNAR and Advance Directives, moving to a consideration of the relevant guidance currently available as issued by the British Medical Association and General Medical Council and ending with the discussion of a central ethical question to which current Law and professional guidance give rise. That is, he asks whether they are ethically inconsistent in opposing the intentional termination of life by an act but not by an omission and by opposing intentional assistance in suicide by an act but not by omission. Many colleagues will find his chapter at once stimulating and emotive.

In Chapter Eighteen, the final chapter of this volume, Ellershaw details his thinking on the clinical usefulness of current clinical pathways for the management of the last 48 hours of life. There is, as this author points out, an increasing movement in health care towards continuous quality improvement and clinical practice guidelines-based care. He notes that while the focus of such initiatives is rightly on the promotion of high quality, efficient, cost-effective care, current systems of monitoring and evaluating outcomes relating to palliative care are poorly developed. The development of multi-professional care pathways has, as Ellershaw observes, proved an innovative way of developing and implementing standards of quality management. Care Pathways are thus used to plan and document care for patients and can provide a method of understanding care across geographical settings and with such benefits in mind he outlines how the Marie Curie Centre Liverpool and the Royal Liverpool University Hospitals have developed the Liverpool Care Pathway for the Dying Patient (LCP). The LCP has now, he reports, been implemented successfully in hospice, hospital, community and nursing home settings and aims to set and maintain standards of excellence in the care of the dying by focusing particular attention on the initial assessment and care of the patient, on ongoing care and on care after death. Having gained Beacon Status for Palliative Care in the Year 2000 its development represents a significant advancement in the clinical care of the dying and we encourage colleagues carefully to consider its structure and utility as part of their own, personal, clinical practice.

In the current age, where doctors and health professionals are increasingly overwhelmed by clinical information, we have aimed to provide a fully current, fully referenced text on the effective prevention and control of common symptoms in cancer that is as succinct as possible but as comprehensive as necessary. Consultants and specialist registrars in palliative medicine will find it of particular use as part of their continuing education and specialist training respectively, and we advance it specifically as an excellent tool for these purposes. We anticipate, however, that the book will prove of considerable use to other members of the clinical team including specialist oncology and palliative care nurses, hospital pharmacists and all those colleagues with a responsibility for, or an interest in, the effective and efficient care of the patient with cancer.

Andrew Hoy FRCP FRCR
Ilora Finlay FRCGP FRCP
Andrew Miles MSc MPhil PhD

PART 1

The prevention and control of weakness and fatigue in cancer

Chapter 1

Pharmacological aspects of cancer-related fatigue

Anne H. Kendall, Patrick Stone and Paul L. R. Andrews

'*For people with cancer, like me, cancer is the C word. What I have discovered is that cancer does not travel alone, but is accompanied by its insidious colleague, namely fatigue, which, for me, is the F word. This profound side effect adds additional disabling restrictions to my struggle against cancer.*'

Robert Wharton MD, 2002

Introduction

Cancer-related fatigue can be defined as 'a subjective state of overwhelming, sustained exhaustion and decreased capacity for physical and mental work that is not relieved by rest'. This last feature can distinguish it from exercise-induced fatigue. As a greater proportion of the cancer population survives their malignancy, increasing attention and emphasis is being placed on long-term sequelae of both cancer and its management. Fatigue is one of the commonest symptoms reported in cancer patients undergoing treatment and is noted by over 75% of patients in most published research trials (Nerenz *et al.* 1982; Jamar *et al.* 1989; Morrow *et al.* 1992; Hickok *et al.* 1996). In one study 54% of patients reported that fatigue was the longest-lasting side effect (Curt *et al.* 2000). It is also described by patients after their treatment has been completed and they are considered to be disease free. Recognition of the importance of fatigue has increased with the development of effective treatments for other debilitating symptoms of cancer and its treatment such as 5-hydroxytryptamine$_3$ (5-HT$_3$) receptor antagonists for chemotherapy-induced emesis. Fatigue has therefore moved up the list of clinical challenges such that there is a new impetus to understand its mechanisms and identify possibilities for therapeutic intervention.

Impact of fatigue on quality of life

Fatigue has been reported to have the greatest impact on quality-of-life scales compared with any other treatment- or disease-related side effect in patients with cancer (Asbury *et al.* 1998; Curt *et al.* 2000). The subjective sensation of fatigue is threefold, with physical (e.g. decreased energy), cognitive (e.g. poor concentration) and affective (e.g. decreased motivation) elements. Fatigue can be so severe and disabling that patients have reported that they wanted to die (Curt *et al.* 2000). In addition, fatigue may interact with other common adverse effects of chemotherapy such as nausea and vomiting, increasing their perceived severity and ultimately leading to a reduced ability to complete treatment. Fatigue is also noted to be a common reason why patients decline enrolment in clinical trials (Kaemper 1982). Sadly, it would appear there are several barriers to recognition and treatment of cancer-related fatigue. In a study conducted by the Fatigue Coalition Group in the USA, 45% of patients thought that nothing could be done, which was echoed at time of consultation by 40% of doctors who gave no recommendation or prescription (Curt *et al.* 2000). Similar findings have been reported in a UK-based survey (Stone *et al.* 2003).

Normal physiological role of fatigue

It is accepted that nausea and vomiting are part of the normal processes of survival and protection. Naturally most toxins are ingested agents which when detected initially result in vomiting and diarrhoea to cleanse the system. In addition, other systemic responses such as fever occur as part of the defence. Aversive responses such as nausea, appetite suppression and conditioned taste aversion occur in an attempt to prevent repeat exposure. Fatigue can be perceived as a further method by which an animal protects itself. Firstly, akin to somatic pain, the sensation of fatigue alerts the animal that a particular physical activity is damaging to them and should be avoided to reduce the possibility of permanent physical injury. Secondly, the feeling of limb weakness associated with fatigue encourages a reduction in activity and refuge-seeking behaviour so as to recover in relative safety.

Normally these responses would be appropriate for survival in the natural environment. Cancer and its treatment can be seen to activate some of these pathways, although in this setting the response is inappropriate and often detrimental. In particular, nausea after cytotoxic agents is the main determinant of future anticipatory emetic responses. Causal agents are not removed by vomiting or diarrhoea because they are in the systemic circulation or other fluid compartments (e.g. cerebrospinal fluid) and it is clear that these are considered side effects of treatment requiring control. However, the role of fatigue is more complex and can be viewed from both standpoints. Its effect on quality of life would lead us to conclude that it should be aggressively treated; however, if it reflects a natural process of recovery from systemic disease then there may be an argument not to treat.

Is it the cancer or the treatment?

Fatigue can occur as a result of the cancer directly and be associated with all treatment modalities given in its treatment (including surgery). Victims of accidental radiation exposure have been shown to experience fatigue and other side effects similar to those attributable to therapeutic radiation in cancer patients (Anno *et al.* 1989). One retrospective review series of 50 men and women receiving radiotherapy for lung cancer found that 78% reported fatigue, and of those there was a linear increase in the severity of fatigue with progressive treatments. There were no significant differences in the level of fatigue experienced between different demographic groups including age, sex, race, work, marital status, disease stage, radiotherapy dose or previous chemotherapy, suggesting that the effect of fatigue was secondary to the cumulative radiotherapy (Hickok *et al.* 1996). Levels of fatigue often increase with treatment duration and with progressive disease (Richardson *et al.* 1996).

Measuring fatigue

There are few research studies at present to clarify the mechanism(s) involved in cancer-related fatigue. In humans, most work has been done in exercise-induced fatigue and chronic fatigue syndromes (CFSs), and extrapolated to cancer. However, as discussed earlier, there are features that suggest this may provide only limited information. Future developments aimed at identifying therapeutic targets based upon an understanding of mechanisms will rely upon a combination of animal and human studies.

Human studies

There are now several questionnaires (e.g. the Functional Assessment Inventory-Fatigue Scale (FACT-F)) that are in use to assess the impact of fatigue on quality of life. Although these help to characterise the phenomenon, they need to be correlated with biochemical and physiological parameters. Taking quantitative measurements of fatigue is difficult, but dynamometers used to measure hand-grip strength have shown a reduction in power with advanced malignancy (Stone *et al.* 1999). A 'wrist watch' actigraph is a monitor used to assess gross movement and has been used to demonstrate sleep disturbance during radiotherapy treatment (Hickok *et al.* 1998). Such techniques provide useful tools with which to correlate biochemical assessments and monitor any therapeutic intervention.

Several studies have investigated the changing profile of cytokines in the plasma of cancer patients. One such report on breast cancer survivors who documented fatigue were found to have higher levels of interleukin-1 (IL-1) and tumour-necrosis factor (TNF-α) when compared with a similarly matched group of women who were also disease free but who did not report fatigue (Bower *et al.* 2002). The search for a single specific biological agent of fatigue might be anticipated to fail because the process is likely to be multi-factorial, and looking for an agent is complex. Levels of an agent in the plasma that correlate with changes in behaviour at the whole body level are difficult to interpret, particularly as most studies measure plasma levels of the substances of interest at single time points, so sampling may have to repeated frequently over a prolonged period (e.g. the duration of chemotherapy) with the attendant ethical and practical problems. Additionally, the plasma may not be the relevant compartment of interest as several pieces of evidence implicate changes in brain neurotransmitters. This could be investigated by using positron emission tomography scans and functional magnetic resonance imaging techniques.

Animal studies

Animal models of fatigue remain in their infancy, although some work has been done in rats after bile duct resection used to mimic cholestatic liver disease, which is frequently associated with fatigue. These animals exhibit features of sickness behaviour with alteration in their locomotor activity within an open field, a marker for stress response (Swain *et al.* 1995). These animals had an altered biochemical profile, with a reduced plasma adrenocorticotrophic hormone (ACTH) response, low background hypothalamic corticotrophin-releasing hormone (CRH) levels, and a blunted CRH response to stress. Such disturbance of the hypothalamic–pituitary–adrenal axis has also been implicated in CFS (Cleare *et al.* 2001). In the study of the rat, it was speculated that such changes were mediated by cytokines such as TNF-a and IL-6. There is evidence to suggest similar cytokine profiles in humans with primary biliary cirrhosis, suggesting that the rat model of bile duct resection may well prove to be a useful tool in the investigation of the genesis of fatigue.

Although not aimed at studying fatigue specifically, there have been many studies in rats of the behavioural responses to infection that have implicated cytokines (e.g. TNF-α, IL-1) in the genesis of 'sickness behaviour'. The cytokines are proposed to influence the brain through activation of abdominal vagal afferents and also through an action on the circumventricular organs of the brain (e.g. area postrema, a region of the dorsal brainstem where the blood–brain barrier is relatively permeable and which has also been implicated in emesis) (Konsman *et al.* 2002).

Hypotheses for the mechanisms of fatigue

By reviewing those conditions with identified pathways of fatigue, for example myasthenia gravis, multiple sclerosis and hypothyroidism, along with those of unclear aetiology such as cancer, chemotherapy, radiation, infections and surgery, it becomes apparent that the mechanisms are multiple and diverse. The mechanisms involved in cancer-related fatigue are largely speculative and open to refutation by experimentation. Four main hypotheses are presented briefly here, and are reviewed more extensively with others by Andrews & Morrow (2001) and Morrow *et al.* (2002).

Anaemia

There are multiple reasons why cancer patients become anaemic, including inadequate erythropoiesis, haemolysis and haemorrhage (Bron 2001). Several pathways have linked cytokines (e.g. TNF-α, interferon-α (IFN-α), IL-1) with reduced erythropoeitin production, impaired iron use and dyserythropoiesis, along with other factors leading to exacerbation of anaemia. There are now several studies showing that there is a gain in the quality of life by maintaining haemoglobin during chemotherapy by the use of recombinant epoetin-α (Glaspy *et al.* 1997; Demetri *et al.* 1998; Gabrilove *et al.* 2001). Although anaemia is commonly found in cancer patients both on and off treatment, what is not clear is how the level of haemoglobin is intrinsically related to the sensation of fatigue, although not surprisingly tissue hypoxia is often given as the mechanism (Mercuriali & Inghilleri 2001); but which tissue(s) is implicated and could this account for all the clinical observations? For example, patients undergoing radiotherapy often report greater levels of fatigue than chemotherapy patients, although anaemia is not as frequent. Clinical experience supports the observation that numerous patients complain of fatigue with normal haemoglobin levels. Is it that the oxygen dissociation curve needs to be revisited in the cancer setting, that other changes in the plasma (e.g. ions) caused by the cancer and treatment alter the functioning of red blood cells or that erythropoietin has other roles beyond maintaining haemoglobin levels? There are anecdotal reports of almost immediate responses to recombinant epoeitin that occur long before a rise in haemoglobin concentration. Apart from its production in the kidney, neurons have been found to synthesise erythropoietin, and erythropoietin receptors are present in brain capillary endothelial cells. Brain erythropoeitin synthesis and receptor expression can be induced by hypoxia. In rat models, exogenous erythropoeitin-α is reported to protect against neuronal damage from ischaemic cerebral events (see Springborg *et al.* (2002) for references).

Hypothalmic–pituitary axis dysregulation

Many of the mechanistic studies of the pathophysiology of fatigue are from studies of CFS. Notable features of CFS include memory and attention deficit, the ability to differentiate symptoms from a major depressive illness, hypofunction of CRH in the hypothalamus, and disturbance in arginine vasopressin (antidiuretic hormone), prolactin and 5-HT-mediated responses (Komaroff *et al.* 1998). Urinary-free cortisol levels were found to be lowered in 121 patients with clinical features of chronic fatigue syndrome when compared with otherwise similarly matched controls (Cleare *et al.* 2001). However, Cleare *et al.* (2001) are keen to point out that it is not known whether this is a primary or secondary phenomenon. Because cortisol is involved with so many physiological processes (maintaining muscle mass and function, modulating emotional well-being and wakefulness among the most relevant) it is conceivable that this plays a significant role in the pathway of fatigue.

Actigraph data in individual patients after radiotherapy have demonstrated marked disruption in sleep patterns. Any impact of radiotherapy on cortisol circadian rhythm may contribute to changes in feelings of well-being. Patients with a more regulated 'normal' circadian rhythm have been found to have reduced symptom severity in terms of fatigue, depression and mood on quality-of-life scales compared with those with a less regular circadian rhythm (Roscoe *et al.* 2002).

Finally, the function of the posterior pituitary has been explored in patients with postviral fatigue syndrome. An inconsistency between plasma osmolality and antidiuretic hormone levels in this group suggests either a problem in posterior pituitary hormone production or a defect in receptors in the hypothalamus (Bakheit *et al.* 1993).

Central 5-HT dysregulation

There are two directions of interest to suggest that central 5-HT regulation is potentially important in fatigue, although the site(s) at which it is involved have not been identified. Firstly, exercise physiologists have recorded an increase in blood tryptophan levels during prolonged exercise. Tryptophan is the amino acid precursor of 5-HT and competes with other branch-chain amino acids to enter the brain during exercise by the same transporter. As branch-chain amino acids are taken up by muscle during exercise, tryptophan is available in relatively higher concentrations to enter the brain and lead to an increase in 5-HT. Because 5-HT is known to be involved with sleep and mood it is thought that this is the mediator of the mental fatigue experienced during and after exercise (Newsholme *et al.* 1995). The ingestion of a solution of branch-chain amino acids in healthy volunteers exercised on a bicycle ergometer reduced the subjects' grading of perceived exertion and mental fatigue (Blomstrand *et al.* 1997).

Further indications of the role of 5-HT have arisen from therapeutic trials using modifiers of brain 5-HT transmission. Paroxetine, a selective 5-HT re-uptake inhibitor given at a single dose of 20 mg, has been shown to reduce the duration of exercise performed in human subjects (Wilson *et al.* 1992). In addition buspirone, a 5-HT_{1A} receptor agonist, had similar effects during exercise, and subjects scored higher on levels of exhaustion (Marvin *et al.* 1997). Jones (1999) reported a substantive benefit in prolonged use of the 5-HT_3 receptor antagonist ondansetron for symptoms of profound fatigue in a patient with chronic liver disease, and more recent studies have reported a benefit of 5-HT_3 receptor antagonists in patients with chronic fatigue syndrome (Spath *et al.* 2000).

Vagal afferent modulation of somatic activity

Skeletal muscle activity has been shown to be modulated by sensory-vagal afferents from pulmonary and abdominal inputs (see Andrews & Morrow (2001) for references) which, after projecting to the brainstem, activate descending inhibitory inputs to the spinal motor neuron pool. In the lungs, it is proposed that this is a mechanism by which afferents induce the sensation of dyspnoea associated with heavy exercise, so as to limit the activity and prevent muscle damage. In animal experiments abdominal vagal afferents have been shown to be activated (directly or indirectly) by a variety of exogenous (chemotherapeutic agents, radiotherapy) and endogenous (5-HT, prostaglandins and cytokines) triggers. Within the cancer setting, neuroactive agents including cytokines are proposed to cause a low level of activation or sensitisation of vagal afferents. This is turn leads to a reflex reduction in somatic motor drive (tone) to skeletal muscles. Consequently there is a perception that it is necessary to exert more 'effort' to accomplish a task than would have been the case in the absence of these stimuli.

Treatment

Traditional therapies have centred around non-pharmacological interventions including patient education, individualised graded exercise programmes, cognitive therapy, sleep management and nutrition. Other approaches include addressing co-existing physical morbidities such as anaemia, cardiac failure, electrolyte imbalances or infection.

The use of pharmacological interventions in the treatment of fatigue is at an early stage. The development of an anti-TNF agent would seem a good target to block the cascade of mechanisms described previously where TNF is implicated. Thalidomide has been shown to improve the sensation of well-being in cancer patients with cancer cachexia and may have some use in cancer-related fatigue (Bruera *et al.* 1999). It is thought to act by inhibiting TNF-α and modulating interleukins. COX-2 inhibitors, which inhibit cytokine action and agents that prevent the release of cytokines (such as pentoxifylline and bradykinin antagonists), are potential future treatments (Burks 2001). Central nervous system stimulants and steroids have also been suggested as potential treatments (see Stone 2002).

Corticosteroids have been shown to reduce fatigue (Bruera *et al.* 1985). The mechanism is unclear and long-term use can, conversely, contribute to fatigue with myopathy, infection and other side effects. A double-blind crossover study of 460 mg/day of megestrol acetate versus placebo in patients with advanced cancer showed a beneficial effect on activity levels after a 10-day treatment course (Bruera *et al.* 1998), although larger, longer duration studies have failed to show any benefit (Simons *et al.* 1996; Westman *et al.* 1999).

Methylphenidate, a psychostimulant, has been shown in a pilot study to produce a beneficial effect on fatigue in 9 out of 11 patients with advanced cancer (Sarhill *et al.* 2001). It has previously been used to treat opiate-induced somnolence, depression and to improve cognitive function, with the advantage of rapid onset of action. Side effects include anxiety, agitation and insomnia. Newer psychostimulants such as modafinil, which report fewer side effects, may have a place in fatigue management. Modafinil has been used for fatigue in patients with multiple sclerosis (Rammohan *et al.* 2002). Interest from the pharmaceutical industry, perhaps in the prophylaxis of fatigue, is likely to prove one of the greatest factors in directing research forward in this area.

Conclusions

There is no doubt about the significant impact of fatigue before, during and after treatment for malignant disease. There are, however, complex mechanisms in the development of fatigue that are not clearly understood. There is evidence from both animal and human studies to suggest that the hypothalamic–pituitary axis, 5-HT and cytokines may all play a role. In addition, anaemia may contribute to fatigue in some patients, but how this mechanistically results in the particular sensation of fatigue is not adequately explained at present. Previous work on exercise-induced fatigue may be worthy of repetition in cancer patients, and the development of animal models is likely to improve our understanding of mechanisms and potential therapeutic targets. There is potential for pharmacological intervention in the treatment of fatigue, with the initial step being identification of the target sites.

References

Andrews, P. L. R. & Morrow, G. R. (2001). Approaches to understanding the mechanisms involved in fatigue associated with cancer and its treatments: a speculative review. In *ESO Scientific Updates*, volume 5 (*Fatigue and Cancer*) (ed. M. Marty & S. Pecorelli), pp. 79–93. Elsevier.

Anno, G. H., Baum, S. J., Withers, H. R. & Young, R. W. (1989). Symptomatology of acute radiation effects in humans after exposure to doses of 0.5–30 Gy. *Health Physics* **56**, 821–838.

Asbury, F. D., Findlay, H., Reynolds, B. & McKerracher, K. (1998). Canadian survey of cancer patients' experiences: are their needs being met? *Journal of Pain and Symptom Management* **16**, 298–306.

Bakheit, A. M. O., Behan, P. O. & Watson, W. S. (1993). Abnormal arginine–vasopressin secretion and water metabolism in patients with postviral fatigue syndrome. *Acta Neurologica Scandinavica* **87**, 234–238.

Blomstrand, E., Hassmen, P., Ekblom, B. & Newsholme, E. A. (1997). Influence of ingesting a solution of branched-chain amino acids on perceived exertion during exercise. *Acta Physiologica Scandinavica* **159**, 41–49.

Bower, J. E., Ganz, P. A., Aziz, N., Fahey, J. L. (2002). Fatigue and proinflammatory cytokine activity in breast cancer survivors. *Psychosomatic Medicine* **64**, 604–611.

Bron, D. (2001). Biological basis of cancer-related anaemia. In *Fatigue and Cancer* (*European School of Oncology Scientific Updates* 5) (ed. M. Marty & S. Pecorelli), pp. 45–50. Elsevier, Amsterdam.

Bruera, E., Roca, E., Cedaro, L., Carraro, S. & Chacon, R. (1985). Action of oral methylprednisolone in terminal cancer patients: a prospective randomised double-blind study. *Cancer Treatment Reports* **69**, 751–754.

Bruera, E., Ernst, S. & Hagen, N. (1998). Effectiveness of megestrol acetate in patients with advanced cancer: a randomised double-blind crossover study. *Cancer Prevention and Control* **2**, 74–78.

Bruera, E., Neumann, C. M., Pituskin, E., Calder, K., Ball, G. & Hanson, J. (1999). Thalidomide in patients with cachexia due to terminal cancer: preliminary report. *Annals of Oncology* **10**, 857–859.

Burks, T. F. (2001). New agents for the treatment of cancer related fatigue. *Cancer* **15** (Suppl. 6), 1714–1718.

Cleare, A. J., Blair, D., Chambers, S., Wessely, S. (2001). Urinary free cortisol in chronic fatigue syndrome. *American Journal of Psychiatry* **158**, 641–643.

Curt, G. A., Breitbart, W., Cella, D., Groopman, J. E., Horning, S. J., Itri, L. M., Johnson, D. H., Miaskowski, C., Scherr, S. L., Potenoy, R. K. & Vogelzang, N. J. (2000). *The Oncologist* **5**, 353–360.

Demetri, G. D., Kris, M., Wade, J., Degos, L. & Cella, D. (1998). Quality of life benefit in chemotherapy patients treated with epoetin alfa is independent of disease response or tumour type. (Procrit study group.) *Journal of Clinical Oncology* **16**, 3412–3425.

Gabrilove, J. L., Cleeland, C. S., Livingston, R. B., Sarokhan, B., Winer, E. & Einhorn, L. H. (2001). Clinical evaluation of once-weekly dosing of epoetin alfa in chemotherapy patients: improvements in haemoglobin and quality of life are similar to three-times-weekly dosing. *Journal of Clinical Oncology* **19**, 2875–2882.

Glaspy, J., Bukowski, R., Steinberg, D., Taylor, C., Tchekmedyian, S. & Vadhan-Raj, S. (1997). Impact of therapy with epoetin alfa on clinical outcomes in patients with non-myeloid malignancies during cancer chemotherapy in community oncology practice. (Procrit study group.) *Journal of Clinical Oncology*, 1218–1234.

Hickok, J. T., Morrow, G. R., McDonald, S. & Bellg, A. J. (1996). Frequency and correlates of fatigue in lung cancer patients receiving radiation therapy: implications for management. *Journal of Pain and Symptom Management* **11**, 370–377.

Hickok, J. T., Roscoe, J. A., Morrow, G. R. & Bushunow, P. (1998). Wrist actigraphy as a measure of fatigue. *Proceedings of the American Society of Clinical Oncology* **17**, 60a.

Jamar, S. C. (1989). Fatigue in women receiving chemotherapy for ovarian cancer. In *Key Aspects of Comfort: Management of Pain, Fatigue and Nausea* (ed. S. Funk, E. Tourniquist, M. Champagne, L. Copp & R. Weise), pp. 224–228. Springer, New York, Berlin & Heidelberg.

Jones, A. E. (1999). Relief from profound fatigue associated with chronic liver disease by long term ondansetron therapy. *The Lancet* **354**, 397.

Kaemper, S. H. (1982). Relaxation training reconsidered. *Oncology Nursing Forum* **9**, 15–18.

Komaroff, A. L. & Buchwald, D. S. (1998). Chronic fatigue syndrome: an update. *Annual Review of Medicine* **49**, 1–13.

Konsman, J. P., Parnet, R. & Dantzer, R. (2002). Cytokine-induced sickness behaviour: mechanisms and implications. *Trends in Neurosciences* **25**, 154–159.

Marvin, G., Sharma, A., Aston, W., Field, C., Kendall, M. J. & Jones, D. A. (1997). The effects of buspirone on perceived exertion and time to fatigue in man. *Experimental Physiology* **82**, 1057–1060.

Mercuriali, F. & Inghilleri, G. (2001). Treatment of anaemia in cancer patients: transfusion of rHuEPO. In *Fatigue and Cancer* (*European School of Oncology Scientific Updates* **5**) (ed. M. Marty & S. Pecorelli), pp. 185–200. Elsevier, Amsterdam.

Morrow, G. R., Andrews, P. L. R., Hickok, J. T., Roscoe, J. A. & Matesson, S. (2002). Fatigue associated with cancer and its treatment. *Supportive Care in Cancer* **10**, 389–398.

Morrow, G. R., Pandya, K., Barry, M., Difino, S., Jennings, P., Flynn, P., Rosenbluth, R. & Dakhil, S. (1992). Chemotherapy-induced fatigue and patient reported psychological depression. *Proceedings of the Annual Meeting of the American Society of Clinical Oncology* **11**, A1329.

Nerenz, D. R., Leventhal, H. & Love, R. R. (1982). Factors contributing to emotional distress during cancer chemotherapy. *Cancer* **50**, 1020–1027.

Newsholme, E. A. & Blomstrand, E. (1995). Tryptophan, 5-hydroxytryptamine and a possible explanation for central fatigue. In *Fatigue. Neural and Muscular Mechanisms* (ed. S. C. Gandevia, R. M. Enoka, A. J. McComas, D. G. Stuart & C. K. Thomas), pp. 315–320. Plenum Press, New York.

Rammohan, K. W., Rosenberg, J. H., Lynn, D. J., Blumenfeld, A. M., Pollack, C. P. & Nagaraja, H. N. (2002). Efficacy and safety of modafinil (Provigil) for the treatment of fatigue in multiple sclerosis: a two centre phase 2 study. *Journal of Neurology, Neurosurgery and Psychiatry* **72**, 179–183.

Richardson, A. & Ream, E. (1996). The experience of fatigue and other symptoms in patients receiving chemotherapy. *European Journal of Cancer Care* **5**, 24–30.

Roscoe, J. A., Morrow, G. R., Hickok, J. T., Bushunow, P., Matteson, S., Rakita, D. & Andrews, P. L. R. (2002). Temporal interrelationships among fatigue, circadian rhythm and depression in breast cancer patients undergoing chemotherapy treatment. *Supportive Care in Cancer* **10**, 329–336.

Sarhill, N., Walsh, D., Nelson, K. A., Homsi, J., LeGrand, S. & Davis, M. P. (2001). Methylphenidate for fatigue in advanced cancer a prospective open label pilot study. *American Journal of Hospital Palliative Care* **18**, 403–407.

Simons, J.-P., Aaronson, N. K., Vansteenkiste, J. F., ten Velde, G. P. M., Muller, M. J., Drenth, B. M., Erdkamp, F. L. G., Cobben, E. G. M., Schoon, E. J., Smeets, J. B. E. *et al.* (1996). Effects of methylprogesterone acetate on appetite, weight, and quality of life in advanced-stage non-hormone-sensitive cancer: a placebo-controlled multicenter study. *Journal of Clinical Oncology* **14**, 1077–1084.

Spath, M., Welzel, D. & Farber, L. (2000). Treatment of chronic fatigue syndrome with 5-HT3 receptor antagonists: preliminary results. *Scandinavian Journal of Rheumatology* **29** (Suppl 113), 72–77.

Springborg, J. B., Ma, X. D., Rochta, P., Knudsen, G. M., Amtorp, O., Paulson, O. B., Juhlier, M. & Olsen, N. V. (2002). A single subcutaneous bolus of erythropoietin normalises cerebral blood flow autoregulation after subarachnoid haemorrhage in rats. *British Journal of Pharmacology* **135**, 823–829.

Stone, P., Hardy, J., Broadley, K., Tookman, A. J., Kurowska, A. & Hern, R. A. (1999). Fatigue in advanced cancer: a prospective controlled cross-sectional study. *British Journal of Cancer* **79**, 1479–1486.

Stone, P. (2002). The measurement, causes and effective management of cancer related fatigue. *International Journal of Palliative Nursing* **8**, 120–128.

Stone, P., Ream, E., Richardson, A., Thomas, H., Andrews, P., Campbell, P., Dawson. T., Goldie, T., Hammick, M., Kearney N. *et al.* (2003). Cancer-related fatigue – a difference of opinion? Results of a multi-centre survey of healthcare professionals, patients and caregivers. *European Journal of Cancer Care* **12**, 20–27.

Swain, M. G. & Maric, M. (1995). Defective corticotrophin-releasing hormone mediated neuroendocrine and behavioural responses in cholestatic rats: implications for cholestatic liver disease-related sickness behaviours. *Hepatology* **22**, 1560–1564.

Westman, G., Bergman., B, Albertson, M., Kadar, L., Gustavsson, G., Thaning, L., Andersson, M., Straumits, A., Jeppson, B., Linden, C.-J. *et al.* (1999). Megestrol acetate in advanced, progressive, hormone-insensitive cancer. Effects on the quality of life: a placebo-controlled, randomised, multicentre trial. *European Journal of Cancer* **35**, 586–595.

Wilson, W. M. & Maughan, R. J. (1992). Evidence for a possible role of 5-hydroxytryptamine in the genesis of fatigue in man: administration of paroxetine, a 5-HT re-uptake inhibitor reduces the capacity to perform prolonged exercise. *Experimental Physiology* **77**, 921–924.

Chapter 2

The management of fatigue and weakness in patients with haematological malignancy

Jens Samol and Tim J. Littlewood

Introduction

Fatigue is a common and often unappreciated problem for patients with malignant disease. A study by Vogelzang (Vogelzang *et al.* 1997) of 400 patients with cancer noted that 60% of the patients considered fatigue to be their single most important symptom, ahead of other important problems such as nausea and pain, whereas the oncologists caring for these patients rated pain and nausea above fatigue in their perception of the major problems for this patient population.

These data were confirmed in another study of patients with cancer (Curt *et al.* 2000) in which 75% of patients reported fatigue as their single most important symptom, and of these patients 59% said that fatigue lasted for a longer period of time and 60% that fatigue had a greater negative impact on quality of life compared with other important symptoms such as pain, nausea and depression.

Fatigue may be caused by many physiological as well as psychological factors. Physiological factors include the impact of the tumour and chemotherapy on the patient's sense of well-being, and these negative influences are commonly exacerbated by symptoms of anaemia.

Anaemia is a major feature in patients with haematological malignancies and can usually be attributed to the anaemia of chronic disease (ACD), to the myelosuppressive effects of the chemotherapy (Spivak 1994) (Table 2.1), to haemolysis in patients with lymphoproliferative disorders, and to tumour infiltration of the bone marrow. The symptoms of chronic anaemia can be very distressing as the patient's quality of life and sense of well-being may be seriously impaired.

Table 2.1 Common causes of anaemia in patients with haematological malignancy

- Anaemia of chronic disease
- Chemotherapy
- Tumour infiltration of the bone marrow
- Haematinic deficiency
- Haemolysis
- Bleeding
- Impaired endogenous erythropoietin production
- Decreased bone marrow response to erythropoietin

The pathophysiology of this type of anaemia is multifactorial but the ACD plays a major role. The ACD is a cytokine mediated, normochromic/normocytic anaemia characterised by reticulocytopenia, hypoferraemia in the presence of adequate iron stores, and a shortened erythrocyte survival of approximately 60–90 days. Cytokines such as tumour-necrosis factor, interferon-γ and interleukin-1 inhibit erythropoiesis both directly by suppressing erythroid colony growth (Kalmanti & Kalmanti 1989) and indirectly by suppressing erythropoietin production. This latter observation is supported by work published by Miller *et al.* (1990), who demonstrated the relative decrease in erythropoietin production that occurs in patients with malignant disease by contrasting serum erythropoietin levels in patients with iron deficiency anaemia with the levels in patients with a variety of cancerous illnesses. Miller *et al.* (1990) showed that for any haemoglobin concentration, serum erythropoietin levels were lower in patients with cancer than for patients with iron deficiency. Although the patients studied had solid tumours, the same relative erythropoietin deficiency has been demonstrated in approximately 75% of patients with haematological malignancies such as chronic lymphocytic leukaemia (CLL), lymphoma and myeloma (Cazzola *et al.* 1997). Thus, in tumour patients, the relative erythropoietin deficiency contributes to the decreased erythropoiesis and the development of ACD (Kasper 2001). Anaemia is commonly treated by blood transfusion, but concerns about adverse effects led to a search for safer and biologically more rational treatment for anaemia. With the availability of recombinant human erythropoietin (rHuEPO) it became standard treatment for the anaemia in chronic renal failure and has been successfully used in anaemia secondary to malignancy.

Incidence and symptoms of anaemia in patients with haematological malignancy

Anaemia is very common in patients with haematological malignancy. For example, in patients with myeloma, around 50% will have a haemoglobin concentration of less than 10.5 g/dl at presentation and most of the remainder will develop anaemia during their initial chemotherapy (San Miguel *et al.* 1995; Kyle 1975). Successful control of the myeloma will usually help to improve the haemoglobin level but anaemia tends to recur with disease progression.

For patients with lymphoma, anaemia (haemoglobin concentration less than 12.0g/dl) is present in around 40% at diagnosis; this figure increases towards 70% after three or four cycles of chemotherapy (Coiffier 2001). Anaemia at diagnosis is also an adverse prognostic factor for many haematological malignancies such as myeloma and chronic lymphatic leukaemia (Coiffier 2000).

Common symptoms of anaemia include fatigue, dyspnoea, anorexia, swollen feet, chest pain and loss of mental acuity.

Treatment of anaemia

The data set out above indicate that anaemia is common in patients with haematological malignancy, that the anaemia may be contributing to the sense of fatigue and that erythropoietin levels are suboptimal for the degree of anaemia in approximately 75% of patients with haematological malignancy such as lymphoma, CLL and myeloma.

The possible treatments for anaemia are to transfuse with red cells or to use rHuEPO. Most anaemic cancer patients do not get treated (Barrett-Lee *et al.* 2000), probably because symptoms of fatigue and lethargy are attributed to the underlying malignancy or treatment or both.

Blood transfusion is the most commonly used treatment modality in patients receiving chemotherapy. The haemoglobin level at which a transfusion will be suggested varies considerably (Barrett-Lee *et al.* 2000). Some doctors will recommend transfusion when the haemoglobin falls below 10.0 g/dl; others believe that transfusion should be withheld until the haemoglobin is less than 8.0 g/dl. Blood transfusion is costly, inconvenient for the patient, usually has to be given in a hospital – with the associated resource implications – and is, of course, not completely safe. However, for most patients, it is an effective way of increasing the haemoglobin concentration relatively safely and improving their sense of well-being. The beneficial effects usually last for two to four weeks, at which point another blood transfusion may be needed. Recombinant human erythropoietin is an alternative treatment option for anaemic patients with haematological malignancy. There are substantial data detailing its use in patients with lymphoproliferative disorders, in myelodysplasia and after bone marrow transplantation. It is not commonly used in patients with acute leukaemia, probably because serum erythropoietin levels tend to be high and because the intensive myelotoxic chemotherapy regimens mitigate against a treatment response.

Recombinant human erythropoietin in patients with haematological malignancy

In 1990 Heinz Ludwig published the first report on rHuEPO treatment of 13 anaemic patients with advanced myeloma (Ludwig *et al.* 1990). The treatment dose of rHuEPO was 150 IU/kg body weight by subcutaneous injection three times per week. The median baseline haemoglobin was 10.2 g/dl; 11 (85%) of the patients responded to treatment, with a haemoglobin rise of more than 2.0 g/dl. The time to response ranged from 3 to 20 weeks, with a median of 5 weeks. In this pilot study, in addition to the beneficial impact on the haemoglobin level, there was no evidence that rHuEPO treatment caused any worsening of the myeloma. As a result of this important initial study several randomised trials were conducted to establish the effectiveness of rHuEPO in anaemic patients with CLL, non-Hodgkin's lymphoma and myeloma.

A summary of the results from five trials is shown in Table 2.2 (Ludwig *et al.* 1990; Cazzola *et al.* 1995; Osterborg *et al.* 1996, 2002; Dammaco *et al.* 2001).

Table 2.2 Clinical studies of rHuEPO in patients with myeloma and lymphoma.

Reference	Patient number	Treatment response (%)	Control response (%)
Ludwig et al. 1990*	13	85	
Cazzola et al. 1995	146	61	7
Osterborg et al. 1996	121	60	24
Dammaco et al. 2001*	145	58	9
Osterborg et al. 2002	349	67	27

* Studies in which only patients with myeloma were investigated.

Response was defined as an increase in haemoglobin of greater than 2.0g/dl above baseline independently of blood transfusion. This was achieved in 58–85% of patients in the treatment arms and 7–27% in the placebo arms. These differences were statistically significant. The proportion of patients requiring transfusion dropped by around 50% in the treatment compared with the placebo arms. Two of these studies randomised patients to different doses of rHuEPO and were able to confirm that a starting dose of, or equivalent to, 150 IU/kg subcutaneously three times per week produced a superior response to a lower starting dose. Doubling the dose to 300 IU/kg after four weeks of treatment in non-responders produces a response in a further quarter of patients. Patients in whom the haemoglobin has risen by less than 1.0 g/dl after eight weeks of treatment should have their erythropoietin stopped. All of the studies confirmed that rHuEPO is safe, with a side effect profile similar to that found with the placebo-treated arms. However, these studies generally recommended a reduction in dose of rHuEPO in responding patients so as to maintain the haemoglobin between 12.0 and 13.0 g/dl. There have been anecdotal reports of venous thrombosis in patients whose haemoglobin rises rapidly and to more than 15.0 g/dl.

An important study was conducted by Rose et al. (1994) in which 221 anaemic patients with CLL were randomised to treatment with rHuEPO or placebo. The baseline haematocrits were 27.5% on the treatment group compared with 27.7% in the placebo group. The mean haematocrit increased by 5.7% in the rHuEPO group compared with 1.5% in the placebo group ($p < 0.0001$); 50% of the rHuEPO group had a haematocrit increase of more than 6 points above baseline compared with 15% of the placebo group ($p < 0.0001$). Quality-of-life scores in this study improved significantly more in the rHuEPO-treated patients compared with the placebo patients, with this response being particularly apparent in those rHuEPO-treated patients whose haematocrit increased to more than 38%.

In an attempt to confirm these important findings, two very large community-based studies were conducted in the USA by Glaspy et al. (1997) and Demetri et al. (1998). Over 4,000 patients were recruited into the two trials. All patients had cancer and were anaemic; they had a mean haemoglobin concentration of 9.2 g/dl in the first study (Glaspy et al. 1997), and 9.3 g/dl in the second (Demetri et al. 1998). They were treated in an open-label fashion with 150 IU/kg rHuEPO subcutaneously three times weekly for four months. Patients in these studies had solid and haematological malignancies and were treated with a variety of cisplatin- and non-cisplatin-containing chemotherapy regimes.

The mean increase in haemoglobin in the Glaspy *et al.* study was 1.8 g/dl; 53.4% of patients responded with a rise in haemoglobin of more than 2.0 g/dl. Sixty-one per cent of patients responded in the Demetri *et al.* study. In both of these trials, need for transfusion decreased by at least 50% from baseline to study completion. Approximately 20% of patients in these trials had a haematological malignancy. The response rate was similar irrespective of the underlying tumour type and independently of whether the patient was treated with platinum-or non-platinum-containing chemotherapy. Other groups have reported similar response rates in patients with myeloma and non-Hodgkin's lymphoma (San Miguel & Garcia-Sanz 1998).

In 2001 the UK Myeloma Forum produced guidelines for diagnosing and treating multiple myeloma. These British Committee for Standards in Haematology (BCSH) Guidelines recommend that a therapeutic trial of rHuEPO should be considered in patients with symptomatic anaemia, and rHuEPO is indicated for the treatment of anaemia in patients with myeloma and chronic renal failure (UK Myeloma Forum 2001). Recently published guidelines from the American Society of Clinical Oncology (ASCO) and the American Society of Hematology (ASH) have recommended that rHuEPO be considered for patients with cancer, receiving chemotherapy, whose haemoglobin is less than 10.0 g/dl. The authors also suggest that consideration for treatment with rHuEPO should be given to those patients whose haemoglobin lies between 10.0 and 12.0 g/dl. (American Society of Clinical Oncology/ American Society of Hematology 2002).

Quality of life

The above studies confirmed that treatment with rHuEPO is safe, would improve the haemoglobin concentration, and reduce the need for transfusion in patients with certain malignant haematological diseases.

Although this is useful, it is important to understand whether a rise in haemoglobin would translate into an improved quality of life for the responding patients. Rose *et al.* (1994) demonstrated an improvement in quality of life in patients treated with rHuEPO who obtained an increase in haematocrit.

Quality of life was addressed by both Glaspy *et al.* (1997) and Demetri *et al.* (1998). Both investigators showed that the quality of life improves with a rise in haemoglobin and, in the latter study, that the improvement in quality of life that occurs as a function of a rise in haemoglobin seems to occur independently of tumour response. A further analysis of these data by Crawford *et al.* (2002) demonstrated a statistically significant, nonlinear relation between haemoglobin level and quality of life. RHuEpo-related increases in haemoglobin were associated with improvements in quality of life for the haemoglobin range 8.0–14.0 g/dl. The largest improvement in quality of life for each 1 g/dl increment in haemoglobin occurred when the haemoglobin increased from 11.0 to 12.0 g/dl.

A large, randomised, placebo-controlled, double-blind trial of rHuEPO in patients with either solid tumours or haematological malignancies (Littlewood *et al.* 2001) has confirmed that treatment with rHuEPO will increase haemoglobin and reduce the need for transfusion, and that a significant improvement in quality of life occurs in patients treated with rHuEPO compared with those treated with placebo.

An important point to remember is that anaemia is just one factor out of many that may be contributing to the patients' impaired quality of life. Correspondingly, correction of anaemia may well improve functional well-being but is unlikely to return the patient to complete normality.

The impact on patient outcomes of correcting anaemia with rHuEPO

Anaemia at presentation has an adverse impact on prognosis for patients with haematological malignancies such as lymphoma, myeloma and CLL. There are several possible explanations why anaemia may be associated with a poor prognosis. Firstly, the anaemia may be a surrogate marker for a more advanced and aggressive malignancy. There are some alternative explanations. Data from patients with solid tumours suggest that many tumours are hypoxic (Molls *et al.* 1998) and that anaemia contributes to that hypoxia (Kelleher 1996). Hypoxic tissues are less radiosensitive than normoxic ones (Hall 1994) and many cytotoxic drugs may be less effective in hypoxic compared with normoxic conditions (Teicher *et al.* 1990). Studies show that, regardless of treatment, patients with hypoxic tumours are likely to have less local disease control and less cure compared with patients with better oxygenated tumours of the same size and stage (Hockel *et al.* 1996; Brizel *et al.* 1997). Three explanations for the adverse impact of tumour hypoxia on survival have been postulated (Hockel *et al.* 1999). Firstly, hypoxia may induce changes within the tumour cells of the expression of oxygen-dependent proteins such as vascular endothelial growth factor (VEGF), which stimulates angiogenesis and increases the potential for tumour growth and metastases. Secondly, ionising radiation results in the formation of free radicals within cells. In the presence of oxygen, the free radicals are fixed and interact with DNA and cell membranes to cause cell death. When cells are hypoxic, free radicals are not fixed and cell death may not occur (Hall 1994). Thirdly, hypoxia may produce a growth advantage for tumour cells that are resistant to apoptosis, with a decrease in the potential for cure or control. In addition, hypoxic tumours may over-express the tumour suppressor gene *p53*, a cell phenotype with a higher malignant potential. Anaemia may also impair survival by diminishing the patient's overall well-being which may, in turn, impact on the delivery of appropriate doses of chemotherapy or radiotherapy or both.

Several non-randomised studies of chemotherapy and radiotherapy in patients with solid tumours have suggested that correcting anaemia during the course of treatment improves prognosis compared with similar patients with anaemia left untreated (Grogan *et al.* 1999; Antonadou *et al.* 1998; Glaser *et al.* 2001).

A large, placebo-controlled, randomised, double-blind clinical trial of erythropoietin was conducted in 375 anaemic patients (baseline haemoglobin less than 10.5 g/dl, or greater than 10.5 but less than 12.0 g/dl after a haemoglobin decrease of more than 1.5 g/dl in the previous month) who received non-platinum chemotherapy for non-myeloid haematological and solid malignancies (Littlewood *et al.* 2001). The original aims of this trial were to assess the effects of erythropoietin on transfusion requirements, haemoglobin level, quality of life, and safety. Before the study was unblinded, an additional aim was included to explore a possible relation between increased haemoglobin and survival. Patients were randomised to receive erythropoietin 150–300 international units per kilogram body weight three times weekly for 12–24 weeks (*n* = 251), or placebo (*n* = 124). Median survival times were 17 months for patients who received erythropoietin, compared with 11 months for the placebo group. The Kaplan-Meier 12-month estimates showed a trend towards better overall survival favouring the erythropoietin group ($p = 0.13$; log rank test). The investigators concluded that although the study was neither designed nor powered for survival as an endpoint, the results suggest a survival benefit with erythropoietin. Further trials are underway to confirm if a survival benefit is apparent, because other uncontrolled variables may have influenced survival, for example tumour stage, intensity of chemotherapy, extent of bone marrow involvement, and disease progression. A small study in patients with CLL has suggested that treatment with rHuEPO can downstage patients in the absence of concomitant chemotherapy and that the downstaged patients have an excellent progression-free survival (Pangalis 2002). One group (Mittelmann *et al.* 2001) has published data suggesting that rHuEPO induces tumour regression in a murine myeloma model. This anti-tumour response is thought to be caused by a tumour-specific immune response mediated by T cells. These are impressive results, which have to be evaluated by further research. However, it might be a reason for prolonged survival as indicated by Littlewood *et al.* (2001).

Although most reports have suggested that correcting anaemia may enhance survival, Henke *et al.* (2003) have reported that in patients with squamous cell tumours of the head and neck treated with radiotherapy, a group treated with epoetin beta had a worse survival than the control group. This result emphasises that the impact of rHuEpo on survival is far from clear and that more well-designed studies are urgently needed.

Predictors of response

Functional iron deficiency is a major factor limiting the efficiency of rHuEPO therapy, and iron supplementation should be considered. A recent study has suggested that intra-venous iron replacement is more effective than oral iron, but this finding requires confirmation (Auerbach 2001). Around 60% of patients will respond to rHuEPO with a haemoglobin increase of greater than 2.0 g/dl. The median time to response is approximately four weeks. Because rHuEPO is an expensive drug, it would be very useful to be able sensitively and specifically to predict those patients most likely to respond. Ludwig *et al.* (1994) showed that if after two weeks of treatment with rHuEPO the serum erythropoietin level was less than 100 international units per millilitre and the haemoglobin concentration had increased by more than 0.5 g/dl, a positive response to treatment could be predicted with 95% accuracy (Ludwig *et al.* 1994). Conversely, in patients meeting neither of those criteria, a lack of response could be predicted with 93% accuracy. Other investigators have shown that low baseline erythropoietin levels (or a low observed: predicted ratio of the erythropoietin level) or a rise in the transferrin receptor level after two weeks of treatment are predictive of patients most likely to respond to treatment with erythropoietin (Adamson *et al.* 1999). A very recent study, however, of 561 patients treated with rHuEPO failed to identify either a single or combination of factors that could sensitively and specifically predict the likelihood of response to treatment (Littlewood *et al.* 2003).

Adverse effects of rHuEPO

Treatment with RHuEPO in anaemic patients with haematological malignancies is generally extremely well tolerated. Pain or erythema at the injection site has been reported. Fever is rare. Hypertension induced by RHuEPO, which occurs most frequently in patients with chronic renal failure who are treated with higher doses, is very uncommon in anaemic patients with haematological malignancies. There are, however, reports that rHuEPO may exacerbate splenomegaly secondary to extramedullary haematopoiesis through stimulation of erythropoiesis in myeloproliferative disorders (Iki *et al.* 1991). In theory, treatment with rHuEPO may stimulate the growth of malignant cells if those tumour cells express surface receptors for erythropoietin. Bauer *et al.* (1992) reported that rHuEPO, either alone or in the presence of other cytokines, does not modulate growth of human cancer cells *in vitro*.

In a recent article (Casadevall *et al.* 2002), rHuEPO-induced pure red cell aplasia secondary to the development of neutralising antierythropoietin antibodies in 13 patients with chronic renal failure was reported. Although rare, this serious event is of concern. One hypothesis is that the antibody is directed against differences in carbohydrate structure between rHuEPO and naturally occurring erythropoietin (Bunn 2002).

Dissenting opinion

The authors believe that rHuEPO is a very useful drug in the management of certain patients with anaemia secondary to malignancy or its treatment, and evidence for this is given above. However, some clinicians and researchers remain sceptical about the benefits of rHuEPO in this setting. A recent report confirming the quality-of-life benefits for patients treated with rHuEpo has largely answered the criticisms of Bottomley and Seidenfield (Fallowfield *et al.* 2002).

Seidenfield *et al.* (2001), in a meta-analysis of randomised trials of rHuEPO, reported that only one patient would avoid transfusion for every five or six patients treated with rHuEPO and that there were insufficient data to recommend the use of rHuEPO in patients with a haemoglobin concentration greater than 10.0 g/dl.

More recently, a further critical review of 13 rHuEPO studies was conducted (Bottomley *et al.* 2002) with a particular emphasis on the quality-of-life issues. The review found that although some studies suggested an improvement in the patients' quality of life after treatment with rHuEPO, there were many methodological limitations in several of the studies which made complete interpretation of the data difficult. Both Seidenfield *et al.* (2001) and Bottomley *et al.* (2002) called for larger and more robustly designed randomised studies.

Conclusions

From the available data there is excellent evidence to recommend the use of erythropoietin in anaemic patients with lymphoproliferative disorders who are receiving chemotherapy, with the aim of maintaining the haemoglobin at greater than 12.0 g/dl (Crawford *et al.* 2002).

The existing data suggest that treating the patient before severe anaemia develops may be the most cost-effective approach, but further studies are needed in this area.

Similarly, most research has been conducted in patients with malignancies who are receiving concurrent chemotherapy or radiotherapy. However, anaemic patients with malignant disease who are not being actively treated may also benefit from treatment with erythropoietin (Quirt *et al.* 2001).

It appears that patients with myelodysplasia respond more readily to a combination of rHuEPO and granulocyte colony-stimulating factor (G-CSF) or granulocyte/macrophage colony-stimulating factor (GM-CSF) than when treated with one human growth factor alone.

There are few data on quality-of-life benefits in myelodysplastic syndrome (MDS) patients treated with erythropoietin/G-CSF, and no studies to determine whether such treatment might have any impact on life expectancy. The lack of such data makes recommendations about the use of rHuEPO in patients with MDS uncertain. Further research is needed.

New drug development has resulted in the design of a novel erythropoiesis-stimulating protein, darbepoetin alpha, which contains five N-linked carbohydrate chains (two more than rHuEPO). This designer drug has a 3-fold longer serum half-life, greater *in vivo* potency, and can be administered less frequently than standard rHuEPO to obtain the same biological response (Egrie & Browne 2001). Clinical trials in patients with anaemia secondary to haematological malignancies and solid tumours indicate that this is a safe and effective agent (Glaspy *et al.* 2002; Hedenus *et al.* 2002).

Many physicians were trained to believe that anaemia is not important in patients with malignant disease until it becomes very severe. This thinking is being challenged by the advent of rHuEPO, but uncertainties about its real worth and high cost still preclude its use in many healthcare systems.

References

Adamson, J. W. & Ludwig, H. (1999). Predicting the hematopoietic response to recombinant human erythropoietin (epoetin alfa) in the treatment of the anemia of cancer. *Oncology* **56**, 46–53.

Antonadou, D., Cardamekis, E., Sarris, V. & Tzigounia, N. (1998). Effect of the administration of recombinant human erythropoietin in patients with pelvic malignancies during radiotherapy. *Radiotherapy and Oncology* **48**, S122.

Auerbach, M., Barker, L., Bahrain, H., Trout, R., McIlwain, M. & Ballard, H. (2001). Intravenous iron (IV Fe) optimises the response to erythropoietin (Epo) in patients with anaemia of cancer and cancer chemotherapy: results of a multicentre, open-label, randomized trial. *Blood* **98**, abstract 3323.

Barrett-Lee, P. J., Bailey, N. P., O'Brien, M. E. R. & Wager, E. (2000). Large scale UK audit of blood transfusion requirements and anaemia in patients receiving cytotoxic chemotherapy. *British Journal of Cancer* **82**, 93–97.

Bauer, E., Danhauser-Riedl, S., De Riese, W., Raab, H. R., Sandner, S., Meyer, H. S., Neuman D., Hanauske U., Freund M., Poliwoda H. *et al.* (1992). Effects of recombinant human eythropoietin on clonogenic growth of primary human tumor specimens in vitro. *European Journal of Cancer* **28**, 1769–1770.

Bottomley, A., Thomas, R., Van, S.K., Flechtner, H. & Djulegovic, B. (2002). Human recombinate erythropoietin and quality of life: a wonder drug or something to wonder about? *Lancet Oncology* **3**(3), 145–153.

Brizel, D. M., Sibley, G. S., Prosnitz, L. R., Scher, R. L. & Dewhirst, M. W. (1997). Tumor hypoxia adversely affects the prognosis of carcinoma of the head and neck. *International Journal of Radiation Oncology Biology Physics* **38**, 285–289.

Bunn, H. F. (2002). Sugar in erythropoietin: clinical and forensic implications. *Blood* **99**(5), 1503.

Casadevall, N., Nataf, J., Viron, B., Kolta, A., Kiladjian, J. J., Martin-Dupont, Ph., Michaud, P., Papo, Th., Ugo, V., Teyssandier, I. *et al.* (2002). Pure red-cell aplasia and antierythropoietin antibodies in patients treated with recombinant erythropoietin. *New England Journal of Medicine* **346**, 469–475.

Cazzola, M., Messinger, D., Battistel, V., Bron, D., Cimino, R., Enller-Ziegel, L., Esser, K., Grell, R., Gross, A., Jager, G. *et al.* (1995). Recombinant human erythropoietin in the anaemia associated with multiple myeloma or non-Hodgkin's lymphoma: dose finding and identification of the predictors of response. *Blood* **86**, 4446–4453.

Cazzola, M., Mercuriali, F. & Brugnara, C. (1997). Use of recombinant human erythropoietin outside the setting of uremia. *Blood* **89**, 4248–4267.

Coiffier, B., Guastalla, J. P., Pujade-Lauraine, E., Bastit, P. (2001). Predicting cancer related anaemia in patients receiving non-platinum chemotherapy; Results of a retrospective survey. *European Journal of Cancer* **37**, 1617–1623

Coiffier, B. (2000). The impact and management of anaemia in haematological malignancies. *Medical Oncology* **17** (Suppl. 1), 2–10.

Crawford, J., Cella, D., Cleeland, C. S. *et al.* (2002). Relationship between changes in haemoglobin level and quality of life during chemotherapy in anemic cancer patients receiving epoetin alfa therapy. *Cancer* **95**, 888–895.

Curt, G. A., Breithart, W., Cella, D. *et al.* (2000). Impact of cancer related fatigue on the lives of patients: new findings from the fatigue coalition. *The Oncologist* **5**, 353–360.

Dammaco, F., Castoldi, G. & Rodjer, S. (2001). Efficacy of epoetin alfa in the treatment of anaemia of multiple myeloma. *British Journal of Haematology* **113**, 172–179.

Demetri, G. D., Kris, M., Wade, J., Degos, L. & Cella, D. (1998). Quality-of-life benefit in chemotherapy patients treated with epoetin alfa is independent of disease response or tumor type: results from a prospective community oncology study. *Journal of Clinical Oncology* **16**(10), 3412–3425.

Egrie, J. C. & Browne, J. K. (2001). Development and characterization of novel erythropoiesis stimulating protein (NESP). *Nephrology, Dialysis, Transplantion* **16** (Suppl. 3), 3–13.

Fallowfield, L., Gagnon, D., Zagari, M. *et al.* (2002). Multivariate regression analyses of data from a randomized, double-blind placebo controlled study confirm quality of life benefit of epoetin alfa in patients receiving non-platinum chemotherapy. *British Journal of Cancer* **87**, 1341–1353.

Glaser, C., Millesi, W., Kornek, G. V., Lang, S., Schull, B., Watzinger, F., Selzer, E. & Lavey, R. S. (2001). Impact of hemoglobin level and use of recombinant erythropoietin on efficacy of preoperative chemotherapy for squamous cell carcinoma of the oral cavity and oropharynx. *International Journal of Radiation Oncology Biology Physics* **3**, 705–715.

Glaspy, J., Bukowski, R., Steinberg, D., Taylor, C., Tchekmedyian, S. & Vadhan-Raj, S. (1997). Impact of therapy with epoetin alfa on clinical outcomes in patients with nonmyeloid malignancies during cancer chemotherapy in community oncology practice. *Journal of Clinical Oncology* **15**(3), 1218–1234.

Glaspy, J. A., Jadeja, J. S., Justice, G., Kessler, J., Richards, D., Schwartzberg, L., Tchekmedyian, N. S., Armstrong, S., O'Byrne, J., Rossi, G. & Colowick, A. B. (2002). Darbepoietin alfa given every 1 or 2 weeks alleviates anaemia associated with cancer chemotherapy. *British Journal of Cancer* **87**, 268–276.

Grogan, M., Thomas, G. M., Melamed, I., Wong, F. L., Pearceym R. G., Josephm P. K., Portelance, L., Crook, J. & Jones, K. D. (1999). The importance of haemoglobin levels during radiotherapy for carcinoma of the cervix. *Cancer* **86**, 1528–1536.

Hall, E. J. (1994). The oxygen effect and reoxygenation. In *Radiobiology for the Radiologist*, 4th edition (ed. E. J. Hall), pp. 133–152. Lippincott, Philadelphia.

Hedenus, M., Hansen, S., Taylor, K., Arthur, C., Emmerich, B., Dewey, C., Watson, D., Rossi, G. & Österborg, A. (2002). Randomized, dose-finding study of darbepoietin alfa in anaemic patients with lymphoproliferative malignancies. *British Journal of Haematology* **119**, 79–86.

Henke, M., Laszig, R., Rube, C. *et al.* (2003). Erythropoietin to treat head and neck cancer patients with anaemia undergoing radiotherapy: randomised, double-blind, placebo-controlled trial. *The Lancet* **362**, 1255–1260.

Höckel, M., Schlenger, K., Arral, B., Mitze, M., Schäffer, U. & Vaupel, P. (1996). Association between tumour hypoxia and malignant progression in advanced cancer of the uterine cervix. *Cancer Research* **56**, 4509–4515.

Höckel, M., Schlenger, K., Hockel, S. & Vaupel, P. (1999). Association between tumor hypoxia and malignant progression: the clinical evidence in cancer of the uterine cervix. In *Tumor Hypoxia* (ed. P. Vaupel & D. K. Kelleher), pp. 65–74. Wissenschaftliche Verlagsgesellschaft MBH, Stuttgart.

Iki, S., Yagisawa, M., Ohbayashi, Y., Sato, H. & Urabe, A. (1991). Adverse effect of erythropoietin in myeloproliferative disorders. *The Lancet* **337**, 187–188.

Kalmanti, M. & Kalmanti, T. (1989). Committed erythroid progenitors and erythropoietin levels in anemic children with lymphomas and tumors. *Pediatric Hematology and Oncology* **6**, 85–93.

Kasper, C. (2001). Recombinant human erythropoietin in the treatment of anemic patients with hematological malignancies. *Annals of Hematology* **80**, 319–329.

Kelleher, D. K., Matthiensen, U., Thews, O. & Vaupel P. (1996). Blood flow, oxygenation and bioenergetic status of tumors after erythropoietin treatment in normal and anemic rats. *Cancer Research* **56**, 4728–4734.

Kyle, R. A. (1975). Multiple myeloma: review of 869 cases. *Mayo Clinic Proceedings* **50**(1), 29–40.

Littlewood, T. J., Bajetta, E., Nortier, J. W. R., Vercammen, E. & Rapoport, B. for the Epoetin Alfa Study Group (2001). Effects of epoetin alfa on hematologic parameters and quality of life in cancer patients receiving nonplatinum chemotherapy: results of a randomized, double-blind, placebo-controlled trial. *Journal of Clinical Oncology* **19**(11), 2865–2874.

Littlewood, T. J., Zagari, M., Pallister, C. & Perkins, A. (2003). Baseline and early treatment factors are not clinically useful for predicting individual response to erythropoietin in anemic cancer patients. *The Oncologist* **8**, 99–107.

Ludwig, H., Fritz, E., Kotzmann, H., Hocker, P., Gisslinger, H. & Barnas, U. (1990). Erythropoietin treatment of anemia associated with multiple myeloma. *New England Journal of Medicine* **322**, 1693–1699.

Ludwig, H., Fritz, E., Leitgeb, C., Pecherstorfer, M., Samonigh, H. & Schuster, J. (1994). Prediction of response to erythropoietin treatment in chronic anemia of cancer. *Blood* **84**, 1056–1063.

Miller, C. B., Jones, R. J., Piantadosi, S., Abelloff, M. D. & Spivak, J. L. (1990). Decreased erythropoietin response in patients with the anemia of cancer. *New England Journal of Medicine* **322**, 1689–1692.

Mittelmann, M., Neumann, D., Peled, A., Kanter, P. & Nechama, H. G. (2001). Erythropoietin induces tumor regression and antitumor immune response in murine myeloma models. *Proceedings of the National Academy of Science of the United States of America* **98**(9), 5181–5186.

Molls, M., Stadler, P., Becker, A., Feldmann, H. J. & Dunst, J. (1998). Relevance of oxygen in radiation oncology. Mechanisms of action, correlation to low hemoglobin levels. *Strahlentherapie Onkologie* **174** (Suppl. IV), 13–16.

Osterborg, A., Boogaerts, M. A., Cimino, R., Essers, U., Holowiecki, J., Julinsson, G,. Jager, G., Najman, A. & Peest, D. (1996). Recombinant human erythropoietin in transfusion-dependent anaemic patients with multiple myeloma and non-Hodgkin's lymphoma – a randomised multicentre study. *Blood* **87**, 2675–2682.

Osterborg, A., Brandberg, Y., Molostova, V., Iosava, G., Abdulkadyrov, K., Hedenus, M. & Messinger, D. (2002). Randomized, double-blind, placebo-controlled trial of recombinant erythropoietin, epoetin beta, in hematologic malignancies. *Journal of Clinical Oncology* **20**, 2486–2494.

Pangalis, G. A., Siakantaris, M. P., Angelopoulou, M. K., Vassilakopoulos, T. P., Dimopoulou, M. N., Kyrtsonis, M. C., Konstantopoulos, K., Tsaftaridis, P., Vaiopoulos, G. A. & Kontopidou, F. N. (2002). Downstaging Rai stage III B-chronic lymphocytic leukemia patients with the administration of recombinant human erythropoietin. *Haematologica* **87**, 500–506.

Quirt, I., Robeson, C., Lau, C. Y., Kovacs, M., Burdette-Radoux, S., Dolan, S., Tang, S. C., McKenzie M. & Couture, F. (Canadian Eprex Oncology Study Group) (2001). Epoetin alfa therapy increases hemoglobin levels and improves quality of life in patients with cancer-related anemia who are not receiving chemotherapy and patients with anemia who are receiving chemotherapy. *Journal of Clinical Oncology* **19**(21), 4126–4134.

Rose, E., Rai, K., Revicki, D., Brown, R. & Reblando, J. (1994). Clinical and health status assessments in anemic chronic lymphocytic leukemia (CLL) patients treated with epoetin alfa (epo). *Journal of the American Society of Hematology* **84**, 526a.

San Miguel, J. F., Garcia-Sanz, R., Gonzalez, M., Moro, M. J., Hernandez, J. M., Ortega, F., Borrego, D., Carnero, M., Casanova, F., Jimenez, R. *et al.* (1995). A new staging system for multiple myeloma based on the number of S-phase plasma cells. *Blood* **85**(2), 448–455.

San Miguel, J. F. & Garcia-Sanz, R. (1998). Recombinant human erythropoietin in the anaemia of multiple myeloma and non-Hodgkin lymphoma. *Medical Oncology* **15**, S29–S34.

Seidenfeld, J., Piper, M., Flamm, C., Hasselblad, V., Armitage, J. O., Bennett, Ch. L., Gordon, M. S., Lichtin, A. L., Wade, J. L. III, Woolf, S. & Aronson, N. (2001). Epoetin treatment of anaemia associated with cancer therapy: a systematic review and meta-analysis of controlled clinical trials. *Journal of the National Cancer Institute* **93**(16), 1204–1214.

Spivak, J. L. (1994). Recombinant human erythropoietin and the anaemia of cancer. *Blood* **84**, 997–1004.

Teicher, B. A., Holden, S. A., al-Achi A. & Herman, T. S. (1990). Classification of antineoplastic treatments by their differential toxicity toward putative oxygenated and hypoxic tumor subpopulations in vivo in the FSaIIC murine fibrosarcoma. *Cancer Research* **50**, 3339–3344.

The UK Myeloma Forum (2001). Guidelines for diagnosis and management of multiple myeloma. *British Journal of Haematology* **115**, 522–540.

Vogelzang, N. J., Breitbart, W., Cella, D., Curt, G. A., Groopman, J. E., Horning, S. J., Itri, L. M., Johnson, D. H., Scherr, S. L. & Portenoy, R. U. (1997). Patient, caregiver and oncologist perceptions of cancer-related fatigue: results of a tripart assessment survey. *Seminars in Haematology* **34** (Suppl. 2), 4–12.

Chapter 3

The management of weakness and fatigue in patients with solid tumours

Richard Booton and Nicholas Thatcher

Introduction

Size of the problem, and predisposing factors

It is now possible to distinguish normal fatigue experienced by the general population from clinical fatigue (asthenia) associated with cancer and its treatments (Cella *et al.* 2002, 2003). Fatigue is a symptom complex and can be associated with specific problems such as lack of energy, weakness, sleepiness, difficulty in concentration, etc. Fatigue is a major problem for patients with cancer, limiting normal functioning and a good quality of life (Vogelzang *et al.* 1997). In 1996, 419 randomly selected patients treated with chemotherapy and/or radiotherapy, primary carers and oncologists were surveyed. The main finding was good agreement between patients and oncologists on the prevalence of fatigue (76% and 78%, respectively); however, 61% of patients said that fatigue affected their lives more than pain, compared with only 37% of oncologists.

In a further survey of 379 patients treated with chemotherapy, about 30% of patients reported feelings of fatigue daily, 59% reported feelings of fatigue weekly or more often, and 76% of patients experienced fatigue at least monthly. Fatigue was more prolonged with therapy, about a third reporting more than two weeks and 45% at least a week (Curt 2000; Curt *et al.* 2000). Criteria have recently been formulated to define clinically relevant fatigue, which may now be described as a multi-dimensional phenomenon developing over time and associated with reduced energy, reduced mental capacity and an impaired psychological profile, i.e. decreased motivation, poor sleep, marked emotional reactivity (sadness, frustration, irritability, etc.) (Cella 1998; Cella *et al.* 2001). These diagnostic criteria for cancer-related fatigue were examined in a sample of cancer survivors (most, 90%, having solid tumours) treated with chemotherapy and with or without radiation therapy. In this survey, 37% of patients reported at least two weeks of fatigue in the previous month. Importantly, 33% reported at least two weeks of fatigue in the month before interview despite having had their last treatment more than five years previously. Cancer-related fatigue can persist well beyond active treatment and requires more attention (Cella *et al.* 2001). Fatigue was the most intrusive side effect of chemotherapy, with a greater effect on quality of life than pain, nausea or depression. Cancer-related fatigue also had important economic consequences: reducing the ability to work and requiring primary carers to take days off or to reduce their responsibilities. Importantly, nearly half the patients thought fatigue was a direct result of their cancer and was untreatable. Recommendations by physicians in response to learning of their patients' fatigue were very non-specific, 40% recommending doing nothing and 37% prescribing a rest (Curt *et al.* 2000).

In a survey of fatigue in 151 ovarian cancer patients, its prevalence was 69%, and about half the patients described the condition as highly distressing (Portenoy *et al.* 1994). When chemotherapy and radiotherapy have been used, the prevalence rate of fatigue can be as high as 96%. It is also very common with biological modifiers such as interferon alpha or interleukin (Portenoy & Itri 1999).

Assessment of fatigue

Appreciation of the likely aetiological factors and the assessment of fatigue are necessary to target therapeutic management. For example, a description of the fatigue in terms of its existence, severity and temporal relationships, and identifying psychosocial problems and abnormal investigations, particularly in diagnosing anaemia, are valuable. A variety of scales are available to document fatigue, for example the NCI CTC scale. Linear analogue scales (LASA) and FACT-An (Functional Assessment of Cancer Therapy – Anaemia, a scale that assesses both anaemia and a subset of questions for fatigue, FACT-F) may be useful for gauging severity, observing changeover time and assessing the effect of therapeutic intervention. The FACT subscales are particularly appropriate as they are cancer specific, haemoglobin sensitive and easily completed by patients. The LASA are available in a variety of languages.

By using these instruments, a clear association between fatigue and anaemia was demonstrated in cancer patients. As an example, haemoglobin levels greater than 12 g/dl correlates with significantly less fatigue and fewer non-fatigue anaemia symptoms and a better quality of life than those with haemoglobin equal to 12 g/dl (Cella 1997).

Anaemia and cancer-related fatigue

Several predisposing factors lead to fatigue, including the underlying disease, treatment, systemic disorders such as anaemia, infection, failure of important organs (i.e. heart, kidney), poor nutrition, sleep disorders, chronic pain, and psychosocial factors such as depression and anxiety (Portenoy & Itri 1999). Cancer-related anaemia can result from blood loss, the tumour itself and a failure to utilise iron and vitamins appropriately (Ludwig & Fritz 1998). Anaemia may also be responsible for several non-fatigue symptoms such as impaired cognitive function, headache, dyspnoea and chest pain (Ludwig & Fritz 1998).

The pathophysiology of chronic anaemia in cancer probably arises from increased levels of inflammatory cytokines that impair differentiation of erythroid precursors, reduce erythropoietin production and iron utilisation (Ludwig and Fritz 1998). Indeed, erythroid progenitor cells are reduced in patients with small-cell lung cancer even before chemotherapy is started (de Campos *et al.* 1995). Moreover, the erythropoietin response to cancer-related anaemia is inappropriately low compared with anaemia due to blood loss or iron deficiency (Miller *et al.* 1990).

To diagnose chronic anaemia of cancer, other causes of anaemia need to be excluded. The finding of normocytic or microcytic red cells, often reduced reticulocytes and normal or increased iron stores with a low transferrin saturation, low serum iron, low transferrin and increased acute phase proteins, supports the diagnosis of chronic anaemia of cancer.

A recent review of common chemotherapy regimens used in common malignancies reported a high rate of mild or moderate anaemia. Moreover, severe anaemia is common during the treatment of lung, breast and ovarian cancer (Groopman & Itri 1999). The large UK audit of blood transfusion requirements in patients receiving chemotherapy revealed differences in the percentage of transfused patients according to tumour type, with lung cancer (43%) and ovarian cancer (41%) being highest and breast cancer less so (19%) (Barrett Lee *et al.* 2000). The high level in lung cancer patients probably represents these patients' sensitivity to mild or moderate anaemia given their high level of co-morbidity. Clinically significant anaemia occurs in up to 25% of patients receiving standard chemotherapy but increases to 63% in those on intensified regimens (Del Mastro *et al.* 1997). Clearly, using transfusions for mild/ moderate anaemia is fraught with logistic difficulty, and despite the causal relationship between even moderate anaemia and fatigue, anaemia is often under-treated until other symptoms appear (Cella 1997; Groopman & Itri 1999; Portenoy 2000; Cella *et al.* 2001, 2003). Nevertheless, this level of anaemia can lead to fatigue and a poorer quality of life. Therefore alternative methods of correcting anaemia have been investigated.

Management strategy

A broad management approach is required, as indicated by Portenoy & Itri (1999). Clearly, it is important to try to correct the causes of cancer-related fatigue including rationalising patients' medication, treatment of sleep problems, metabolic abnormalities and relieving depression. Several non-pharmacological interventions include patient education, individualised exercise programmes, modification of activity, specified rest patterns, management of stress, and a variety of cognitive therapies together with adequate nutrition. Pharmacological therapies have not been evaluated comprehensively in controlled trials. However, there is some evidence that psychostimulants such as methylphenidate may have a place in the treatment of opioid-related somnolence and cognitive impairment. Indeed, a well-written patient view has recently been published (Wharton 2002) which also illustrates the problems the patient has from fatigue. There is also some support for the use of low-dose corticosteroids in patients with advanced cancer and multiple symptoms (Inui 2002). Anaemia, an important contributor to cancer-related fatigue, remains crucial to identify.

The value of erythropoietin therapy in cancer patients

The FACT-An scale was completed by 50 cancer patients and differentiated between patients with low and high haemoglobin levels. The lower haemoglobin levels corresponded with greater fatigue, poorer overall quality of life and a decreased ability to work (Cella 1997). The correction of anaemia, confirmed by a recent meta-analysis of controlled erythropoietin trials, demonstrated the benefit of erythropoietin in terms of increasing the haemoglobin, reducing blood transfusion and improving quality of life when used at haemoglobin concentrations of 10 g/dl or below (Siedenfeld *et al.* 2001). There is additional evidence to suggest that the greatest incremental improvement in quality of life occurred when haemoglobin levels rose from 11 to 12 g/dl (Crawford *et al.* 2002).

Treatment for anaemia and cancer-related fatigue

Patients with symptomatic anaemia should be treated but this is often inadequate. Part of the problem is that moderate anaemia is not considered important, and there may be particular transfusion policies in place limiting the availability of red cell transfusion.

Several concerns, including potential transmission of human immunodeficiency virus and more recently prion disease, have moved the threshold from giving red cell transfusions from 10 g/dl or below in the 1980s to 7–8 g/dl or less in the 1990s (Surgenor *et al.* 1988, 1990; Welch 1992). Nevertheless, we should be optimistic that when appropriate emphasis has been placed on other serious symptoms, for example pain, nausea and vomiting associated with cancer, management improves.

Several studies have now investigated the effects of correcting the underlying anaemia with recombinant human erythropoietin. Many were controlled against the standard treatment of blood transfusion, and assessments were made of quality of life. These critical studies have be summarised (Booton & Thatcher 2004; Seidenfeld *et al.* 2001) (see Tables 3.1–3.4). Interestingly, anaemia might be a contributory factor to the wasting seen in cachetic patients as anaemia increases energy expenditure similar to systemic inflammation (Lundholm *et al.* 1994; Daneryd *et al.* 1998). In the Daneryd study, 108 patients with progressive cachexia due to solid tumours (mainly gastrointestinal cancer) were randomised either to receive an anti-inflammatory drug (indomethacin) or indomethacin and erythropoietin. Erythropoietin prevented the development of anaemia during the observation period and was associated with a significantly better maximum exercise capacity and other energy parameters compared with control patients.

Table 3.1 Erythropoietin: no chemotherapy (studies with more than 50 patients)

Number of patients	Randomised	Performance status better	Quality of life
118 (68%)	Yes	—	LASA ↑ (Abels 1993)
180 (prostate)	Yes for dose	—	EORTC ↑ if Hb ≥ 2 g (Johansson et al. 2001)
67 (40%)	No	Yes	(↑) (Ludwig et al. 1993)
183 (60%)	No	Yes	LASA, FACT-An ↑ (Quirt et al. 2001)

Figure in parenthesis is the percentage of solid cancer patients.
↑, Quality of life improved. EORTC, European Organisation for the Research and Treatment of Cancer.

Table 3.2 Erythropoietin: prophylaxis on chemotherapy (studies with more than 50 patients)

Number of patients	Randomised	Chemotherapy	Quality of life
62 (breast)	Yes	Cyclophosphamide epirubicin, fluorouracil	no difference (del Mastro et al. 1997)
84 (gastrointestinal)	Yes for dose	Non-Pt	EORTC Fatigue ↑ (Glimelius et al. 1998)
130 (small cell lung cancer)	Yes	Pt based	no difference (Thatcher et al. 1999)

Pt, platinum.
↑, Quality of life improved.

Table 3.3 Erythropoietin: chemotherapy-induced anaemia (randomised studies with more than 200 patients)

Number of patients	Solid tumours (percentage in study)	Epo response versus control	Quality of life
278	68%	48% versus 7%	LASA ↑ (Abels 1993)
359	54%	66% versus 21%	LASA ↑, FACT-An ↑ (Littlewood et al. 2001)
320	Lung	66% versus 24%	FACT fatigue ↑ (Vansteenkiste et al. 2002)

Table 3.4 Erythropoietin: chemotherapy-induced anaemia (non-randomised studies with more than 200 patients)

Number of patients	Solid tumours (percentage in study)	Epo response versus control	Quality of life
2289	78%	60%	LASA ↑, FACT-An↑ (Demetri et al. 1998)
2030	77%	53%	LASA ↑ (Glaspy et al. 1997)
2964	81%	49%	LASA ↑, FACT-An ↑ (Gabrilove et al. 2001)
218	67%	63%	LASA ↑ (Quirt et al. 2001)

(a) The use of erythropoietin in cancer patients not receiving cytotoxic chemotherapy

In non-randomised trials significant responses to erythropoietin, defined as an increase in haemoglobin of 2 g/dl over the study period, were identified with a reduction in transfusion requirements and improved performance status and quality of life (Ludwig et al. 1993, 1995; Leitgeb et al. 1994). A randomised double-blind placebo controlled study of erythropoietin in cancer patients not receiving chemotherapy also demonstrated significant increases in the haematocrit, correction of anaemia and quality of life improvement compared with placebo (Abels 1993), though the transfusion reductions did not reach statistical significance. In a study of patients with gastrointestinal cancer, erythropoietin was associated with improved quality of life (Glimelius et al. 1998), and in hormone refractory prostate cancer significant reductions in transfusions and improvements in quality of life were seen with a high erythropoietin dose (5,000 units three times a week) compared with a lower dose of 1,000 units three times a week (Johansson et al. 2001).

(b) Prophylactic use of erythropoietin with cytotoxic chemotherapy

Several randomised trials have demonstrated the possibility of preventing anaemia in patients undergoing chemotherapy (Table 3.2). In advanced gastrointestinal cancer, a faster and greater increase in haemoglobin was achieved with erythropoietin at 500 U/kg than at 1000 U/kg three times a week. Furthermore, fatigue and tiredness in daily activities significantly improved in patients whose haemoglobin rose by 1 g/dl (Glimelius et al. 1998). Other studies used dosages of either 150 U/kg or 300 U/kg three times a week, which ameliorated the haemoglobin drop with chemotherapy compared with control groups (Dunphy et al. 1997, 1999; Levine et al. 1999).

In a randomised controlled study of prophylactic erythropoietin in small-cell lung cancer, a significant reduction in patients becoming anaemic was demonstrated, i.e.

no erythropoietin (66%) versus 150 U/kg (48%; $p < 0.05$) versus 300 U/kg (39%; $p = 0.005$). There was also a significant reduction in blood transfusion requirement: placebo 59% versus 150 U/kg (45%; $p < 0.05$) versus 300 U/kg (20%; $p = 0.05$) (Thatcher *et al.* 1999). Patients with ovarian cancer receiving platinum-based chemotherapy in a placebo controlled trial also demonstrated a significantly longer time to first transfusion, and fewer episodes of a nadir haemoglobin of less than 10 g/dl (ten Bokkel *et al.* 1998). Other randomised trials also indicated reductions in transfusions, but not all studies routinely assessed quality of life. In the small-cell lung cancer study, LASA was used to evaluate energy level, daily activity and overall quality of life. There were no marked changes from baseline at the end of therapy in the three cohorts other than a significant improvement in overall quality of life in those patients receiving the 150 U/kg dose. However, supplemental iron was not routinely given and therefore at the end of the study period (when quality of life measurements were taken) several patients had failed to continue to respond to erythropoietin because of lack of available iron (Thatcher *et al.* 1999).

(c) Erythropoietin and chemotherapy-induced anaemia

Several randomised trials have investigated whether erythropoietin in patients who are anaemic on chemotherapy can restore the haemoglobin level, reduce transfusion requirement and maintain or improve the patients' quality of life (Table 3.3). Patients receiving either platinum-based chemotherapy ($n = 125$) or non-platinum-based chemotherapy ($n = 153$) for a variety of malignancies were randomised to placebo versus erythropoietin 150 U/kg three times a week. There was a significant increase in haematocrit, and a reduction in the number of patients requiring transfusion on platinum-based chemotherapy compared with placebo. However, no decreases in transfusion requirements were noted for patients receiving non-platinum chemotherapy in this particular study (Henry and Abels 1994). There was improvement in the QoL measures, including the ability to do daily activities, and increased energy levels in erythropoietin-treated patients compared with placebo. The large study by Littlewood *et al.* (2001) (mainly of patients with breast cancer and non-myeloid haematological malignancy receiving non-platinum chemotherapy) demonstrated reduction in the numbers of patients requiring transfusion, and a significant rise in haemoglobin from baseline compared with placebo. Quality of life was carefully measured by using FACT-G, FACT-F, FACT-An and LASA assessment scales. Each of the FACT scores, as well as the LASA scores, revealed an improvement in patients receiving erythropoietin compared with placebo. Furthermore, there was a significant correlation between increase in haemoglobin level and improvement in quality of life score (Fallowfield *et al.* 2002). In two other placebo-controlled studies, erythropoietin was investigated in patients undergoing chemotherapy for gynaecological or malignant bone tumours (Kurz *et al.* 1997; Wurnig *et al.* 1996). Again, there was a significant reduction in transfusion requirements and, in the gynaecological cancer group, significant improvements in quality of life in responders.

Other studies using erythropoietin for chemotherapy-induced anaemia have been done in a community setting and have supported the results of controlled randomised trials in a general cancer population. These have included many patients with breast, bronchial and gynaecological cancers, and are shown in Table 3.4 (Glaspy *et al.* 1997; Demetri *et al.* 1998; Quirt *et al.* 2001; Gabrilove *et al.* 2001). A significant increase in haemoglobin, a reduction in transfusion requirements, and an improvement in quality of life were noted in all trials. The changes in quality of life correlated with changes in haemoglobin levels: the greatest incremental improvement in quality of life occurred when the haemoglobin increased from 11 to 12 g/dl (Crawford *et al.* 2002). Interestingly, there was a trend (although not significant) towards improved quality of life, even in those patients with progressive disease, providing there was an erythropoietin response (Demetri *et al.*1998; Glaspy *et al.* 1997). Gabrilove *et al.* (2002) demonstrated that a once weekly rather than the traditional three times a week dose of erythropoietin was just as effective. A formal phase III trial comparing the alternative regimens is probably required (Nguyen 2002; Gabrilove *et al.* 2002).

(d) The use of erythropoietin with radiotherapy

A large volume of literature is available about the relation between tumour oxygenation and response primarily to radiotherapy but also to some chemotherapeutic agents. It is therefore appealing to correct anaemia in an attempt to improve tumour oxygenation and treatment outcomes (Hockel & Vaupel 2001; Langer *et al.* 2003). The tumours investigated, mainly by obtaining pO_2 tumour measurements, have been cervical carcinoma and head and neck tumours. In a randomised phase II trial, erythropoietin significantly improved haemoglobin concentration and quality of life compared with controls (Sweeney *et al.* 1998). However, most of these studies were more concerned with loco-regional tumour control, the disease-free survival and tumour response rather than quality of life.

Darbepoetin is a hyperglycoslyated analogue of erythropoietin, with approximately a threefold longer half-life, which only needs to be administered on a once weekly basis (Heatherington *et al.* 2001). It was shown to be effective in patients with non-myeloid malignancy who had not received chemotherapy. In this non-randomised study erythropoietin increased haemoglobin, reduced transfusion rates and patient-reported fatigue (FACT-F scale) (Smith *et al.* 2001).

The efficacy and safety of darbepoetin (2.25 µg/kg/week) has been confirmed in a large randomised placebo-controlled trial in lung cancer patients on chemotherapy. Patients who received darbepoetin required fewer transfusions, fewer units of red cells per patient, and more haemoglobin increases in the absence of red cell transfusions than those receiving placebo. Improvement of the FACT-F was significantly better with darbepoetin than placebo. There was some suggestion of a median survival difference (46 weeks, 95% confidence interval 39–53, versus 34 weeks, 95% confidence interval 29–39) in favour of the darbepoetin-treated group (Vansteenkiste *et al.* 2002).

Conclusion

Patients suffer from a wide variety of problems as a result of their cancer or treatment. Fatigue is a major symptom for which anaemia is an important cause. The use of recombinant human erythropoietin in correcting anaemia has beneficial effects not only in reducing transfusion requirements but also in improving quality of life, including fatigue. Future work should involve reducing the need for thrice weekly to weekly administration, perhaps to frequencies as low as once every three or four weeks. Higher initial loading doses may reduce the lag period for the erythropoietin–haemoglobin response. Furthermore, the use of erythropoietin response predictors and the effect of maintaining or increasing the haemoglobin level during treatment on survival require additional attention. Much work, therefore, needs to be performed on attaining the maximum benefits of erythropoietin and improving therapeutic outcomes.

References

Abels, R. (1993). Erythropoietin for anaemia in cancer patients. *European Journal of Cancer* **29A** (Suppl. 2), S2–S8.

Barrett-Lee, P. J., Bailey, N. P., O'Brien, M. E. & Wager, E. (2000). Large-scale UK audit of blood transfusion requirements and anaemia in patients receiving cytotoxic chemotherapy. *British Journal of Cancer* **82**, 93–97.

Booton, R. & Thatcher, N. (2004). The value of erythropoietin therapy in cancer patients. *American Journal of Cancer.* (In the press.)

Cella, D. (1997). The Functional Assessment of Cancer Therapy-Anemia (FACT-An) scale: a new tool for the assessment of outcomes in cancer anemia and fatigue. *Seminars in Hematology* **34** (Suppl. 2), 13–19.

Cella, D. (1998). Factors influencing quality of life in cancer patients: anemia and fatigue. *Seminars in Oncology* **25** (Suppl. 7), 43–46.

Cella, D., Davis, K., Breitbart, W. *et al.* (2001). Cancer-related fatigue: prevalence of proposed diagnostic criteria in a United States sample of cancer survivors. *Journal of Clinical Oncology* **19**, 3385–3391.

Cella, D., Lai, J. S., Chang, C. H., Peterman, A. & Slavin, M. (2002). Fatigue in cancer patients compared with fatigue in the general United States population. *Cancer* **94**, 528–538.

Cella, D., Zagari, M. J., Vandoros, C., Gagnon, D. D., Hurtz, H.-J. & Nortier, J. W. R. (2003). Epoetin alfa treatment results in clinically significant improvements in quality of life in anemic cancer patients when referenced to the general population. *Journal of Clinical Oncology* **21**, 366–373.

Crawford, J., Cella, D., Cleeland, C. S., Cremieux, P. Y., Demetri, G. D., Sarokham, B. J., Slavin, M. B. & Glaspy, J. A. (2002). Relationship between changes in hemoglobin level and quality of life during chemotherapy in anemic cancer patients receiving epoetin alfa therapy. *Cancer* **95**, 888–895.

Curt, G. A. (2000). The impact of fatigue on patients with cancer: Overview of FATIGUE 1 and 2. *The Oncologist* **5** (Suppl. 2), 9–12.

Curt, G. A., Breitbart, W., Cella, D., Groopman, J. E., Horning, S. J., Itri, L. M., Johnston, D. H., Miaskowski, C., Scherr, S. L., Portenoy, R. K. *et al.* (2000). Impact of cancer-related fatigue on the lives of patients: new findings from the fatigue coalition. *The Oncologist* **5**, 353–360.

Daneryd, P., Svanberg, E., Korner, U., Lindholm, E., Sandstrom, R., Brevinge, H., Pettersson, C., Bosaeus, I. & Lundholm, K. (1998). Protection of metabolic and exercise capacity in unselected weight-losing cancer patients following treatment with recombinant erythropoietin: a randomised prospective study. *Cancer Research* **58**, 5374–5379.

de Campos, E., Radford, J., Steward, W., Milroy, R., Dougal, M., Swindell, R., Testa, N., & Thatcher, N. (1995). Clinical and in vitro effects of recombinant human erythropoietin in patients receiving intensive chemotherapy for small-cell lung cancer. *Journal of Clinical Oncology* **13**, 1623–1631.

Del Mastro, L., Venturini, M., Lionetto, R., Garrone, O., Melioli, G., Pasquetti, W., Sertoli, M. R., Bertelli, G., Canvese, G., Costantini, M. *et al.* (1997). Randomized phase III trial evaluating the role of erythropoietin in the prevention of chemotherapy-induced anemia. *Journal of Clinical Oncology* **15**, 2715–2721.

Demetri, G. D., Kris, M., Wade, J., Degos, L. & Cella, D. (1998). Quality-of-life benefit in chemotherapy patients treated with epoetin alfa is independent of disease response or tumor type: results from a prospective community oncology study for the Procrit Study Group. *Journal of Clinical Oncology* **16**, 3412–3425.

Dunphy, F. R., Dunleavy, T. L., Harrison, B. R., Boyd, J. H., Varvares, M. A., Dunphy, C. H., Rodriguez, J. J., McDonough, E. M., Minster, J. R. & McGrady, M. D. (1997). Erythropoietin reduces anemia and transfusions after chemotherapy with paclitaxel and carboplatin. *Cancer* **79**, 1623–1628.

Dunphy, F. R., Harrison, B. R., Dunleavy, T. L., Rodriguez, J. J., Hilton, J.G. & Boyd, J. H. (1999). Erythropoietin reduces anemia and transfusions: A randomized trial with or without erythropoietin during chemotherapy. *Cancer* **86**, 1362–1367.

Fallowfield, L., Gagnon, D., Zagari, M., Cella, D., Bresnaham, B., Littlewood, T. J., McNulty, P., Gorzegno, G. & Freund, M. (2002). Multivariate regression analysis of data from a randomised, double-blind, placebo-controlled study confirm quality of life benefit of epoetin alfa in patients receiving non-platinum chemotherapy. *British Journal of Cancer* **87**, 1341–1353.

Gabrilove, J. L., Cleeland, C. S., Livingston, R. B., Sarokham, B., Winer, E. & Einhorn, L. H. (2001). Clinical evaluation of once-weekly dosing of epoetin alfa in chemotherapy patients: improvements in hemoglobin and quality of life are similar to three-times-weekly dosing. *Journal of Clinical Oncology* **19**, 2875–2882.

Gabrilove, J., Sarokhan, B. & Cremieux, P. (2002). Statistical explanations for a community-based study of once-weekly epoetin alpha therapy in patients receiving chemotherapy. *Journal of Clinical Oncology* **20**, 27–57.

Glaspy, J., Bukowski, R., Steinberg, D. *et al.* (1997) Impact of therapy with epoetin alfa on clinical outcomes in patients with nonmyeloid malignancies during cancer chemotherapy in community oncology practice. Procrit Study Group. *Journal of Clinical Oncology* **15**, 1218–1234.

Glimelius, B., Linne, T., Hoffman, K., Larsson, L., Svensson, J. H., Nasman, P., Svensson, B. & Helmers, C. (1998). Epoetin beta in the treatment of anemia in patients with advanced gastrointestinal cancer. *Journal of Clinical Oncology* **16**, 434–440.

Groopman, J. E. & Itri, L. M. (1999). Chemotherapy-induced anemia in adults: incidence and treatment. *Journal of the National Cancer Institute* **91**, 1616–1634.

Heatherington, A. C., Schuller, J. & Mercer, A. J. (2001). Pharmacokinetics of novel erythropoiesis stimulating protein (NESP) in cancer patients: preliminary report. *British Journal of Cancer* **84** (Suppl. 1), 11–16.

Henry, D. H. & Abels, R. I. (1994). Recombinant human erythropoietin in the treatment of cancer and chemotherapy-induced anemia: results of double-blind and open-label follow-up studies. *Seminars in Oncology* **21** (Suppl. 3), 21–28.

Hockel, M. & Vaupel, P. (2001). Tumor hypoxia: definitions and current clinical, biologic, and molecular aspects. *Journal of the National Cancer Institute* **93**(4), 266–276.

Inui, A. (2002). Cancer anorexia–cachexia syndrome: current issues in research and management. *CA: A Cancer Journal for Clinicians* **52**, 72–91.

Johansson, J. E., Wersall, P., Brandberg, Y., Andersson, S. O. & Nordstrom, L. (2001). Efficacy of epoetin beta on hemoglobin, quality of life, and transfusion needs in patients with anemia due to hormone-refractory prostate cancer–a randomized study. *Scandinavian Journal of Urology and Nephrology* **35**, 288–294.

Kurz, C., Marth, C., Windbichler, G., Lahousen, M., Medl, M., Vavra, N. & Sevelda, P. (1997). Erythropoietin treatment under polychemotherapy in patients with gynecologic malignancies: a prospective, randomized, double-blind placebo-controlled multicenter study. *Gynecologic Oncology* **65**, 461–466.

Langer, C., Hirsch, F. R., Cortes-Funes, H., Sawyer, S. T. & Thatcher, N. (2003). Targeted molecular mechanisms of epoetin alfa. *Lung Cancer* **41**(Suppl. 1), S133–S145.

Leitgeb, C., Pecherstorfer, M., Fritz, E., & Ludwig, H. (1994). Quality of life in chronic anemia of cancer during treatment with recombinant human erythropoietin. *Cancer* **73**, 2535–2542.

Levine, E. A., Laborde, C., Hambrick, E., McKnight, C. A. & Vijayakumar, S. (1999). Influence of erythropoietin on transfusion requirements in patients receiving preoperative chemoradiotherapy for rectal cancer. *Diseases of the Colon and Rectum* **42**, 1065–1069; discussion 1069–1071.

Littlewood, T. J., Bajetta, E., Nortier, J. W., Vercammen, E. & Rapoport, B. (2001). Effects of epoetin alfa on hematologic parameters and quality of life in cancer patients receiving non-platinum chemotherapy: results of a randomized, double-blind, placebo-controlled trial. *Journal of Clinical Oncology* **19**, 2865–2874.

Ludwig, H., Leitgeb, C., Fritz, E., Krainer, M., Kuhrer, I., Kornek, G., Sagaster, P. & Weissmann, A. (1993). Erythropoietin treatment of chronic anaemia of cancer. *European Journal of Cancer* **29A** (Suppl. 2), S8–S12.

Ludwig, H. & Fritz, E. (1998). Anemia in cancer patients. *Seminars in Oncology* **25** (Suppl. 7), 2–6

Ludwig, H., Sundal, E., Pecherstorfer, M. *et al.* (1995). Recombinant human erythropoietin for the correction of cancer associated anemia with and without concomitant cytotoxic chemotherapy. *Cancer* **76**, 2319–2329.

Lundholm, K., Gelin, J., Hyltander, A. *et al.* (1994). Anti-inflammatory treatment may prolong survival in undernourished patients with metastatic solid tumors. *Cancer Research* **54**, 5602–5606.

Miller, C. B., Jones, R. J., Piantadosi, S. Abeloff, M. D. & Spivak, J. L. *et al.* (1990). Decreased erythropoietin response in patients with the anemia of cancer. *New England Journal of Medicine* **322**, 1689–1692.

Nguyen, T. V. & Trinh, G. N. (2002). Clinical evaluation of once-weekly and three-times-weekly dosings of epoetin alfa in chemotherapy patients: problems of study design and interpretation. *Journal of Clinical Oncology* **20**, 878.

Portenoy, R. K., Kornblith, A. B., Wong, G., Vlamis, V., Lepore, J. M., Loseth, D. B., Hakes, T., Foley, K. M. & Hoskins, W. J. (1994). Pain in ovarian cancer patients. Prevalence, characteristics and associated symptoms. *Cancer* **74**, 907–915.

Portenoy, R. K. & Itri, L. M. (1999). Cancer-related fatigue: Guidelines for evaluation and management. *The Oncologist* **4**, 1–10.

Portenoy, R. K. (2000). Cancer-related fatigue: An immense problem. *The Oncologist* **5**, 350–352.

Quirt, I., Robeson, C., Lau, C. Y., Kovacs, M., Burdette-Radoux, S., Dolan, S., Tang, S. C., McKenzie, M. & Couture, F. (2001). Epoetin alfa therapy increases hemoglobin levels and improves quality of life in patients with cancer-related anemia who are not receiving chemotherapy and patients with anemia who are receiving chemotherapy. *Journal of Clinical Oncology* **19**, 4126–4134.

Seidenfeld, J., Piper, M., Flamm, C., Hasselblad, V., Armitage, J. O., Bennett, C. L., Gordon, M. S., Lichtin, A. E., Wade, J. L., 3rd, Woolf, S. *et al.* (2001). Epoetin treatment of anemia associated with cancer therapy: a systematic review and meta-analysis of controlled clinical trials. *Journal of the National Cancer Institute* **93**, 1204–1214.

Smith, R. E. Jr, Jaiyesimi, I. A., Meza, L. A., Tchekmedyian, N. S., Chan, D., Griffith, H., Brosman, S., Bukowski, R., Murdoch, M., Rarick, M. *et al.* (2001). Novel erythropoiesis stimulating protein (NESP) for the treatment of anaemia of chronic disease associated with cancer. *British Journal of Cancer* **84** (Suppl. 1), 24–30.

Surgenor, D. M., Wallace, E. L., Hale, S. G. & Gilpatrick, M. W. (1988). Changing patterns of blood transfusions in four sets of United States hospitals, 1980–1985. *Transfusion* **28**, 513–518.

Surgenor, D., Wallace, E., Hao, S. & Chapman, R. (1990). Collection and transfusion of blood in the United States, 1982–1988. *New England Journal of Medicine* **322**, 1646–1651.

Sweeney, P. J., Nicolae, D., Ignacio, L., Chen, L., Roach, M., 3rd, Wara, W., Marcus, K. C. & Vijayakumar, S. (1998). Effect of subcutaneous recombinant human erythropoietin in cancer patients receiving radiotherapy: final report of a randomized, open-labelled, phase II trial. *British Journal of Cancer* **77**, 1996–2002.

ten Bokkel Huinink, W. W., de Swart, C. A., van Toorn, D. W., Morack, G., Breed, W. P., Hillen, H. F., van der Hoeven, J. J., Reed, N. S., Fairlamb, D. J., Chan, S. Y. *et al.* (1998). Controlled multicentre study of the influence of subcutaneous recombinant human erythropoietin on anaemia and transfusion dependency in patients with ovarian carcinoma treated with platinum-based chemotherapy. *Medical Oncology* **15**, 174–182.

Thatcher, N., De Campos, E. S., Bell, D. R., Steward, W. P., Varghese, G., Morant, R., Vansteenkiste, J. F., Rosso, R., Ewers, S. B., Sundal, E. *et al.* (1999). Epoetin alpha prevents anaemia and reduces transfusion requirements in patients undergoing primarily platinum-based chemotherapy for small cell lung cancer. *British Journal of Cancer* **80**, 396–402.

Vansteenkiste, J., Pirker, R., Massuti, B., Barata, F., Font, A., Fiegl, M., Siena, S., Gateley, J., Tomita, D., Colowick, A. B. *et al.* (2002). Double-blind, placebo-controlled, randomized phase III trial of darbepoetin alfa in lung cancer patients receiving chemotherapy. *Journal of the National Cancer Institute* **94**, 1211–1120.

Vogelzang, N. J., Breitbart, W., Cella, D., Curt, G. A., Groopman, J. E., Horning, S. J., Itri, L. M., Johnson, D. H., Scherr, S. L. & Portenoy, R. K. (1997). Patient, caregiver, and oncologist perceptions of cancer-related fatigue: results of a tripart assessment survey. *Seminars in Hematology* **34**, 4–12.

Wharton, R. H. (2002). Sleeping with the enemy: treatment of fatigue in individuals with cancer. *The Oncologist* **7**, 96–99.

Welch, H. G., Meehan, K. R. & Goodrough, L. T. (1992). Prudent strategies for elective red blood cell transfusion. *Annals of Internal Medicine* **116**, 393–402.

Wurnig C, Windhager R, Schwameis E., Kotz, R., Zoubek, A., Stockenhuber, F & Kurz, R. W. (1996). Prevention of chemotherapy-induced anemia by the use of erythropoietin in patients with primary malignant bone tumors (a double-blind, randomized, phase III study). *Transfusion* **36**, 155–159.

Chapter 4

Blood transfusion in the treatment of weakness and fatigue in cancer

Aleksandar Mijovic

Anaemia is common in cancer patients: haemoglobin concentrations less than 11 g/dl are found in 50–60% of patients with lung cancer (Langer *et al.* 2002); 45% of multiple myeloma patients have a haemoglobin concentration of less than 10 g/dl, and 21% a haemoglobin concentration of less than 8.5 g/dl (Ludwig *et al.* 2002). One of the highest prevalences of anaemia is found in myelodysplastic syndromes (MDS), with about 80% patients being anaemic (Mijovic 2002). Pathogenesis of the anaemia in cancer is complex, comprising suppression of erythropoiesis by cytokines (tumour necrosis factor, interleukin-1, interferons), blunted erythropoietin response to anaemia, retention of iron by the macrophages and impaired internalisation of iron (Means 1999). Anaemia is occasionally exacerbated by blood loss and nutritional deficiencies and, importantly, chemotherapy and radiotherapy.

Rates of red cell transfusion in solid tumours vary between 19% and 43% (Barrett-Lee *et al.* 2000). These rates are higher in haematological malignancies: nearly all patients with acute leukaemia receive transfusions at some stage of their disease. Increased intensity of chemotherapy, wider use of haemopoietic stem cell transplantation, and prolonged survival contribute to increased blood component usage. A recent UK audit of the use of red cell transfusions has shown that 15.5% of red cell units were transfused into haematological patients (Wells *et al.* 2002).

Fatigue is a common symptom in cancer patients. Causes of fatigue are multiple (pain, depression, adverse effects of treatment), but anaemia may also contribute. Recent studies of quality of life in oncology patients have shown, somewhat unexpectedly, that moderate anaemia (haemoglobin 9–11 g/dl) may be associated with impaired quality of life, and that the greatest quality of life improvements may be achieved by the correction of haemoglobin values of 10–11 g/dl (Glaspy *et al.* 1997; Demetri *et al.* 1998; Cleeland *et al.* 1999).

Since its successful introduction for the anaemia of renal failure, erythropoietin has been used to improve anaemia in a variety of malignant disorders. Not surprisingly, because of the multifactorial nature of anaemia in cancer, its overall efficacy in this setting is 50–60%. Several studies in multiple myeloma have shown efficacies of around 60% (Dammacco *et al.* 2001; Cazzola *et al.* 1995). A study of 221 patients with chronic lymphocytic leukaemia (Rose *et al.* 1994) had a response rate (6-point increase in haematocrit) of 47%. In MDS, a paradigm disease with long-term transfusion dependence, correction of anaemia was achieved in 37% of patients by using a high erythropoietin dose (150 U/kg/day for at least 8 weeks) (Italian Cooperative Group 1998). The importance of prolonged administration (up to 26 weeks) of erythropoietin was demonstrated again in a phase II study in which complete and partial responses were achieved in up to 58% of patients (Terpos *et al.* 2002).

Erythropoietin has not been the sole agent used to treat anaemia in MDS. Modest reductions in transfusion dependence have been reported with amifostine (with or without steroids) and thalidomide (Raza *et al.* 2001).

Because of the uncertain effect of erythropoietin (and other anti-anaemic agents), the interval of several weeks that it takes to exert its effect, and the need for prolonged administration of higher doses, red cell transfusions remain widely used to treat anaemia in cancer. Transfusion owes its appeal to a prompt and assured effect. Since the outbreak of the AIDS epidemics in 1980s, however, blood safety has been in focus, prompting various measures to reduce transfusion-related complications. As a result, the risk of infectious complications declined due to better donor selection, donation testing, and implementation of good manufacturing principles. Current estimated risks of transfusion-transmitted viral disease in the UK are 1 in 4 million transfused units for HIV, 1 in 3 million for hepatitis C, and between 1 in 100,000–400,000 for hepatitis B. Life-threatening, non-infectious transfusion complications are relatively rare. The commonest one is transfusion-associated acute lung injury, with an estimated incidence of 1 in 50,000–200,000 transfusions, and mortality around 5–15% (Serious Hazards of Transfusion Report 2000/2001). At the time of writing, concerns about transmission of variant Creutzfeldt–Jakob disease (vCJD) through blood products continue but have not been corroborated. The National Blood Service has traced the blood components made from ten donors who later developed vCJD. No recipient developed neurological disease. On the other hand, four vCJD patients had received a total of 117 blood products before developing disease. Of the 111 donors who supplied these products, none developed vCJD (P. Hewitt, personal communication 2002). However, risks of vCJD transmission remain unknown, albeit probably low.

For patients on regular transfusion programmes, iron overload remains a problem. Although clinical problems are rarely encountered with ferritin values below 2,500 ng/ml (Gordon-Smith & Marsh 2000), this degree of iron overload can be reached after one or two years of regular red cell transfusions. Desferrioxamine is the only well-established iron chelator in use, but its use is marred with inconvenience of subcutaneous infusions and high cost. Wider experience with the available oral iron chelator, deferiprone, in managing transfusion iron overload is urgently needed.

Finally, detailed economic studies comparing blood transfusion and erythropoietin in cancer patients are still lacking.

Red cell transfusions remain the mainstay of treatment of anaemia in malignant disease. Decision to transfuse should always be based on clinical judgement, but transfusion is usually necessary when haemoglobin falls below 8.5–9.0 g/dl, especially in the elderly, who are most cancer patients. It is important to adjust volume and frequency of transfusions to ensure optimal quality of life. Transfusion at higher baseline haemoglobin concentrations, i.e. 9.0–11.0 g/dl, may be warranted depending on clinical and other (e.g. social) circumstances.

References

Barrett-Lee, P. J., Bailey, N. P., O'Brien, M. E. R. & Wager, E. (2000). Large-scale UK audit of blood transfusion requirements and anaemia in patients receiving cytotoxic chemotherapy. *British Journal of Cancer* **82**, 93–97.

Cazzola, M., Messinger D., Battistel, V., Bron, D., Cimino, R., Enller-Ziegler, L., Essers, U., Greil, R., Grossi, A., Jager, G. *et al.* (1995). Recombinant human erythropoietin in the anemia associated with multiple myeloma and non-Hodgkin's lymphoma: dose finding and identification of predictors of response. *Blood* **86**, 4446–4453.

Cleeland, C. S., Demetri, G. D. *et al.* (1999). Identifying hemoglobin level for optimal quality of life: results of an incremental analysis. *Proceedings of the American Society of Clinical Oncology* **18**, 574A (no.2215).

Dammacco, F., Castoldi, G. & Roedjer, S. (2001). Efficacy of epoetin alfa in the treatment of anaemia of multiple myeloma. *British Journal of Haematology* **113**, 172–179.

Demetri, G. D., Kris, M.,Wade, J., Degos, L. & Cella, D. (1998). Quality-of-life benefit in chemotherapy patients treated with epoetin alpha is independent of disease response or tumor type: results from a prospective community oncology study. Procrit Study Group. *Journal of Clinical Oncology* **16**, 3412–3425.

Glaspy, J., Bukowski, R., Steinberg, D., Taylor, C., Tchekmedyian, S. & Vadhan-Raj, S. (1997). Impact of therapy with epoetin alpha on clinical outcomes in patients with nonmyeloid malignancies during cancer chemotherapy in community oncology practice. *Journal of Clinical Oncology* **15**, 1218–1234.

Gordon-Smith, E. C. & Marsh, J. C. W. (2000). Management of acquired aplastic anemia. *Reviews in Clinical and Experimental Hematology* **4**, 260–278.

Italian Cooperative Study Group (1998). A randomized double-blind placebo-controlled study with subcutaneous recombinant human erythropoietin in patients with low-risk myelodysplastic syndromes. *British Journal of Haematology* **103**, 1070–1074.

Langer, C. J., Choy, H., Glaspy, J. A. & Colowick, A. (2002). Standards of care for anemia management in oncology. *Cancer* **95**, 613–623.

Ludwig, H., Rai, K., Blade, J., Dammacco, F., Degos, L., Itri, L., Kyle, R., Liso, V., Littlewood, T. J., Mandelli, F. *et al.* (2002). Management of disease-related anemia in patients with multiple myeloma or chronic lymphocytic leukemia: epoetin treatment recommendations. *Haematology Journal* **3**, 121–130.

Means, R. T. Jr (1999). The anemia of chronic disorders. In *Wintrobe's clinical haematology*, 10th edn (ed. G. R. Lee, J. Foerster *et al.*), pp. 1011–1021. Williams & Wilkins, Baltimore.

Mijovic, A. (2002). Blood transfusion in patients requiring long-term support. In *Transfusion medicine in practice* (ed. J. Duguid, L. T. Goodnough & M. J. Desmond), pp. 49–72. Martin Dunitz, London.

Raza, A., Meyer, P., Dutt, D., Zorat, F., Lisak, L., Nascimben, F., du Randt, M., Kaspar, C., Goldberg, C., Loew, J. *et al.* (2001). Thalidomide produces transfusion independence in long-standing refractory anaemias of patients with myelodysplastic syndromes. *Blood* **98**, 958–965.

Rose, E., Rai, K., Revicki, D., Brown, R. & Reblando, J. (1994). Clinical and health status assessments in anemia chronic lymphocytic leukemia (CLL) patients treated with epoetin alfa (EPO). *Blood* **84** (Suppl.), 526A.

Serious Hazards of Transfusion Report 2000/2001. (www.shot-uk.org)

Terpos, E., Mougiou, A., Kouraklis, A., Chatzivassili, A., Michalis, E., Giannakoulas, N., Manioudaki, E., Lazaridou, A., Bakaloudi, V., Protopappa, M. *et al.* (2002). Prolonged administration of erythropoietin increases erythroid response rate in myelodysplastic syndromes: a phase II trial in 281 patients. *British Journal of Haematology* **118**, 174–180.

Wells, A. W., Mounter, P. J., Chapman, C. E., Stainsby, D. & Wallis, J. P. (2002). Where does blood go? Prospective observational study of red cell transfusions in north England. *British Medical Journal* **325**, 803–804.

Chapter 5

Increasing tumour oxygenation before radiation as a mechanism for maximising response to treatment

Nick Reed

Introduction

That tumour hypoxia has an impact on the efficacy of radiotherapy and even chemotherapy and surgery is not a new discovery. It has been recognised for several years that cancer patients with anaemia have a worse prognosis. For many years this was thought to represent a surrogate for other adverse risk factors such as advanced stage, bleeding tumours, greater risk of metastasis and bone marrow infiltration. However, it has emerged that there may be other factors that make this an independent risk factor. Recent recognition of molecular mechanisms that underplay the consequences of anaemia and hypoxia in the tissues has led to a resurgence of interest in this area, particularly in the past five years. Furthermore, the availability of new products such as the erythropoietin derivatives has led to new applications and new approaches.

Other issues that need to be considered are the relationship between anaemia, haemoglobin level and hypoxia and the oxygen carrying capacity of the blood. Is hypoxia simply a consequence of a low haemoglobin concentration, which reflects anaemia? Again the answer is not as simple as it might first seem, reflecting the fact that there are molecular changes that may account for the consequences of anaemia. It is reported that in 1909 Gottwald Schwartz first noted that hypoxia rendered skin resistant to ionising radiation, but the seminal work was the publication of a series of papers in the 1950s by Thomlinson, Gray and Read (Thomlinson *et al.* 1955) that tumours could be demonstrated to have hypoxic micro-regions (Figure 5.1). They elegantly showed that around the intact blood vessels there was a good circulation and oxygen supply, but surrounding occluded blood vessels there were hypoxic cells. Furthermore, as one moves distantly from the vascular supply the pO_2 significantly falls. They and others (Elkind *et al.* 1965) went on to show, through a series of classical studies, that the radio-sensitivity of cells in oxygen was significantly higher than the radio-sensitivity of hypoxic cells, leading to the formulation of the oxygen enhancement ratio (OER), in other words that hypoxic cells need additional radiation dose to achieve the same level of cell kill. Over the years several important clinical studies demonstrated that various chemicals known as hypoxic cell sensitisers could reverse the negative effect on hypoxic cells, but unfortunately in clinical practice this has proved to be disappointing because of the side effects of these substances (Figure 5.2).

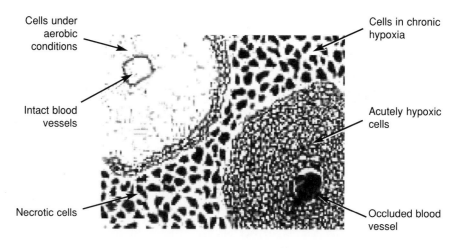

Cells under aerobic conditions

Intact blood vessels

Necrotic cells

Cells in chronic hypoxia

Acutely hypoxic cells

Occluded blood vessel

Figure 5.1 Hypoxic and aerobic cells surrounding blood supply

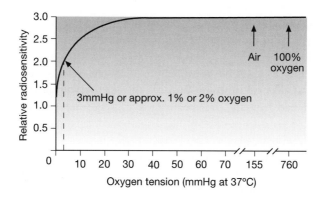

Figure 5.2 Radiosensitivity of cells in differing oxygen tensions

It was initially assumed that cancer cells that were rapidly dividing would use up more oxygen and nutrients and that as the tumour grows and outgrows its blood supply, hypoxia is a simple reflection of the inadequate circulation and lack of nutrients; however, it can also be demonstrated that there are irregularities of the vascular tree, which may lead to non homogenous perfusion. It was traditionally perceived that anaemia simply reduced the oxygen carrying capacity of the blood, but recent evidence has suggested that it is not simply a macroscopic effect due to the lack of oxygen in the blood, and that as a consequence of hypoxia there are changes in the tumour micro-environment which lead to changes in the tumour phenotype. This genetic instability can lead to the greater risk of tumour metastasis and implantation.

There is evidence of up-regulation of tumour promoter genes and down-regulation of the tumour suppressor genes, which in turn lead to the greater risk of metastatic change and a worsening of the malignant phenotype (Figure 5.3). It is also evident that there are changes in p53 and activation of hypoxia inducible factor 1 (HIF1) and changes in the level of vascular endothelial growth factor (VEGF) (Wang & Semenza 1993; Marme 1996; Kieser *et al.* 1994; Brown & Garcia 1998; Graeber *et al.* 1996).

Summary of effects of tumour hypoxia

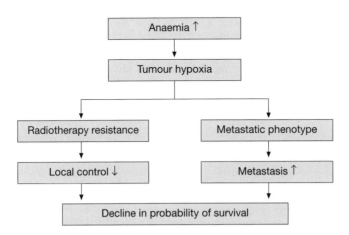

Figure 5.3 Diagram of possible links between anaemia and hypoxia

All these changes are more evident in more hypoxic tissues. Thus it becomes evident that the consequences of hypoxia lead to the promotion of malignant change in the cell to a more aggressive type, with the additional benefit to the cancer cell of a greater likelihood of metastasis and implantation in distant tissues. The major question is which is the chicken and which is the egg in this process? What perhaps remains in doubt is the timing of all these changes. At the moment it is suggested that the increasing development of hypoxia in the tumour micro-regions promotes these negative effects as the tumour grows, but it is conceded that some of these changes may occur at an earlier stage, leading to these bad risk cancers having a poorer prognosis from the outset, maybe before we, as clinicians, can influence the outcome i.e. before the anaemia is clinically detected.

What has led to a major change in the past decade has been the ability to measure the oxygen saturation in the tissues. The development of the Eppendorf probe has allowed researchers like Vaupel and Hoeckel (Kallinowski *et al.* 1990; Vaupel *et al.* 1998) to carry out key studies demonstrating that normal breast tissue and normal cervix tissue has a much higher level of well-oxygenated cells compared with malignant tissues, which have a greater likelihood of hypoxic cells. Subsequent to this, several researchers have shown that the oxygenation status in the tissues is an important predictor of loco-regional control. Much of the work has come from squamous head and neck cancers by Nordsmark *et al.* (1996) and Brizel *et al.* (1995). They have shown that the overall survival and disease-free survival for the patients with better oxygenated tumours was much higher, with a more than doubling of the survival. They also demonstrated in those patients who went on to have post-radiation surgery that those tumours with an initially increased fraction of hypoxic cells were more likely to contain residual disease at the time of post-radiation neck dissection (Brizel 1999). Interestingly, there are also some data to suggest that tumours treated exclusively with surgery had worse outcomes if they had more hypoxic cells at the initial time of diagnosis; hence this issue is important to all oncologists.

So just how serious is the problem? How much of a clinical issue is it in practice? It has been demonstrated by Vaupel and Hoeckel (Hoeckel *et al.* 1996) that patients with cervical cancer and a higher haemoglobin concentration have higher levels of pO_2 in the tissues and also have a lower proportion of hypoxic cells. Several surveys have been done that examine the incidence of anaemia in patients coming for treatment (Groopman & Itri 1999; Barrett-Lee *et al.* 2000). Harrison *et al.* (2000), in a survey from Massachusetts, showed that in a series of over 420 patients there was a range of 8–76% who had a haemoglobin concentration less than 12 g/dl at the beginning of treatment. This was highest in the patients with cervical cancer at 76%, followed by lung cancer and breast and colorectal cancer; it was significantly lower in prostate and head and neck cancers. By the end of treatment there had been a significant rise in all tumour types with cervical, lung and colonic cancers all exceeding 60%.

As has already been hinted at, is anaemia an independent risk factor or is it simply a surrogate for some of the other adverse risk factors? Several people have looked at this. Studies by Frommhold, for example (Frommhold *et al.* 1998) would seem to indicate that anaemia is an independent risk factor. Not surprisingly, in a group of patients with head and neck cancer, the use of definitive radiation treatment, T stage and nodal stage were important, but haemoglobin level emerged as an independent risk factor. Similarly, in work from Hsu and Girinski (Hsu 1998; Girinski *et al.* 1998) in cervical cancer, parametrial involvement, hydronephrosis and the haemoglobin level emerged as the three most important risk factors. Much of the clinical trial work has been done in Canada, and the work of Ray Bush followed by other investigators has demonstrated the importance of low levels of haemoglobin. In 1986 Bush (Bush *et al.* 1978) indicated that patients with cervical cancer who commenced therapy with a haemoglobin greater than 12.5 g/dl had local control for stage 2b and stage 3 disease of the order of 78% whereas those patients who commenced therapy with a haemoglobin level of less than 12.5 g/dl which was not maintained achieved local control of the order of only 56%. In the group where the haemoglobin was boosted to greater than 12.5 g/dl the percentage local control rose to 85% and the confidence level was very significant. Michelle Grogan, on behalf of the Canadian Co-operative Group (Grogan *et al.* 1999; Thomas 1999), published a paper in 1999 looking at an audit of three years (1989, 1990 and 1992) in which they reviewed virtually all the patients treated with radiation only, at the eight regional cancer centres in Canada. They were able to study very substantial numbers of patients (about 475), and probably the most important additional factor to emerge was in relation to the maintenance of the haemoglobin level greater than 12 g/dl. Previously, it had been thought that the haemoglobin level at the start of treatment was the important factor, but in this study Grogan *et al.* showed that in those patients who commenced therapy with a high haemoglobin level but where there was a failure to maintain it, outcome from treatment fell to match those who commenced therapy with a haemoglobin concentration below 12 g/dl and where it was similarly not maintained. Thus, regular attention to the haemoglobin level during the course of treatment and intervention led to a significant improvement in the outcome. The authors suggested the expression 'the average weekly nadir haemoglobin' (AWNH) to reflect the haemoglobin level during the course of treatment. The three principal risk factors that emerged from their survey were the average haemoglobin level during treatment, the stage of disease and the use of brachytherapy, all with probability values of 0.0001 or less.

Around this time several clinical trials were developed. Dusenbery *et al.* (1994) reported on patients with stage 1b–3 cervical cancer with a haemoglobin less than 12.5 g/dl who were treated with pelvic and para-aortic node irradiation and brachytherapy and who also received recombinant human erythropoietin (rh-EPO) and iron supplements. Those patients who received both rh-EPO and iron had the highest haemoglobin levels and the highest rise from the baseline. Those who had iron only had a modest rise but those who had neither rh-EPO nor iron had the lowest levels. This confirmed the benefit of rh-EPO in this group of patients. Robert Lavey on behalf of the South West Oncology Group (SWOG) (Lavey & Dempsey 1993; Lavey *et al.* 2000) group reported their SWOG-9318 trial which compared patients receiving concomitant chemo/radiotherapy who were randomised to receive either additional rh-EPO or no treatment. Importantly, these patients were also given iron supplements. The main endpoint was the rise in haemoglobin level to greater than 12.5 g/dl during treatment with a secondary endpoint of survival. Not surprisingly, those patients who started with a low haemoglobin had a significant rise so that by the end of the treatment 46% of patients in the EPO arm had a haemoglobin level greater than 12.5 g/dl. There was a correlation between the rate of haemoglobin increase and baseline iron stores. Toxicity was acceptable although there was a small incidence of deep vein thromboses.

Finally, one other trial was conducted, again in Canada: the CX2 study by the National Cancer Institute of Canada (NCIC) (Pearcey *et al.* 2002). This was a study that compared conventional concomitant chemo/radiotherapy with radiation alone. This study was not published until 2002 and not until after the results of the five North American studies which had led to the NCI consensus statement (Thomas 1999) about patients set to receive radiotherapy, which indicated that consideration should be given to using chemotherapy concomitantly in these individuals.

This Canadian study showed no significant difference in the outcome between those patients randomised to radiation alone or radiation and chemotherapy. A lot of detailed analysis has been performed to try to explain why this study proved negative in the wake of the five previous positive studies. Although there is a chance that this could be a statistical fluke, the explanation that has emerged and which seems most credible is that the patients receiving the concomitant chemo/radiotherapy had a significant fall in the haemoglobin level during treatment which was not seen in the patients receiving radiation only. This study was conducted before Grogan's work had been published and reflected the historical view that haemoglobin levels at the time of diagnosis were more important. The mean difference in haemoglobin level was such that a significant number of patients in the concomitant arm had a haemoglobin level under 12 g/dl, and it has therefore been suggested that this fall in the haemoglobin level may have counteracted any benefit expected by the addition of chemotherapy. It is also worth pointing out that the radiation schedule used in this study was a short course lasting four weeks only, and most patients completed their treatment within seven days of the planned treatment course; it has been suggested that this may also have contributed to the favourable results seen in the radiation-only arm. This contrasts with much longer courses of radiation and often more intervals and gaps seen in the USA studies. Nevertheless, this does seem to lend significant evidence to support the belief that haemoglobin level and indirectly hypoxia are important determinants of the outcome of cervical cancer treatment and that this finding is probably applicable to a whole range of tumours.

Options: blood transfusions, EPO alpha and beta, darbepoetin, CERA newer agents

Finally, there are several studies that have recently been conducted or are underway using epoetin alpha (Eprex), epoetin beta (NeoRecormon) and darbepoetin (Aranesp). Some preliminary data are emerging from these studies. For example, the NeoRecormon Once Weekly (NOW) study has shown that once weekly scheduling is equally as beneficial as thrice weekly. The rationale for thrice weekly scheduling seems to have been derived from treatment of renal dialysis patients, who were administered their injection of rh-EPO to coincide with their episode of haemodialysis. Shifting to a once weekly schedule is far more convenient, and there are newer compounds such as darbepoetin and the Roche long-acting formulation CERA (continuous erythropoiesis receptor activator) which may allow scheduling every three weeks, which fits more conveniently with many chemotherapy schedules. One final note of caution is that pure red cell aplasia (PRCA) has been reported recently, and at the end of 2002, for example, there were around 140 cases reported worldwide in the literature. Virtually all PRCA has been observed in patients undergoing renal dialysis and at the time of writing the incidence in oncology patients has not been an issue. Furthermore, most of the patients in whom PRCA has been seen have been treated with the European preparation of alpha recombinant erythropoietin (Eprex), and PRCA has been a very rare consequence of treatment in the USA preparation of alpha rh-EPO preparation (Procrit). Nor has it been seen significantly with beta rh-EPO (NeoRecormon). Clearly, vigilance is required in monitoring ongoing developments in this context. Nevertheless, in conclusion, it should be stated that the rh-EPO products do offer a safe and simple alternative to blood transfusion and blood products. Furthermore, as the expected looming crisis in blood transfusion safety and availability develops, and as we see the pool of potential donors diminishing, it may well be that rh-EPO products and their newer derivatives acquire central relevance in the management and control of anaemia in this group of patients both for symptom relief and, more importantly, for improvement in clinical outcome from cancer treatment.

References

Barrett-Lee, P. J., Bailey, N. P., O'Brien, M. E. & Wager, E. (2000). Large-scale UK audit of blood transfusion requirements and anaemia in patients receiving cytotoxic chemotherapy. *British Journal of Cancer* **82**, 93–97.

Brizel, D. M., Rosner, G. & Dewhirst, M. W. (1995). An evaluation of patterns and variability of tumour oxygenation in human soft tissue sarcomas, cervical carcinomas and lymph node metastases. *International Journal of Radiation Oncology, Biology, Physics* **32**, 1121–1125.

Brown, J. M. & Garcia, A. J. (1998). The unique physiology of solid tumours: opportunities and problems for cancer therapy. *Cancer Research* **58**, 1408–1416.

Bush, R. S., Jenkin, R. D. T., Allt, W. E. C. *et al*. (1978). Definitive evidence for hypoxic cells influencing cure in cancer therapy. *British Journal of Cancer* **37**, 302–306.

Dusenbery, K. E., McGuire, W. A., Holt, P. J. *et al*. (1994): Erythropoietin increases haemoglobin during radiation therapy for cervical cancer. *International Journal of Radiation Oncology, Biology, Physics* **29**, 1079–1084.

Elkind, M. M., Swain, R. W., Alescio, T., Sutton, H. & Moses, W. B. (1965). Oxygen, nitrogen, recovery and radiation therapy. In *Cellular radiation biology*, pp. 442–461. Williams and Wilkins, Baltimore.

Frommhold, H., Guttenberger, R. & Henke, M. (1998). The impact of blood haemoglobin content on the outcome of radiotherapy. The Freiburg experience. *Strahlentherapie und Onkologie* **174** (Suppl. 4), 31–34.

Girinski, T, Pejovic-Lenfant, M. H., Bourhis, J. *et al*. (1989). Prognostic value of haemoglobin concentrations and blood transfusions in advanced carcinoma of the cervix treated by radiation therapy: Results of a retrospective study of 386 patients. *International Journal of Radiation Oncology, Biology, Physics* **16**, 37–42.

Graeber, T. G., Osmanian, C., Jacks, T., Housman, D. E., Koch, C. J., Lowe, S. W. & Giaccia, A. J. (1996). Hypoxia-mediated selection of cells with diminished apoptotic potential in solid tumours. *Nature* **379**, 88–91.

Grogan, M., Thomas, G.M., Melamed, I. *et al*. (1999). The importance of haemoglobin levels during radiotherapy for carcinoma of the cervix. *Cancer* **86**, 1528–1536.

Groopman, J. E. & Itri, L. M. (1999). Chemotherapy-induced anaemia in adults; incidence and treatment. *Journal of the National Cancer Institute* **91**, 1616–1634.

Harrison, L. B, Shasha, S., Shiaova, L. *et al.* (2000). Prevalence of anemia in cancer patients undergoing radiotherapy (abstract 1849). *Proceedings of the American Society of Clinical Oncology* **19**, 471a.

Hoeckel, M., Schlenger, K., Aral, B., Mitze, M., Schaffer, U. & Vaupel, P. (1996). Association between tumour hypoxia and malignant progression in advanced cancer of the uterine cervix. *Cancer Research* **56**, 4509–4515.

Hsu, H. C. (1998). Prognostic factors for control of cervix cancer by radiation therapy. *International Journal of Radiation Oncology, Biology, Physics* **40**, 405–409.

Kallinowski, F., Zander, R., Hoeckel, M. & Vaupel, P. (1990). Tumour oxygenation as evaluated by computerised pO_2–histography. *International Journal of Radiation Oncology, Biology, Physics* **19**, 953–962.

Kieser, A., Weich H. A., Brandner, G., Marme, D. & Kolch, W. (1994). Mutant p53 potentiates protein kinase C induction of vascular endothelial growth factor expression. *Oncogene* **9**, 963–969.

Lavey, R. S. & Dempsey, W. H. (1993). Erythropoietin increases haemoglobin in cancer patients during radiation therapy. *International Journal of Radiation Oncology, Biology, Physics* **27**, 1147–1152.

Lavey, R. S., Liu, P. Y., Greer, B. E. *et al.* (2000). Recombinant human erythropoietin (EPO) as an adjunct to concurrent radiation therapy (RT) and cisplatin for stage IIb–IVa carcinoma of the cervix: a Southwest Oncology Group study (abstract 330). *Radiotherapy and Oncology* **56** (Suppl. 1), s92.

Marme, D. (1996). Tumour angiogenesis: the pivotal role of vascular endothelial growth factor. *World Journal of Urology* **14**, 166–174.

Nordsmark, M., Overgaard, J. & Overgaard, M. (1996). Pre-treatment oxygenation predicts radiation response in advanced squamous cell carcinomas of the head and neck. *Radiotherapy and Oncology* **41**, 31–39.

Pearcey, R., Brundage, M., Drouin, P., Jeffrey, J., Johnston, D., Lukka, H., MacLean, G., Souhami, L., Stuart, G. & Tu, D. (2002). Phase III trial comparing radical radiotherapy with and without cisplatin chemotherapy in patients with advanced squamous cell cancer of the cervix. *Journal of Clinical Oncology* **20**, 966–972.

Thomas, G. M. (1999). Improved treatment for cervical cancer – concurrent chemotherapy and radiotherapy. *New England Journal of Medicine* **340**, 1198–1200.

Thomlinson, R. H. & Gray, L. (1955). The histological structure of some human lung cancers and the possible implications for radiotherapy. *British Journal of Cancer* **9**, 539–549.

Vaupel, P. Thews, O., Kelleher, D. K. & Hoeckel, M. (1998). Oxygenation of human tumours: the Mainz experience. *Strahlentherapie und Onkologie* **174** (Suppl. 4), 6–12.

Wang, G. L. & Semenza, G. L. (1993). Characterization of hypoxia-inducible factor 1 and regulation of DNA binding activity by hypoxia. *Journal of Biological Chemistry* **268**, 21513–21518.

Chapter 6

Measurement of symptom improvement and survival in cancer

Alastair G. Smith, Rachel Newman and Shirley E. Crofts

Introduction

In developed countries approximately one in three individuals will develop a malignancy during their lifetime; approximately 50% of cancer patients will die of their disease. Until the latter half of the 20th century, a diagnosis of cancer was accepted as inevitably fatal. Treatment was palliative. Physical measures such as radiotherapy and surgery were aimed at managing local tumour-associated complications. Essentially, however, the focus of care was on dealing with symptomatic discomfort and prolonging survival wherever possible, without causing undue distress to the patient and his or her family. This remains the fundamental approach for most forms of cancer despite advances in our knowledge of causation and biology of cancer, and availability of newer drugs and other therapeutic agents.

Chemotherapy for cancer promised much but has, in reality, made an impact on survival and curability in relatively few specific tumour types. Combinations of chemotherapy with radiotherapy and stem-cell transplantation techniques have similarly resulted in long-term survival and cure in few clinical situations. Such gains and overall clinical experience have been achieved at the expense of significant treatment-related toxicity. Much effort in the past 25 years has also been in the field of managing and limiting the unpleasant side effects of the more intense and toxic chemotherapy and radiotherapy treatments. Significant success has been achieved, for example, in the development of effective anti-emetics and marrow growth factors.

It is perhaps unsurprising that initial research into cancer treatment moved from palliative intent to more determined efforts at tumour eradication with outcome assessments of tumour response, 'disease-free' survival and treatment-related mortality. Some assessments of treatment morbidity and toxicity were also considered and studied. Efforts to prolong survival assumed this was the sole objective. Quality-of-life (QoL) benefits for the patient were assumed and not measured in any systematic way, other than the use of determinants such as 'performance status' (e.g. the Karnofsky scale (Karnofsky & Burchenal 1949)) as a treatment outcome assessment; improved performance status was generally taken to imply a gain in QoL.

Measuring duration of survival in malignant disease is straightforward. Similarly, symptomatic improvement can be assessed quite easily by means of questionnaires on specific symptoms. Such information is important in assessing outcomes, but does not adequately convey the whole picture for patient groups undergoing different forms of therapy. The combined effect of the symptomatic problems, the underlying condition, and other factors, influence what life is like for the individual patient. It is the combination that determines his or her QoL. Being able to measure QoL should therefore be a potentially valuable part of overall symptomatic improvement in managing cancer.

Features contributing to symptoms associated with malignant disease can be categorised as shown in Table 6.1. Personal effects are, by definition, individual and relevant to the individual patient; the others are of more generalised nature. QoL for the individual will therefore be a function of the local and systemic tumour and treatment effects, together with the personal factors.

As the successes and limitations of the various forms of anti-cancer therapies have become better understood there has been an increased understanding of the need to develop broader, patient-focused outcome measures in developing and assessing treatments. These measures assess symptom control, and seek to assess broader facets of patient experience. Thus the concepts of health status, health-related QoL and global QoL have been developed and expanded in the past 20 years; there is an increasing amount of published research on the development of 'tools' to measure these (Garratt *et al.* 2002).

Table 6.1 Classification of symptomatic effects of cancer

Tumour effects	local	e.g. presenting symptoms in colorectal cancer
	systemic	e.g. anorexia and weight loss, fatigue
Treatment (iatrogenic) effects	local	e.g. significant change in bodily appearance e.g. mastectomy; local side effects of radiotherapy
	systemic	e.g. side effects of chemotherapy regimens: alopecia, nausea and vomiting, susceptibility to infection; fatigue, etc.
Personal effects	these can be directly or indirectly related to tumour, treatment, both of these and/or other factors	e.g. psychological impact of diagnosis of cancer, knowledge of mortality; changes in body image; changes in role (in work, family); loss of control (including possible dependency on others); effects on lifestyle and choices; financial impacts; changes in relationships (including work, family, sexuality etc); potential impacts on beliefs, values, etc.

Defining quality of life

Perhaps the simplest definition of QoL is that advanced by Calman (1984). He described it as: 'The measure of the difference at a particular time point between the hopes and expectations of the individual and that individual's present experiences'. This definition has the merit of simplicity; it also embodies the fundamental intrinsic concept that QoL is determined by the individual.

Subsequent theories and research have recognised the changing nature of an individual's QoL status. It is a 'dynamic construct' (Allison *et al.* 1997), whereby an individual adapts to circumstances over time, causing a 'response shift' in their reporting of QoL, when to an observer little may have changed. Also there is observation of the 'disability paradox'. This is demonstrated when an individual with apparently severe disabilities, or nearing the end of life, nevertheless reports good QoL. In this context Albrecht and Devlieger (1999). reported this as showing that QoL is expressed in terms of 'balance between body, mind and spirit, and relationships to their external environment'. Perhaps it is most useful to think, in broad terms, that a measure of QoL attempts to measure those qualities, which render life (and survival) valuable to the individual.

The World Health Organization QoL Group's definition attempts to recognise some of these broader aspects, and the need for a balanced approach incorporating positive as well as negative aspects. They define QoL as: 'an individual's perception of their position in life in the context of the culture and value systems in which they live, and in relation to their goals, expectations, and standards and concerns' (World Health Organization 1993).

Underpinning most QoL measurement instruments are questions to the patient, which try to assess the impact of disease. QoL instruments directly ask about the impact of the disease on physical, psychological, social and occupational and role functions (e.g. sickness impact profile (Bergner *et al.* 1981), SF-36 medical outcomes scale (Ware & Sherbourne 1992), and the Nottingham health profile (Hunt *et al.* 1985)). QoL questionnaires undergo a rigorous validation process to ensure their validity in the setting in which they will be used. Analysis of the answers in the questionnaires will generally derive scores for particular aspects or 'domains' of QoL for the individual, which can then be recorded and used as numerical data capable of statistical analysis in outcome assessment.

Measurement of quality of life

Sanders *et al.* (1998). reviewed the frequency of measurement of QoL in cancer trials and observed that fewer than 10% of randomised controlled trials in cancer reported on QoL. Many of the published reports were inadequate. An underlying problem at that time and which is still unresolved is the lack of standardisation of instruments used to measure QoL. There are an ever-increasing number of questionnaire tools available to measure QoL (Garratt *et al.* 2002). Not all are validated. Currently there is no single, 'correct', QoL instrument.

The context in which QoL is being measured, the nature of the disease or health problem under study, and whether aggregated data from large patient groups or individual data are required, determine the form of instrument used. Different measures address different aspects of health status, or QoL, and are used for different purposes. Furthermore, the choice of measure may be influenced by a perceived need to meet other people's priorities (e.g. those of politicians or managers rather than clinical ones). There is thus the problem of knowing what to measure, how to measure it, and how to interpret and use the resulting information. We have a growth in QoL instrument development but no standardisation (Garratt *et al.* 2002). Some of the key aspects involved in QoL measurement are summarised in Table 6.2.

Table 6.2 Aspects of quality of life measurement

dimension specific	particular aspects of health
disease specific	aspects of health relative to a particular condition
generic measures	can be used in differing populations; ask more general questions
individualised measures	respondents report and weight aspects of their own life
utility measures	are focused more on health economics
time period assessed	usually limited, e.g. during the previous week, etc.
'user friendliness'	ease of completion, ease of analysis, timeliness of analysis
q-twist methodology	attempts to incorporate time with treatment related toxicity, disease free survival and overall survival
interpretation of changes in scores	comparison with previous data or normative data
longitudinal measurement	methodology for repeated measurement; effects of 'response shift' and 'disability paradox'

In terms of assessing QoL, the great variety of measures available may assess or measure any or all of the following. These have been recently reviewed (Bowling 2002; Higginson & Carr 2001, 2002; Addington-Hall & Kalra 2001, 2002).

- Health status
- Health-related QoL
- Global QoL
  - Measures being used for different purposes
  - To evaluate treatment toxicity (e.g. Murray & Cole 2000)
  - To monitor symptom changes (e.g. Bruera *et al.* 1991; Bruera & MacDonald 1993; McCorkle & Young 1978, de Haes *et al.* 1990)
  - To evaluate clinical services (e.g. Ellershaw *et al.* 1995)
  - To plan and prioritise healthcare services
  - As a health economics tool (see Hearn & Higginson 1997)
- QoL in different populations and at different times: different cancers, stages of disease e.g. early, potentially curable phases as opposed to advanced or terminal phases (Aaronson *et al.* 1993; Morris *et al.* 1986)

- QoL in different settings, e.g. research, developed for use in clinical trials, versus clinical practice (Aaronson *et al.* 1993; Association for Palliative Medicine 2001), primary care as opposed to hospital or specialist palliative care unit (Paterson 1996; Ellershaw *et al.* 1995; Morris *et al.* 1986)
- Measures designed to be completed by different people (e.g. health professionals, patients, family and carers, see Hearn & Higginson 1997)

There are a range of different QoL measures available which do not all measure the same thing and are not all useful in every setting or context. In using any measure, it is essential to know the purpose for which QoL measurement will be used, so that an appropriate instrument is used for the setting, patient population, disease and stage of illness. In clinical research settings QoL measures should be employed as study endpoints, which then provide informative data for healthcare professionals and patients alike, and will thus contribute to treatment decisions and choices, as well as influencing treatment questions in future research.

Why such little information?

The lack of standardisation in the use and application of QoL instruments is clearly one factor contributing to the relative lack of published data on QoL as an outcome in cancer treatment. There are other factors that contribute to the deficiency which reflect technical difficulties as well as cultural, organisational and scientific ones.

Limited clinical continuity in the total care

In the much used phrase, the patient's 'cancer journey', there is generally no means or tradition of looking at the whole course of events. Different professional groups are involved at different stages in diagnosis and treatment. The tendency is to look at outcomes at the beginning and very end but not what goes on in between. Patients themselves live with a cancer illness from diagnosis to cure or eventual death, but during that time may only have very intermittent contact with healthcare services. By necessity, healthcare professionals, responding to need, focus on the care of the ill–at diagnosis and initial treatment, at relapse or progression of disease, and in the terminal phase. Patients often perceive a lack of interest, and experience a sense of abandonment when relatively well, e.g. during periods of remission. There is simply no means or tradition of looking at the whole course of events.

The agenda and objectives of patients and different healthcare teams varies

As the objective of treatment moves from curative to palliative in malignant disease, there tends to be a resultant shift of focus in the clinical care to more personal issues, such as improving communication and relationships between family members. Spiritual aspects also often assume a greater priority in the later phases of cancers and, indeed, other chronic illnesses. This may result in choices by the patient which may be at variance with the recommendations of the specialist team; where the patient may have moved to a level of acceptance of their illness as terminal at a faster pace than the doctor, whose focus remains more technical as opposed to pastoral. The converse also happens, where medical opinion has moved to focus on palliation and the patient still has hopes of a cure.

Research has traditionally been limited to biological endpoints, clinical markers and molecular pathology

Even after recognition of the need for some form of QoL measure as an endpoint in clinical trials, the measures adopted have tended to concentrate on symptoms, side effects and toxicity of treatments, or changes in functional status, rather than broader (or individualised) measures. In some areas this has been beneficial, for example, certain symptoms have been better defined, and effects of specific treatments researched and monitored (e.g. pain, nausea and vomiting) resulting in improved control of these symptoms. The drawback of focusing only on specific symptoms, and not utilising broader QoL measures, is that only these symptoms are studied; other significant QoL issues are missed. For example, the impact and incidence of fatigue in cancer patients has largely been ignored; recent studies from the USA and UK have demonstrated the relevance of fatigue to the cancer patient in terms of their QoL and the differing priorities given to it by health professionals (Vogelzang *et al.* 1997; Stone *et al.* 2000, 2003).

Time-scales in research are dictated by priorities other than those directly related to the condition being studied

For example, time may be restricted to a particular researcher's availability (e.g. a trainee in clinical research) or may be limited to a certain limited time period funded by a grant awarding body or commercial sponsor. Cancer survivals often extend over many years; research is commonly funded for short periods, typically two to three years for individuals as part of their career development. This agenda also fits with grant-awarding bodies, whether charitable or commercial. As a result, sustained study of QoL, as an outcome over time in cancer patients, simply does not happen. Qualitative research, although gaining respectability, is still often not seen as a clinical priority, as often the data generated are not perceived as 'hard' or 'reliable'. There is still a perceived difficulty in gaining training in qualitative research, and as it often requires increased commitment both in time and in money, it can be more difficult to gain the necessary funding and support personnel to carry it out.

Lack of standardisation of methods

As discussed above, this remains a major problem, but is probably lessening with increasing use of standardised, validated cancer QoL questionnaires such as EORTC

QLQ C30 or FACT (Aaronson *et al.* 1993; Cella *et al.* 1993). Interpretation and analysis of data are also not straightforward.

Cost and time-scale

Systematically measuring and coordinating QoL measurement in the discipline of trials, or at specific time points in the management and follow up of cancer patients, requires a robust administrative process. It also needs to run for significant time periods if other than just initial treatment and outcome data are to be collected.

No external quality standard required

From the point of view of both society and healthcare-funding bodies there is no single quality standard required or available. In the UK NHS, for example, process markers such as waiting times for consultations are used as implied markers of quality.

QoL versus health economics

Improving QoL does not necessarily or demonstrably increase survival. The individual patient, his family and friends may gain quality whether or not life expectancy is increased. QoL measurement thus does not have an overt gain in terms of health economics; over time there is more incentive for healthcare providers to understand the economic issues surrounding cancer management; QoL would represent only one group of variables in this respect.

The 'disability paradox' and response shift

It is a common assumption that increasing symptoms are associated with a decrease in QoL, and that symptom improvement is therefore likely to be associated with a gain in QoL. This has been somewhat challenged by the 'disability paradox' theory referred to earlier, and some research suggesting that even very near the end of life, patients may report a good QoL (Albrecht & Devlieger 1999; Addington-Hall & Kalra 2001, 2002). Patients assess their QoL in terms of their present context, as this changes so does their evaluation of their current QoL which produces this response shift.

Quality of life scores

These will certainly improve with symptom improvement if they incorporate a scoring system heavily weighted towards experiences in the physical domain. These QoL measures (e.g. McCorkle & Young 1978; de Haes *et al.* 1990; Bruera *et al.* 1991), are therefore most likely to be a valid measurement of symptom improvement, whereas individualised measures (e.g. the SEIQoL (O'Boyle *et al.* 1994)), where patients choose and weight their own domains, may not throw any light on the symptom experience.

Symptomatic improvement and survival: currently available information

Information on symptomatic improvement and survival quality currently available is derived from a range of sources. which include the following.

Individual accounts

These may range from the 'self-help' or 'support' publication, detailing how to defeat your cancer, to descriptive accounts of the 'the cancer journey' The latter may incorporate stories of coping (or not) with the illness, accepting or rejecting treatments conventional or otherwise, and exploring emotions, personal reactions, experiences of healthcare, and changes in values and priorities over time. News headlines and press reports of individual cases (or treatments) may be very misleading and lead people to seek an unrealistic cure.

The accounts of 'celebrities' e.g. John Diamond's column and book (Diamond 1999), may achieve some insight into that individual's personality and coping strategies, but may have no relevance to another's experience and may make them feel inadequate or a failure if they are not responding in a similar manner. These reports are easily and commonly accessible to the public and do have an impact on patients and how they perceive their condition, its treatment, and the role of their doctors.

The public (i.e. current and future patients) is exposed to an enormous range of different sources of information on cancer. Available information is focused on a great variety of different 'endpoints' which vary from the very narrow and specific, to the global but potentially confusing. Nowadays, a large amount of this information is accessible on the Internet. Unfortunately much of the Internet information is unregulated and has no accountability. The effects of these accounts and such available information influence patients' expectations. By definition, this will shape the context in which the individual assesses his or her QoL.

Biological endpoints are readily measurable

Pathological, haematological, biochemical and radiological measures are most useful in assessing 'disease status', and are commonly measured in clinical trials. Simple monitoring of performance status (using such scales as the Karnofsky performance status), or physical functioning, may give prognostic information either at pre-treatment levels or in the terminal phase (Vigano *et al.* 2000). The rate of change of performance status or physical functioning may be more informative than a single measure at a specific point in time. These scales use a professional-rated assessment, not a patient-rated one. Historically, improvements in performance status were assumed to indicate QoL improvements. Research has shown that this is not the case (Albrecht & Devlieger 1999), and that performance status cannot be used as a surrogate measurement of QoL. Similarly, doctors' assessments of patients' QoL have been shown to be unreliable (Slevin *et al.* 1988).

Survival

It is assumed that an increase in disease-free survival or overall survival will automatically translate into improved QoL. This may not be the case as an individual's expectations will correspondingly change, and they may rate their QoL as reduced if it fails to live up to expectations. In a specific example from the Nordic myeloma group, they showed that although the time to disease progression was delayed by four to five months using interferon-α maintenance, this was not associated with improved QoL (Wisloff *et al.* 1996a,b).

Measurement of quality of life in cancer trial research

The search for the 'cure' in cancer has generally resulted in more radical and intensive treatments, particularly as technological advances make the range of possible interventions ever wider. These different or new therapeutic approaches need comprehensive study in their own right and in comparison to established regimens. The latter is achieved through randomised clinical trials comparing the efficacy and tolerance of the newer approaches with the established ones. So far, improved response rates and survival have largely been assumed to equate with improved QoL, but this has yet to be proved. Increasingly intensive approaches in cancer management need to be evaluated in terms of their impact on QoL as well as on response rates, survival and the traditional clinicopathological measures.

Where there is little or no difference in survival duration from different treatment regimes QoL data become increasingly important. Doctors and patients faced with the decision as to which treatment to select or recommend at present mostly lack this additional knowledge, which can help the decision-making process for the individual patient. Research should therefore be aiming to record QoL data, which can then inform patients (for whom it matters most), doctors and other clinical professionals, service providers and the direction of future research. Where 'cure' is unlikely, a key focus for treatment needs to be on maximising the QoL as a therapeutic outcome. This becomes increasingly important as patients approach the terminal stages of their condition.

In this context, QoL measurement needs to be an intrinsic component of outcome measures in cancer treatment. Sanders *et al.* (1998). have drawn attention to the paucity of information on QoL in cancer trials before 1997: under 10% of studies reported on QoL. In 48 randomised controlled trials reporting on QoL, 62 instruments were used highlighting methodological difficulties as a factor contributing to the relative lack of data. The type and choice of instrument are important. To assess cancer-related QoL, a disease-specific instrument is required; such instruments focus on the impact of the condition and are thus more likely to discriminate between specific patient groups and to be responsive to changes (Robinson *et al.* 2002).

EORTC QLQ-C30: a specific example

QLQ-C30 is a questionnaire developed by the European Organisation for Research and Treatment of Cancer (EORTC) (Aaronsen *et al.* 1993). It is a generic questionnaire designed to cover common aspects of QoL for all types of cancer. It contains several questions that assess function in five areas: physical, cognitive, emotional, role and social. It includes three symptom scales that measure pain, fatigue, nausea and vomiting and a global QoL and health scale, and six single-item scales that assess constipation, diarrhoea, dysnoea, appetite, sleep and finances.

The questionnaire is easily completed by patients, within 10–12 minutes. It is available in the main European languages, except Icelandic. Since there is variation in the problems posed by different tumour types and treatment regimens, the approach has been adopted whereby the core questionnaire is supplemented with an additional disease-specific questionnaire.

'Add-on' disease-specific modules have been developed for specific tumour types, including lung (QLQ-LC13) (Bergman *et al.* 1994) breast (QLQ-BR23) (Sprangers *et al.* 1996) and head and neck cancer (QLQ-H&N35) (Bjordal *et al.* 1999). These have been validated. Other modules are currently undergoing validation such as the myeloma-specific module (QLQ-MY24; Stead *et al.* 1999). The addition of disease-specific 'add-ons' enables research specifically to assess the effect that different treatments have on QoL generally, and on particular aspects of QoL relevant to the tumour type being studied. QoL can be measured during treatment and more longitudinally (Osoba *et al.* 1998). QoL assessment can either explore individual differences or different population measures against time. Normative data sets are available for many questionnaires, e.g. EORTC and FAC, and comparison with these allows the significance of any change in QoL scores to be evaluated. Ease of analysis needs to be considered, especially in small trials where little statistical help is available, but for many questionnaires is quite straightforward.

Q-TWiST (quality-adjusted time without symptoms and toxicity) analysis represents another method of looking at QoL in cancer treatment. It represents a technique of survival analysis, taking into account the fact that patients will experience differing health states during their period of survival. It seeks to weight time periods related to: time with toxicity, time without disease relapse or toxicity, and time following disease relapse/progression. Through a mathematical function, data can be derived that can compare the impact of different treatments (Glasziou *et al.* 1990; Cole *et al.* 1995).

Quality of life in cancer management guidelines

As well as providing research information, QoL data can inform evidence-based recommendations for clinical guidelines; multiple myeloma is taken as an example of this process.

Myeloma is a plasma cell tumour accounting for 1–2% of adult cancers, the median age at diagnosis is 62 yrs with a 3–5 year average survival. The condition appears incurable with current therapies. It poses a range of clinical problems. Bone pain, fractures and vertebral collapse are major problems for myeloma patients, as are anaemia and fatigue. Until recently efficacy had been evaluated by tumour response rates, remission duration and survival. There was little evidence relating to the effect of therapy on QoL.

Using experience in the management of multiple myeloma as a paradigm for other cancers is informative in looking at the influence of measured QoL data, and proven symptomatic gains, in deriving management guidelines. Current treatment options include a range of chemotherapy regimens from simple to complex, including options for stem-cell transplantation. There are also important supportive and maintenance treatment issues.

Guidelines on the diagnosis and management of multiple myeloma have recently been published (UKMF 2001). Information on published QoL data formed a helpful part of the evidence base and contributed to some of the key recommendations. With, as yet, no clear impact on curability, and so far modest survival differences in the chemotherapy plus stem-cell transplantation options, QoL implications assume greater importance in helping both patient and physician select appropriate therapy.

Published trial data are now showing a clearer survival advantage for high-dose chemotherapy and peripheral blood stem-cell transplantation. The gain in survival is supported by QoL data, showing a favourable profile for this more intensive approach in patients up to the age of 60 years old (Lenhoff *et al.* 2000, Gulbrandsen 2001a,b). Similarly, using Q-TWiST analysis to address the same issue in two trials of conventional versus high-dose therapy, there was a favourable effect on offering high-dose therapy at an early stage in treatment, compared with offering it at disease progression. However, there was no overall survival difference for the two approaches (Porcher *et al.* 2002).

On the basis of a high incidence of unacceptable side effects, high cost and no QoL benefit in a range of studies (Wisloff *et al.* 1996), the UK Myeloma guidelines concluded, 'careful consideration should be given as to whether interferon therapy should be continued in the face of side effects which impair QoL' (UK Myeloma Forum 2001). This recommendation is further backed up by data using Q-TWiST analysis, which found in a study of interferon maintenance that, although patients on interferon gained an average of 5 months of overall survival, they suffered an average of 4.1 months of moderate or worse toxicity (Zee *et al.* 1998). Wisloff *et al.* (1999) demonstrated an unfavourable pharmaco-economic profile for interferon.

Direct QoL data on bisphosphonates are lacking, but interpretation of specific morbidity information shows a favourable effect for maintenance treatment on the incidence of bony morbidity and the use of analgesia (Berenson *et al.* 1996, 1998; McCloskey *et al.* 1998). These are reasonable markers of symptomatic benefit and therefore the use of bisphosphonates is recommended. There is now a substantial body of evidence to support the effectiveness of erythropoietin as treatment for the anaemia associated with myeloma and its therapy. The evidence confirms its ability to improve haemoglobin levels and improve patient QoL (Osterborg *et al.* 1996; Demetri *et al.* 1998; Dammacco *et al.* 2001). Guidelines support its use, but with no clear survival gain there are service cost issues which currently limit its widespread uptake.

Why measure quality of life? Clinical practice

In busy clinical practice, specialist cancer care tends to a more technical than holistic focus; the diagnosis, what is going to be done, what changes there are in the results of imaging or pathological tests, etc. The impact of specific symptoms such as pain, nausea and vomiting will generally be assessed. Patients will usually be asked, 'How are you?'. More often than not the answer will be 'fine', 'I'm getting on quite well' or a general statement that things are acceptable. The pressures in the clinic and the dynamic of the consultation combine not to ask further; sometimes patients simply give the answer they think 'the doctor' wants to hear when the reality may be quite different. The use of QoL assessment in clinical practice can be very helpful in counteracting this tendency.

Using QoL measures in the clinical setting offers a way of including the personal and social effects of the condition and its treatment; Higginson & Carr (2001, 2002) have summarised the potential uses, which include:

- Identification and prioritisation of problems; a broader assessment of issues can be achieved by use of an appropriate QoL measurement tool. Identified problems can be prioritised, and factors identified which may impair the individual's ability to cope with the disease and its treatment.
- Achieving better communication and understanding between patients and doctors, doctors and nurses, patients and nurses, as well as between the patient and family/ friends.
- Helping identify patient preferences in respect of their aspirations or goals of treatment.
- A means to monitor the effects of treatment on other than the progress made as indicated from clinical laboratory or radiological findings.

Further, QoL measures are useful in clinical practice in that they provide a framework for clinical professionals to become, and remain, better trained in broader aspects of clinical assessment. This occurs through appreciation of the facets that contribute to the well-being and QoL of the individual patient. In terms of clinical governance, QoL assessment offers more direct means to address patient and carer satisfaction issues; data from QoL also will contribute to clinical audit.

There is, however, no 'gold standard' measure of QoL in the clinical setting. There are a range of instruments available, so that the difficulty is to choose one that is appropriate. There are differences in applying QoL measurement in the clinic setting as opposed to trials. In the clinic, measures need to be more focused on the individual patient, whereas in trials the need is to obtain data converted into numeric form from groups of patients with the condition under study. The clinic QoL instrument needs to be relevant to the problem being assessed, acceptable and practical to use, reliable in respect of its ability to produce consistency in results in an unchanged population, and responsive in its ability to detect clinically meaningful changes (Carr & Higginson 2001). User friendliness is also fundamental in terms of ease of use by the patient and ease and/or rapidity of analysis. Touch-screen computer technology offers a means for rapid collection and analysis of data; some pilot work is under way using such approaches (Velikova 2001).

Increasing use and understanding of QoL measurement seems to be a desirable goal in respect of quality and satisfaction. QoL measurement in the clinic setting also enables more patient-centred care, and complements the data on the more technical aspects of clinical progress. There is no evidence currently available to suggest that life expectancy is increased through the utility of QoL assessment. Improved quality of care, and patient/carer satisfaction, are likely outcomes through better communication. Intuitively there would appear potential service and system gains from improved communication between doctors, nurses and patients. So far, however, evidence of change in practice is lacking (Higginson & Carr 2002), although identifying potential and actual problems ought to be a valid first step in such a process if change is indeed needed.

Measurement of QoL nevertheless needs to be realistic in its objectives and purpose. Much time and effort in compiling, completing and analysing questionnaires to produce data are not ends in themselves. This applies particularly to clinical practice. QoL assessment is an adjunct to communication, not a substitute for it. Before embarking on such attempted measurements it is essential to be clear about their purpose, and for whom the data are being collected (e.g., for the patients, to justify clinical practice, to gain resources, or to fulfil the demands of the heathcare system— which, inevitably, includes political priorities). Also, at a very basic level, some of the improvements sought by the patient and carers are not covered in QoL analysis; some are more at the consumer level, some are simply practical and include nothing more profound than anxieties, concerns and frustrations over car parking facilities.

It also is important to retain a sense of perspective. Not everything done in medicine can or should be measured. Writing in the journal of the Royal College of Physicians of London, the Archbishop of Canterbury reminds us that the practice of medicine lies somewhere between science, as we normally understand it, and art. He also points out that humanity nowadays is 'hasty, anxious, obsessed with measurable success, deeply embarrassed by failure and death' and that 'the rules of our humanity are apparently being rewritten to suit the imperatives of management and profit.' (Williams 2002) It also needs to be recognised and accepted that, in dealing with cancer illnesses, death is often inevitable, and should not be perceived as failure. Many reported important aspects of QoL are shared with the perceived aspects of 'a good death' (Smith 2000). Improving patients QoL may therefore improve the experience of death for them and their families.

Summary and conclusions

Cancer illnesses will increase in their incidence in Westernised societies as result of increasing life expectancy. The word still carries the stigma of inevitable death despite significant advances in diagnosis, biological understanding and management. This perception was used to justify the radical approaches adopted to find a 'cure' over the past few decades. Such approaches often have dramatic effects on QoL, which initially were simply accepted as the price that had to be paid for the chance of cure and increased longevity.

With better understanding of likely overall and disease-free survival in cancers, allied to a more questioning society, there is now an increasing focus on the QoL obtained or expected in these conditions. Survival and improvement in specific symptoms are generally well covered in published literature. The impact of the diagnosis of cancer and the effects of therapy have a significant impact on QoL. QoL can be variously defined, but can be summarised as: 'The measure of the difference at a particular time point between the hopes and expectations of the individual and that individual's present experiences'. Through the development of structured questionnaires many facets of QoL can now reliably be measured. There is no standard QoL measurement and an appropriate questionnaire 'tool' to the problem being studied must be used.

In comparison to clinical and pathological outcome measures, the measurement of QoL remains at a disappointingly low level. The main reasons for this are the lack of standardised instruments to measure QoL, and intrinsic scientific and organisational difficulties in the processes involved. Standardised QoL instruments are being used increasingly in cancer trials, the data obtained are informing the direction of future research and contributing evidence to management guidelines in several cancers of which multiple myeloma is one.

At a clinical level, there is the potential to incorporate the measurement of QoL in to the clinic setting; the instruments used have a different orientation and purpose compared with those used for trials. QoL information obtained has the potential to improve quality for the patient through improved communication and understanding of issues.

References

Aaronson, N. K., Ahmedzai, S., Bergman, B., Bullinger, M., Cull, A., Duez, N. J., Filiberti, H., Flechtner, H., Fleischman, S. B., de Haes, J. C. J. M. *et al.* for the European Organisation for Research and Treatment of Cancer Study Group on QOL (1993). The European Organisation for Research and Treatment of Cancer QLQ-C30: a quality-of-life instrument for use in international clinical trials in oncology. *Journal of the National Cancer Institute* **85**, 365–376.

Addington-Hall, J. & Kalra, L. (2001). Who should measure quality of life? *British Medical Journal* **322**, 1417–1420.

Addington-Hall, J. & Kalra, L. (2002). Who should measure quality of life? In *Quality of life* (ed. I. Higginson, A. Carr & P. Robinson), pp. 1–8. BMJ Books.

Albrecht, G. L. & Devlieger, P. J. (1999). The disability paradox: high quality life against all odds. *Social Science and Medicine* **48**, 977–988.

Allison, P. J., Locker, D. & Feine J. S. (1997). Quality of life: a dynamic construct *Social Science and Medicine* **45**, 221–230.

Association for Palliative Medicine of Great Britain and Ireland (2001). *The 'Which Tool' guide: preliminary review of tools to measure clinical effectiveness in palliative care.* Southampton.

Berenson, J. R., Lichtenstein, A., Porter, L., Dimopoulos, M. A., Bordoni, R., George, S., Lipton, A., Keller, A., Ballester, O., Kovacs, M. *et al.* (1996). Efficacy of pamidronate in reducing skeletal events in patients with advanced multiple myeloma. Myeloma Aredia Study Group. *New England Journal of Medicine* **334**, 488–493.

Berenson J. R., Lichtenstein, A., Porter, L., Dimopoulos, M. A., Bordoni, R., George, S., Lipton, A., Keller, A., Ballester, O., Kovacs, M. *et al.* (1998). Long-term pamidronate treatment of advanced multiple myeloma patients reduces skeletal events. Myeloma Aredia Study Group. *Journal of Clinical Oncology* **16**, 593–602.

Bergman, B., Aaronson, N. K., Ahmedzai, S., Kaasa, S. & Sullivan, M. (1994). The EORTC QLQ-LC 13: a modular supplement to the EORTC core QoL questionnaire (QLQ-C30) for use in lung cancer clinical trials. *European Journal of Cancer* **30A**, 635–642.

Bergner, M., Bobbitt, R. A., Carter, W. B. & Gilson, B.S. (1981). The Sickness Impact Profile: development and final revision of a health status measure. *Medical Care* **19**, 787–805.

Bjordal, K., Hammerlid, E., Ahlner-Elmqvist, M. de Graeff, A., Boysen, M., Evensen, J. F., Biorklund, A., de Leeuw, J. R., Fayers, P. M., Jannert, M. *et al.* (1999). Quality of life in head and neck cancer patients: validation of the EORTC QoL questionnaire-H&N35. *Journal of Clinical Oncology* **17**, 1008–1019.

Bowling, A. (2002). Current state of the art in Quality of Life measurement. In *Quality of life* (ed. I. Higginson, A. Carr & P. Robinson), pp. 1–8. BMJ Books.

Bruera, E., Kuehn, N., Miller, M. J. *et al.* (1991). The Edmonton Symptom Assessment Schedule (ESAS): a simple method for the assessment of palliative care patients. *Journal of Palliative Care* **7**, 6–9.

Bruera, E. & MacDonald, S. (1993). Audit methods: the Edmonton Symptom Assessment System in clinical audit. In *Palliative care* (ed. I. Higginson), pp. 34–47. Oxford: Radcliffe Medical Press.

Calman, K. C. (1984). Quality of life in cancer patients; a hypothesis. *Journal of Medical Ethics* **10**, 124–129.

Carr, A. J. & Higginson, I. J. (2001). Are quality of life measures patient-centred? *British Medical Journal* **322**, 1357–1361.

Cella, D. F., Tulsky, D. S., Gray, G., Sarafian, B., Linn, E., Bonomi, A., Silberman, M., Yellen, S.B., Winicour, P., Brannon, J. *et al*. (1993). The functional assessment of cancer therapy scale: development and validation of the general measure. *Journal of Clinical Oncology* **11**, 570–579.

Cole, B. F., Gelber, R. D. & Goldhirsch, A. (1995). A quality-adjusted survival meta-analysis of adjuvant chemotherapy for pre-menopausal breast cancer. International Breast Cancer Study Group. *Statistics in Medicine* **14**, 1771–1784.

Dammacco, F., Castoldi, G. & Rodjer, S. (2001). Efficacy of epoetin alfa in the treatment of anaemia of multiple myeloma. *British Journal of Haematology* **113**, 172–179.

Demetri, G., Kris, M., Wade, J., Degos, L. & Cella, D. for the Procrit Study Group (1998). Quality-of-life benefit in chemotherapy patients treated with epoetin alfa is independent of disease response or tumour type: results from a prospective community oncology study. *Journal of Clinical Oncology* **16**, 3412–3425.

Diamond, J. (1999). *Because cowards get cancer too*. London: Vermilion Books.

Ellershaw, J. E., Peat, S. J. & Boys, L. C. (1995). Assessing the effectiveness of a hospital palliative care team. *Palliative Medicine* **9**, 145–152.

Garratt, A., Schmidt, L., Mackintosh, A. & Fitzpatrick, R. (2002). Quality of life measurement; bibliographic study of assessed health outcome measures. *British Medical Journal* **324**, 1417.

Glasziou, P. P., Simes, R. J. & Gelber, R. D. (1990). Quality adjusted survival analysis. *Statistics in Medicine* **9**, 1259–1276.

Gulbrandsen, N., Wisloff, F., Nord, E., Lenhoff, S., Hjorth, M. & Westin, J. (2001a). Cost-utility analysis of high-dose melphalan with autologous blood stem cell support vs. melphalan plus prednisone in patients younger than 60 years with multiple myeloma. *European Journal of Haematology* **66**, 328–336.

Gulbrandsen, N., Wisløff, F., Brinch, L., Carlson, K., Dahl, I. M., Gimsing, P., Hippe, E., Hjorth, M., Knudsen, L., Lamvik, J. *et al*. Nordic Myeloma Study Group. (2001b). Health-related quality-of-life in multiple myeloma patients receiving high dose chemotherapy with autologous blood stem cell support. *Medical Oncology* **18**, 65–77.

de Haes, J. C. J. M., van Knippenberg, F. C. E. & Neijt, J. P. (1990). Measuring psychological and physical distress in cancer patients: structure and application of the Rotterdam Symptom Checklist. *British Journal of Cancer* **62**, 1034–1038.

Hearn, J. & Higginson, I. J. (1997). Outcome measures in palliative care for advanced cancer patients: a review. *Journal of Public Health Medicine* **19**, 193–199.

Higginson, I. J. & Carr, A. J. (2001). Using quality of life measures in the clinical setting. *British Medical Journal* **322**, 1297–1300.

Higginson, I. J. & Carr, A. J. (2002). The clinical utility of QoL measures. In *Quality of life* (ed. I. Higginson, A. Carr & P. Robinson), pp. 63–78. BMJ Books.

Hunt, S. M, McEwen, J. & McKenna, S. P. (1985). Measuring health status: a new tool for clinicians and epidemiologists. *Journal of the Royal College of General Practitioners* **35**, 1191–1194.

Karnofsky, D. A. & Burchenal, J. H (1949). The clinical evaluation of chemotherapeutic agents in cancer. In *Evaluation of chemotherapeutic agents* (ed. C. M MacLeod), p. 196. New York: Columbia Press.

Lenhoff, S., Hjorth, M., Holmberg, E., Tureson, I., Westin, M., Nielsen, J. L., Wisloff, F., Brinch, L., Carlson, K., Carlsson, M. *et al*. (2000). Impact on survival of high-dose therapy with autologous stem cell support in patients younger than 60 years with newly diagnosed multiple myeloma: a population based study. *Blood* **95**, 7–11.

McCloskey, E. V., MacLennan, I. C. M., Drayson, M. T. *et al.* (1998). A randomised trial of the effect of clodronate on skeletal morbidity in multiple myeloma. *British Journal of Haematology* **100**, 317–325.

McCorkle, R. & Young, K. (1978). Development of a symptom distress scale. *Cancer Nursing* **1**, 373–378.

Morris, J. N., Suissa, S., Sherwood, S., Wright, S. M. & Greer, D. (1986). Last days: a study of the QoL of terminally ill cancer patients. *Journal of Chronic Disease* **39**, 47–62.

Murray, S. & Cole, B. (2000). Variance and sample size calculations in quality-of-life-adjusted survival analysis (Q-TwiST). *Biometrics* **56**, 173–182.

O'Boyle, C. A., McGee, H. & Joyce, C. R. B. (1994). Quality of life: assessing the individual. *Advances in Medical Sociology* **5**, 159–180.

Osterborg, A., Boogaerts, M. A., Cimino, R., Essers, U., Holowiecki, J., Juliusson, G., Jager, G., Najman, A. & Peest, D. (1996). Recombinant human erythropoietin in transfusion-dependent anaemic patients with multiple myeloma and non-Hodgkin's lymphoma. *Blood* **87**, 2675–2682.

Osoba, D., Rodrigues, G., Myles, J., Zee, B. & Pater, J. (1998). Interpreting the significance of changes in health-related quality of life scores. *Journal of Clinical Oncology* **16**, 139–144.

Paterson, C. (1996). Measuring outcomes in primary care: a patient generated measure, MYMOP, compared with the SF-36 health survey. *British Medical Journal* **312**, 1016–1020.

Porcher, R., Levy, V., Fermand, J.P., Katshahian, S., Chevret, S. & Ravaud, P. (2002). Evaluating high dose therapy in multiple myeloma: use of quality-adjusted survival analysis. *Quality of Life Research* **11**, 91–99.

Robinson, P. G., Carr, A. J. & Higginson, I. J. (2002). How to choose a quality of life measure. In *Quality of life* (ed. I. Higginson, A. Carr & P. Robinson), pp. 63–78. BMJ Books.

Sanders, C., Egger, M., Donovan, J., Tallon, D. & Frankel, S. (1998). Reporting on Quality of Life in randomised controlled trials; bibliographic study. *British Medical Journal* **317**, 1191–1194.

Slevin, M. L., Plant, H., Lynch, D., Drinkwater, J. & Gregory W. M. (1988). Who should measure quality of life, the doctor or the patient? *British Journal of Cancer* **57**, 109–12

Smith, R. J. (2000). A good death. *British Medical Journal* **320**, 129–130.

Sprangers, M. A. G., Groenvold, M., Arraras, J. I., Frankilin, J., te Velde, A., Muller, M., Franzini, L., Williams, A., de Haes, H. C., Hopwood, P. *et al.* (1996). The EORTC breast cancer-specific QoL questionnaire module: first results from a three-country field study. *Journal of Clinical Oncology* **14**, 2756–2768.

Stead, M., Brown, J. M., Velikova, G., Kaasa, S., Wisloff, F., Child, J. A., Hippe, E., Hjorth, M., Sezer, O. & Selby, P. (1999). Development of an EORTC questiooaire module to be used in health-related quality-of-life assessment for patients with multiple myeloma. European Organization for Research and Treatment of Cancer Study Group on Quality of Life. *British Journal of Haematology* **104**, 605–611.

Stone, P., Ream, E., Richardson, Thomas, H., Andrews, P., Campbell, P., Dawson, T., Edwards, J., Goldie, T., Hammick, M. *et al.* (2003). Cancer-related fatigue – a difference of opinion? Results of a multicentre survey of healthcare professionals, patients and caregivers. *European Journal of Cancer Care (England)* **12**, 20–27.

Stone, P., Richardson, A., Ream, E., Smith, A.G., Kerr, D.J., Kearney, N. (2000). Cancer-related fatigue; inevitable, unimportant and untreatable? Results of a multi-centre patient survey. Cancer Fatigue Forum. *Annals of Oncology* **11**, 971–975.

UK Myeloma Forum (2001). Guidelines on the diagnosis and management of multiple myeloma. *British Journal of Haematology* **115**, 522–540.

Velikova, G. (2001). Quality of life measures in oncology practice – getting some early answers? *British Medical Journal* **322**, 1297.

Vigano, A., Dorgan, M., Buckingham, J., Bruera, E., Suarez-Almazor, M. E. (2000). Survival prediction in terminal cancer patients: a systematic review of the medical literature. *Palliative Medicine* **14**, 363–374.

Vogelzang, N. J., Breitbart, W., Cella, D., Curt, G. A., Groopman, J. E., Horning, S. J., Itri, L. M., Johnson, D. H., Scherr, S. L. & Portenoy, R. K. (1997). Patient, caregiver and oncologist perceptions of cancer-related fatigue; results of a tripart assessment survey, The Fatigue Coalition. *Seminars in Hematology* **34** (Suppl. 2), 4–12.

Ware, J. E. & Sherbourne, C. D. (1992). The MOS 36-item Short-form Health Survey (SF-36). 1. Conceptual framework and item selection. *Medical Care* **30**, 473–483.

Williams, R. (2002). On the edge of faith. *Clinical Medicine* **2**, 495.

Wisloff, F., Eika, S., Hippe, E., Hjorth, M., Holmberg, E., Kaasa, S., Palva, I. & Westin, J. (1996a). Measurement of health-related QOL in multiple myeloma. Nordic Myeloma Study Group. *British Journal of Haematology* **92**, 604–613.

Wisloff, F., Gulbrandsen, N. & Nord, E. (1999). Therapeutic options in the treatment of multiple myeloma: pharmacoeconomic and quality of life considerations. *Pharmacoeconomics* **16**, 329–341.

Wisloff, F., Hjorth, M., Kaasa, S. & Westin, J. (1996b). Effect of interferon on the health-related Quality of Life of multiple myeloma patients: results of a Nordic randomised trial comparing melphalan-prednisolone to melphalan-prednisolone + alpha-interferon. The Nordic Myeloma Study Group. *British Journal of Haematology* **94**, 324–332.

World Health Organization (1993). Measuring quality of life; the development of the World Health Organization QOL Instrument (WHOQOL). Geneva: World Health Organization.

Zee, B., Cole, B., Li, T., Browman, G., James, K., Johnston, D., Sugano, D. & Pater, J. (1998). Quality-adjusted time without symptoms or toxicity analysis of interferon maintenance in multiple myeloma. *Journal of Clinical Oncology* **16**, 2834–2839.

PART 2

The prevention and control of pain in cancer

Chapter 7

Bone pain: the evidentiary basis of current management strategies

Peter J. Hoskin

Introduction

Metastatic bone pain is a significant burden for many patients with advanced cancer. It is a feature of the common cancers arising in breast, lung and prostate, together with less common sites in the thyroid and kidneys; and on occasions can be associated with most other primary sites. Management is based on both non-specific pharmacological manipulation of the pain process and specific oncological treatment of the bone metastasis using radiotherapy, chemotherapy, hormone therapy and surgery. The bisphosphonates have in addition provided a major new treatment option for patients with metastatic bone pain. An overall schema for the management of metastatic bone pain is shown in Figure 7.1.

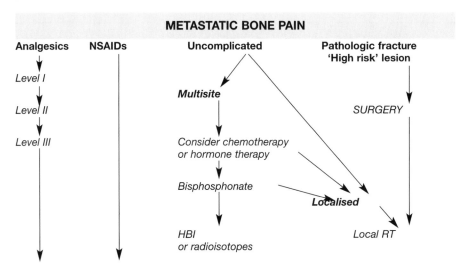

Figure 7.1 Overview of the management of metastatic bone pain

Analgesics and non-steroidal anti-inflammatory drugs

As with any cancer pain scenario, the fundamentals of analgesic use in metastatic bone pain should follow the World Heath Organization (WHO) analgesic ladder escalating from level I, through level II to level III analgesia, on a regular basis. Level

I analgesia includes the use of non-steroidal anti-inflammatory drugs (NSAIDs) which may also be maintained through the other levels of the ladder as an adjuvant analgesic by their anti-inflammatory action. The use of simple analgesics in a general population of patients with cancer pain has been reviewed. When the analgesic ladder is applied strictly, only 11% are found to have adequate analgesia on level I (Ventafridda et al. 1987). In populations of patients with bone pain referred for radiotherapy in randomised trials the incidence of level I analgesic use varies from 13% to 38% (Nielsen et al. 1998; Bone Pain Trial Working Party 1999; Steenland et al. 1999). It may, however, be deduced that because of referral for radiotherapy, pain control in these patients is not satisfactory with level I analgesia and that most patients with metastatic bone pain require level II or III analgesia.

Single agent data for the efficacy of NSAIDs in metastatic bone pain is limited, but early studies suggest that the actual response rate for pain relief may be as low as 20% with indomethacin, aspirin or flurbiprofen (Coombes et al. 1979).

A meta-analysis of the use of NSAIDs in cancer patients reviewed the results of 25 randomised controlled trials which evaluated 16 different drugs in a total of 15,445 patients (Eisenberg et al. 1994). Of the 25 trials, pain related to bone metastasis was described in only 7, of which only 3 were specific studies in bone metastasis alone, the other 4 including other types of pain. Of the 3 trials specific for bone metatasis, only 2 reported analgesic efficacy data. The first of these was a single-dose, randomised, placebo-controlled crossover study of ketoprofen reporting a peak pain intensity difference (PPID) of 40–50% and summed pain intensity difference (SPID) of 34–45%. The second trial was a multiple dose study of two dose levels of naproxen comparing 275 mg with 550 mg; the overall PPID for naproxen was 23–33%.

There are even fewer published data for response rates to level II and level III analgesia from metastatic bone pain. Anecdotally, bone pain is often quoted as being 'relatively resistant' to opioids but specific clinical data are lacking to support this statement. There may be additional complications with metastatic bone pain, where incident pain may be prominent and a neuropathic component may also be a major feature of the pain picture.

In summary, therefore, there are limited data to confirm the efficacy of the WHO analgesic ladder for metastatic bone pain as a specific entity. The results for NSAIDs as single agents suggest a response rate for metastatic bone pain of between 20% and 40%.

Surgery

The role of surgery in metastatic bone pain has also suffered from a paucity of published data evaluating its efficacy and relative place in the management of these patients. It is the recommended treatment for pathological fractures of long bones, and both anecdotally and intuitively the management by internal fixation of a pathological fracture seems the optimal approach. There are, however, few published data on this scenario specifically, either in established pathological fracture or as a prophylactic procedure. There are no randomised controlled trials comparing surgery with alternative local treatment, for example radiotherapy.

Chemotherapy

For chemotherapy-responsive tumours, then metastatic bone pain can respond well to systemic chemotherapy. The common scenarios are breast and lung cancer. In breast cancer the complete response rate for bone pain is reported in between 0% and 84% of patients; the median time to response may be some weeks, quoted figures being of the order of 32 weeks (Whitehouse 1985). There is no clear evidence that any one chemotherapy regime recognised for metastatic breast cancer has advantages in metastatic bone pain over any other scenario where it may be indicated.

Response rates for bone pain specifically in studies of lung cancer are difficult to find in the published literature. The main focus in these studies is on quality of life questionnaires where there is an undoubted improvement in scores for patients receiving chemotherapy compared with best supportive care in both non-small-cell lung cancer (NSCLC) and small-cell lung cancer (SCLC).

Multiple myeloma, although a relatively rare malignancy compared with lung, prostate and breast cancers, is particularly associated with metastatic bone pain. The mainstay of treatment is chemotherapy using alkylating agents or high-dose steroid combinations. Chemotherapy has an important role in the control of skeletal disease in these patients. A reduction in severity of bone pain and overall incidence is seen; at presentation it is a feature in 75% of patients, falling to less than 15% in plateau phase, representing the time of maximal response to chemotherapy. Response rates are greater for rib and back pain than limb pain (Kanis & McCloskey 1998).

Hormone therapy

Prostate and breast cancers commonly metastasise to bone and are hormone sensitive. Hormone therapy for prostate cancer is in the form of anti-androgen treatment with either luteinising hormone releasing hormone (LHRH) analogues such as goserelin, peripheral anti-androgens such as bicalutamide or flutamide or surgical orchidectomy. The response rates for any of these manoeuvres are high, with no difference between them. Responses for metastatic bone pain from anti-androgen therapy are reported in the range 90–95%, with a median duration of 18–24 months (Ventafridda *et al.* 1990). Pain relief may be rapid after orchidectomy or introduction of an anti-androgen drug. On relapse, however, second responses to hormone therapy are unusual and rarely durable.

Hormone therapy for metastatic breast cancer is well established, using an anti-oestrogen such as tamoxifen (Nolvadex), progestogen such as megestrol acetate (Megace), or aromatase inhibitors such as anastrozole (Arimidex), letrozole (Femara). In the population of patients with predominantly bone metastases, hormone treatment is the most common systemic therapy. Responses to first- or second-line hormone therapy are in the range of 20–35% (Smith & Macaulay 1985), although rates of around 50% are seen when 'stable disease' is included in the response criteria (Plunkett et al. 2000). Few other cancers are reliably hormone sensitive. Endometrial cancer is one other example where bone metastases are occasionally seen and in which responses to progestogens or LHRH analogues are seen in around 30% of patients (Cohen 1992).

Radiotherapy

Radiotherapy is often regarded as one of the most effective treatments for metastatic bone pain. For localised pain then external beam radiotherapy is indicated; for more widespread sites of pain then wide-field external beam radiotherapy or systemic radioisotope therapy has an important role.

Localised radiotherapy

Localised radiotherapy for metastatic bone pain has been the subject of many studies in the literature. Single-arm, single-centre reports in over 3,000 patients using varying definitions of pain relief and methods of assessment have consistently reported response rates of around 80%. There are 14 published randomised controlled trials that confirm the efficacy of radiotherapy in this setting. Most of these have investigated different radiation doses and no consistent evidence for a radiation dose response for pain relief has emerged. Absolute response rates are difficult to compare in this setting and this is exemplified in the Danish Bone Pain Trial (Nielsen et al. 1998) in which very thorough assessments including pain scores, analgesic use and a quality-of-life score were determined for patients. By using these different endpoints it was possible to define a complete response of 25% with a simple pain score of 0, 12% when the definition was a pain score of 0 with no morphine, but only 4% when the definition of complete response included complete well-being on the quality-of-life scale.

This has been the subject of two Cochrane reviews, the first of which identified 13 trials and included one hemibody fractionation study and four isotope studies in this total (McQuay et al. 2000) The overall analysis resulted in a number needed to treat (NNT) value for complete pain relief of 3.9 (3.5–4.4) and partial pain relief of 3.6 (3.2–3.9). A more recent Cochrane review of 12 trials selected on the basis of reporting overall pain response as one of the outcomes representing a total of 3,621 patients on which a meta-analysis was performed quotes complete pain responses of 34% for single fraction radiotherapy and 32% for multifraction radiotherapy, with overall pain responses of 60% and 59% respectively (Sze et al. 2003). A higher re-treatment rate of 21.5% after single doses of radiotherapy was noted compared with 7.4% after multifraction radiotherapy. There was a suggestion that the pathological fracture rate may also be higher after single doses than multiple doses (3% compared with 1.6%). No difference in the incidence of spinal cord compression was seen and the overall conclusion from these data is once again to confirm the efficacy of radiotherapy for pain relief, to refute any suggestion that there is a significant dose response above single doses of 8 Gy, but to recognise that after single doses of radiotherapy there may be a higher incidence of further re-treatment usually with another single dose.

There remain uncertainties over the role of radiotherapy for certain scenarios in metastatic bone pain, in particular its role in neuropathic bone pain and the most appropriate dose in this setting (Roos *et al.* 2000), and similarly its value in pathological fracture particularly after surgical fixation.

Wide-field radiotherapy

Wide-field radiotherapy, or hemibody radiotherapy as it is often termed, has been subject to several single arm studies. Twelve of these can be identified in the literature that confirm efficacy similar to external beam radiotherapy but with some different features, in particular a more rapid response reported within the first 24 h in up to 25% of patients. Two randomised controlled trials have been performed (Poulter *et al.* 1992; Salazar *et al.* 2002), the first addressing the question of its role as prophylaxis and the second comparing different dose levels in a multicentre international study of 156 patients encompassing treatment centres in Brazil, Cameroon, Pakistan, Peru, Spain and the USA. This confirmed the efficacy of hemibody radiotherapy for pain relief, with an overall response rate of 91%, of whom 45% were complete and 46% partial responders. Toxicity was considered acceptable: it was recorded as mild/ moderate in 50% and severe but transitory in 12%. An important outcome measure in this group of patients who have a short life expectancy is the proportion of their remaining survival that is pain free. In this study the mean overall survival was 174 days and the mean pain-free survival was 122 days; thus 70% of the remaining survival time was 'pain free' from the radiotherapy treatment. It is important to recognise that the actuarial analysis method used here censors patients once their pain has returned and does not detect further successful pain control from additional measures; this does not imply that 30% of patients died with pain.

Radioisotope therapy

Radioisotope therapy seeks to treat all sites of bone metastases by systemic administration of a radioisotope which will be concentrated at the site of bone invasion. The ideal isotope will deliver short range beta radiation as its main decay but also some gamma irradiation for imaging to track the distribution of the isotope where necessary. In the past phosphorus (^{32}P) has been used, but the most common radioisotope in use currently is strontium (^{89}Sr). This is targeted to sites of increased bone mineralisation, being metabolised in the same way as calcium. Two other compounds are available which are targeted to areas of bone remineralisation through conjugation with a phosphonate compound: these are samarium (^{153}Sm–EDTMP) and rhenium (^{186}Re–HEDP).

The advantage of radioisotopes is that they require a single intravenous injection, which can usually be given as an outpatient to deliver systemic radiotherapy. Their toxicity is low, the major impact usually being bone marrow toxicity. In therapeutic doses this is rarely of clinical significance, being exemplified by modest falls in haemoglobin, white count and platelets, and a few patients requiring blood transfusion before recovery is seen within 4–6 weeks of the isotope administration.

Their toxicity and efficacy has been carefully defined in phase I, phase II and phase III trials. The greatest body of evidence is for strontium. Phase I/II dose escalation studies have defined the optimal therapeutic dose to be 150 MBq, above which platelet toxicity is seen (Laing et al. 1991). Phase III placebo-controlled randomised trials have demonstrated its efficacy over placebo for pain relief in metastatic bone pain from prostate cancer (Lewington et al. 1991). Two studies have compared strontium with external beam radiotherapy. The first was a case-control study against hemibody radiotherapy which confirmed equivalent efficacy and a lower requirement for blood transfusion in the radioisotope group compared with the wide-field radiotherapy group (Dearnaley et al. 1992). A randomised controlled trial of 284 patients with either local pain or scattered pain compared external beam radiotherapy using either a local field for patients with local pain or wide field for those having scattered pain with ^{89}Sr (Quilty et al. 1994). Pain relief was seen in 65–70% of patients with no difference between the randomisation arms, and although there was a higher level of platelet toxicity observed in the strontium arms of 6.9% compared with 3.4% and a higher level of white cell toxicity of 3.1% compared with 0, no neutropenic sepsis events were seen in the patient population and no blood transfusions were given.

Samarium has also been carefully investigated in phase I/II dose escalation studies, defining the optimal clinical dose at 1 mCi/kg (Resche et al. 1997). A phase III placebo-controlled randomised trial in metastatic prostate cancer has again confirmed its efficacy over placebo (Sartor et al. 1997).

Bisphosphonates

Bisphosphonates act by inhibiting osteoclast activity. One of the fundamental pathological events in the establishment and maintenance of a bone metastasis is osteoclast activation by chemotactic factors released by the tumour cells. Therefore the use of an osteoclast inhibitor is a rational approach to altering their pathophysiology. They have been shown in several phase III trials to be effective in reducing bone morbidity events when used prophylactically in high-risk patients with breast cancer and myeloma (Bloomfield 1998; Hoskin 2003). There are fewer data on their role as therapeutic agents for metastatic bone pain, but there are now seven randomised controlled trials that have compared them with placebo or best supportive care which confirm superior efficacy to this control arm. A Cochrane review of the role of bisphosphonates in breast cancer identified four studies in which there were significant improvements in pain control with the use of bisphosphonates for metastatic bone pain (Pavlakis & Stockler 2002). Three other randomised trials in lung and prostate cancer have confirmed activity with improved pain control compared with placebo (Ernst *et al.* 1992; Coleman *et al.* 1995; Robertson *et al.* 1995).

The emergence of bisphosphonates as useful agents for metastatic bone pain has raised the question of their relative role compared with chemotherapy, hormone therapy or radiotherapy. One study has evaluated the addition of pamidronate to chemotherapy in 295 randomised patients with breast cancer and bone metastasis (Conte *et al.* 1996). Bone pain was present in 85% of these patients at their baseline pain assessment; the number of patients having marked pain improvement defined as a 2 point reduction on a 6 point pain scale for at least six weeks was 30% in the chemotherapy alone arm and 44% in the combined chemotherapy and bisphonate arm. This was statistically significant ($p = 0.025$). There is therefore a suggestion that the combination of chemotherapy with bisphosphonate may be more effective against bone pain than chemotherapy alone in carcinoma of the breast. The relative role of bisphosphonates in the setting of local radiotherapy for bone pain is currently the subject of a randomised controlled trial in the UK, the RIB trial comparing single-dose radiotherapy with a single infusion of ibandronate.

Summary

There is a considerable choice of treatment available for patients with metastatic bone pain. No single treatment can claim overall superiority, most patients being best served by a combination of non-specific analgesic medication, specific chemoradiation or hormone interventions and, increasingly, the addition of bisphosphonates. In terms of the evidentiary basis, it is interesting to note that this is most robust for the more recent treatments, in particular radioisotopes and bisphosphonates whereas the established traditional treatments using the analgesic ladder, NSAIDs and surgery have limited published evidence to define their efficacy.

References

Bloomfield, D. J. (1998). Should bisphosphonates be part of the standard therapy of patients with multiple myeloma or bone metastases from other cancers? An evidence-based review. *Journal of Clinical Oncology* **16**, 1218–1225.

Bone Pain Trial Working Party (1999). 8 Gy single fraction radiotherapy for the treatment of metastatic skeletal pain: randomised comparison with a multifraction schedule over 12 months of patient follow-up. *Radiotherapy and Oncology* **52**, 111–121.

Cohen, C. J. (1992). Advanced and recurrent carcinoma of the endometrium. In *Gynecologic Oncology* (ed. M. Coppleston), 2nd edition, vol. 2, pp. 795–797. Edinburgh: Churchill Livingstone.

Coleman, R. E., Vinholes, J., Abbey, M. E., Purohit, O. P. (1995). Double blind randomised trial of pamidronate for the palliative treatment of metastatic bone pain. *Journal of Clinical Oncology* **15**, 528.

Conte, P. F., Latreille, J., Mauriac, L., Calabresi, F., Santos, R., Campos, D., Bonneterre, J., Francini, G., Ford, J. M. *et al.* (1996). Delay in progression of bone metastases in breast cancer patients treated with intravenous pamidronate: results from a multinational randomised trial. *Journal of Clinical Oncology* **14**, 2552–2559.

Coombes, R. C., Munro Neville, A., Gazet, J.-C., Ford, H. T., Nash, A. G., Baker, J. W., Powles, T. J. (1979). Agents affecting osteolysis in patients with breast cancer. *Cancer Chemotherapy and Pharmacology* **3**, 41–44.

Dearnaley, D. P., Bayley, R. J., A'Hern, R. P., Gadd, J., Zivanaic, M. M., Lewington, V. J. (1992). Palliation of bone metastases in prostate cancer. Hemibody irradiation or strontium-89. *Clinical Oncology* **4**, 101–107.

Eisenberg, E., Berkey, C. S., Carr, D. B., Mosteller, F. & Chalmers, T. C. (1994). Efficacy and safety of nonsteroidal anti-inflammatory drugs for cancer pain: a meta-analysis. *Journal of Clinical Oncology* **12**, 2756–2765.

Ernst, S. D., MacDonald, N., Paterson, A., Jensen, J., Bruera, E. *et al.* (1992). A double blind cross over trial of intravenous clodronate in metastatic bone pain. *Journal of Pain and Symptom Management* **7**, 4–11.

Hoskin, P. J. (2003). Bisphosphonates and radiation therapy. *Cancer Treatment Reviews* **29**, 321–327.

Kanis, J. A. & McCloskey, E. V. (1998). Disorders of calcium and skeletal metabolism. In *Myeloma: biology and management* (ed. J. Malpas, D. Bergasel, R. Kyle & K. Anderson), 2nd edition, pp. 372–373. Oxford: Oxford University Press.

Laing, A. H., Ackery, D. M., Bayly, R. J., Lewington, V. J., McEwan, A. J. B., Macleod, P. M., Zivanovic, M. A. (1991). Strontium 89 chloride for pain palliation in prostatic skeletal malignancy. *British Journal of Radiology* **64**, 816–822.

Lewington, V. J., McEwan, A. J., Ackery, D. M., Bayly, R. J., Keeling, D., Macleod, P. M., Porter, A. T., Zivanovic, A. M. (1991). A prospective randomized double-blind crossover study to examine the efficacy of strontium-89 in pain palliation in patients with advanced prostate cancer metastatic to bone. *European Journal of Cancer* **27**, 954–958.

McQuay, H. J., Collins, S. L., Carroll, D. & Moore, R. A. (2000). Radiotherapy for the palliation of painful bone metastases: a systematic review. *Cochrane Database Systematic Reviews* (2), CD001793.

Nielsen, O. S., Bentzen, S. M., Sandberg, E., Gadeberg, C. C., Timothy, A. R. (1998). Randomized trial of single dose versus fractionated palliative radiotherapy of bone metastases. *Radiotherapy and Oncology* **47**, 233–224.

Pavlakis, N. & Stockler, M. (2002). Bisphosphonates for breast cancer. *Cochrane Database Systematic Reviews* (1), CD003474 UI: 11869664.

Plunkett, T. A., Smith, P. & Rubens, R. D. (2000). Risk of complications from bone metastases in breast cancer: implications for management. *European Journal of Cancer* **36**, 476–482.

Poulter, C. A., Cosmatos, D., Rubin, P., Urtasun, R., Cooper, J. S., Kuske, R. R., Hornback, N., Coughlin, C., Weigensberg, I. & Rotman, M. (1992). A report of RTOG 8206: a Phase III study of whether the addition of single dose hemibody irradiation to standard fractionated local field irradiation is more effective than local field irradiation alone in the treatment of symptomatic osseous metastases. *International Journal of Radiation Oncology, Biology, Physics* **23**, 207–214.

Quilty, P. M., Kirk, D., Bolger, J. J., Dearnaley, D. P., Lewington, V. J., Mason, M. D., Reed, N. S. E., Russell, J. M., Yardley, J. (1994). A comparison of the palliative effects of strontium-89 and external beam radiotherapy in metastatic prostate cancer. *Radiotherapy and Oncology* **31**, 33–40.

Resche, I., Chatal, J.-F., Pecking, A., Ell, P., Duschesne, G., Rubens, R., Fogelman, I., Housten, S., Fauser, A., Fischer, M., Wilkins, D. (1997). A dose-controlled study of 153 Sm-ethylenediaminetatramethylenephosphate (EDTMP) in the treatment of patients with painful bone metastases. *European Journal of Cancer* **33**, 1583–1591.

Robertson, A. G., Reed, N. S. & Ralston, S. H. (1995). Effect of oral clodronate on metastatic bone pain: a double blind placebo controlled trial. *Journal of Clinical Oncology* **13**, 2427–2430.

Roos, D. E., O'Brien, P. C., Smith, J. G., Spry, N. A., Hoskin, P. J., Burmeister, B. H., Turner, S. L, Bernshaw, D. M. (2000). A role for radiotherapy in neuropathic bone pain: preliminary response rates from a prospective trial (TROG 96.05). *International Journal of Radiation Oncology, Biology, Physics* **46**, 975–981.

Salazar, O. M., Sanhu, T., Da Motta, N. W., Esantia, M. A. P., Lanzos-Gonzales, E., Mouelle-Sane, A., Moscol, A., Zaharia, M. & Zaman, S. (2001). Fractionated half body irradiation (HBI) for the rapid palliation of widespread symptomatic metastatic disease: a randomised phase III trial of the International Atomic Energy Agency. *International Journal of Radiation Oncology, Biology, Physics* **50**, 765–775.

Sartor, O., Quick, D., Reid, R., Hoskin, P., Duschesne, G. *et al.* (1997). A double blind placebo controlled study of 153 samarium EDTMP for palliation of bone pain in patients with hormone-refractory prostate cancer. *Journal of Urology* **157**, 321.

Smith, I. E. & Macaulay, V. (1985). Comparison of different endocrine therapies in management of bone metastases from breast carcinoma. *Journal of the Royal Society of Medicine* **78** (Suppl. 9), 15–21.

Steenland, E., Leer, J., van Houwelingen, H., Post, W. J., van den Hout, W. B., Kievit, J., de Haes, H., Martijn, H., Oei, B., Vonke, E. *et al.* (1999). The effect of a single fraction compared to multiple fractions on painful bone metastases: a global analysis of the Dutch Bone Metastasis Study. *Radiotherapy and Oncology* **52**, 101–109.

Sze, W.-M., Sheley, M. D., Held, I. & Mason, M. D. (2003). Palliation of metastatic bone pain: a single fraction versus multifraction radiotherapy – a systematic review of randomised trials. *Clinical Oncology* **15**, 345–352.

Ventafridda, V., Tamburini, M., Caraceni, A., De Conno, F. & Naldi, F. (1987). A validation study of the WHO method for cancer pain relief. *Cancer* **59**, 850–856.

Ventafridda, V., Sbanotto, A. & Dconno, F. (1990). Pain in prostatic cancer. *Palliative Medicine* **4**, 173–184.

Whitehouse, J. M. A. (1985). Site-dependent response to chemotherapy for carcinoma of the breast. *Journal of the Royal Society of Medicine* **78** (Suppl.9),18–22.

Chapter 8

Cancer-induced bone pain: mechanisms and novel therapeutics

Catherine E. Urch

Introduction

Pain arising within a bone either from a primary bone sarcoma or metastatic spread from a carcinoma is a common sequel in disease progression. Indeed, up to two-thirds of patients with breast or prostate carcinoma will develop bone metastases, with a significant proportion suffering pain (Coleman 1997; Mercadante & Arcuri 1998). Bone pain has been shown to correlate with an increased morbidity, reduced performance status, increased anxiety and depression, and reduced quality of life (Portenoy & Hagen 1990; Portenoy *et al.* 1999; Bruera *et al.* 1995). Although bone-related pains have been recognised for a considerable time, the terminology remains confused (Mercadante *et al.* 2002). Pain arising from within the bone comprises a triad of tonic (background) ache/pain, spontaneous pain and movement-induced pain (Mercadante & Arcuri 1998; Janjan 2001). Although occasionally the triad is referred to as incident pain, often it is just the movement induced or weight-bearing component that is termed incident pain. In addition, the movement-induced pain is often referred to as breakthrough pain. Breakthrough pains are heterogeneous and must be distinguished from recurrent acute pain, fluctuations in chronic pain, classic 'end of dose' failure, spontaneous pain and movement-related pains (Portenoy & Hagen 1990; Portenoy *et al.* 1999). Despite the clinical importance of movement related pain, information is lacking in defining the subtypes of breakthrough pain in the medically ill patient, where numerous pains may be present. The Breakthrough Pain Questionnaire (Portenoy *et al.* 1999) attempts to characterise the acute pain flares, thereby allowing sub-analyses of movement-induced, spontaneous or end-of-dose failure pains. However, this questionnaire is not validated and there is some way to go before a readily useable clinical tool becomes available.

Breakthrough pain is relatively common, with more than 60% of cancer inpatients reporting acute flares of pain, and up to 90% of ambulatory cancer patients attending a pain clinic reported pain on movement (Portenoy & Hagen 1990; Banning *et al.* 1991). The presence of breakthrough pain has been demonstrated to reduce the efficacy of opioid analgesia (Mercadante *et al.* 1992; Bruera *et al.* 1995). Within a hospice population, 93% of 242 consecutive admissions reported episodic, weight-bearing pain, more than one-third were due to concurrent non-cancer diagnoses, and satisfactory analgesia was achieved in only 54% of cases (Swanwick *et al.* 2001).

Analgesic therapies for bone-mediated pain are multi-modal and include systemic analgesics (opioids, non-steroidal anti-inflammatory drugs (NSAIDs)), bisphosphonates, anti-tumour chemotherapy, radiotherapy, systemic radio-isotopes, local surgery and anaesthesia (McQuay *et al.* 2000; Serafini 2001; Mercadante *et al.* 2002; Wong & Wiffen 2002). No single modality is effective in all patients or for a prolonged length of time, and all treatments have limiting side-effects. Although there have been improvements on the old, standard analgesics, there have been no novel therapeutic approaches to the persistent problem of movement-induced bone pain. This is in part due to a lack of data on the mechanisms underlying the pathophysiology of bone-induced pain.

Animal models

Until the late 20th century all animal models of cancer-induced bone pain had relied on the systemic injection of carcinoma cells, which resulted in systemically unwell animals and random and multiple-sited bone deposits. Schwei *et al.* (1999) reported the intra-medullar injection of an osteolytic sarcoma cell line in mice. The sarcoma cells were injected into the medulla at the distal end of the mouse femur, with control groups of sham operated (media only injected) and sarcoma cells injected into the surrounding quadriceps muscle. Over the subsequent 21 days the animals with either sham medulla injection or sarcoma into the quadriceps displayed no behavioural sign of ongoing, spontaneous or movement-induced pain. However, the animals receiving the intra-medullar injection of sarcoma cells displayed progressively severe nocifensive behaviour which correlated with a progressive destruction of the femur (Schwei *et al.* 1999). The animals remained well, with good weight gain. Furthermore, the type of pain behaviours exhibited (progressive limping, guarding, spontaneous flinching and vocalisation on palpation, reduced movement, secondary hyperalgesia and allodynia) were similar to those seen in humans (Honore *et al.* 2000a). The bone destruction also paralleled the human case progressing from a small lytic lesion with minimal derangement of the medulla through to pathological fractures in a grossly destroyed bone (Honore *et al.* 2000a). In addition, the response to systemic opioids in the mouse model was similar to that found in humans: when compared with inflammation-induced pain the attenuation with morphine was reduced (Luger *et al.* 2002). Based on the original work, alternative models have been developed: breast carcinoma cells within the rat tibia, or fibrosarcoma or melanoma cells within the mouse humerus (Medhurst *et al.* 2002; Wacnik *et al.* 2003). The development of reproducible, locally contained cancer-induced bone destruction has allowed the elucidation of the neurochemical changes both locally (within the bone medulla) and centrally (within the dorsal horn).

Why is tumour-induced bone destruction painful?

In the past it was suggested that tumour-induced bone pain may be due to vascular occlusion, compression of the bone or peripheral nerve or due to mechanical instability. However, these failed to consider the basic mechanisms of nociceptor activation, transmission, or primary and secondary sensitisation.

Bones are richly innervated by primary afferent and sympathetic neurons (SNS). The periosteum is densely innervated with broadly similar afferents to the mineralised bone, especially around the blood vessels and Haversian canals (Hohmann *et al.* 1986; Hill & Elde 1991; Hukkanen *et al.* 1992). The primary afferents are predominately neuropeptidergic C fibres (expressing calcitonin gene related peptide (CGRP) and vallinoid receptor (VR1) channels), not isolectin (IB4) positive C fibres, Aδ and sympathetic fibres expressing neuropeptide Y (NPY) and vasoactive intestinal peptide (VIP) (Bjurholm *et al.* 1988; Goto *et al.* 1998; Mach *et al.* 2002). Neonatal injection of capsaicin or guanethidine ablates C fibres and SNS respectively and resulted in a 21% and 45% reduction in bone surface osteoclasts (Hill *et al.* 1991). The means by which these neurons interact and influence osteoclast action is unknown, but may be influenced by blood flow. Neuropeptides such as VIP, CGRP and substance P (SP) have been implicated in bone metabolism. VIP has been demonstrated to stimulate bone resorption *in vitro*, through VIP receptors on osteosarcoma cells, whereas CGRP at high doses can inhibit osteoclast action *in vitro* (Hill & Elde 1991). In addition, glutaminergic nerve terminals have been demonstrated in the vicinity of bone cells. Glutamate released from nerve terminals may act on the NMDA receptors expressed by osteoclasts; alternatively glutamate released from bone cells may activate nerve terminals (Chenu *et al.* 1998; Serre *et al.* 1999).

Tumours invading and growing within the medullary space of the bone interact and activate primary afferent fibres, alter osteoblast/osteoclast balance and induce a pronounced inflammatory infiltrate. Tumour cells have been shown to release a host of growth factors (i.e. nerve growth factor, NGF), cytokines (i.e. tumour necrosis factor (TNF), interleukin (IL)-1, IL-6), chemokines, prostanoids, endothelins, reduce the pH to below 5 in their vicinity and directly deform primary afferents (Griffiths 1991; Suzuki & Yamada 1994; Watkins *et al.* 1994; Safieh-Garabedian *et al.* 1995; Sorkin *et al.* 1997; Woolf *et al.* 1997). The paracrine interactions between tumours and peripheral nerves are crucial to understand the mechanisms of peripheral nociceptor activation. Studies using *in vitro* cancer cell lines, or assays on animal or human cancers and occasionally from *in vivo* animal or human cancers have provided most information about substances released by tumours (see Figure 8.1) (Wacnik *et al.* 2000).

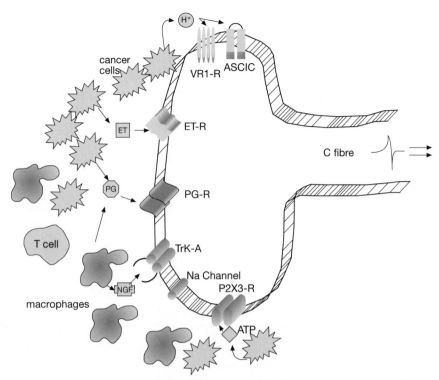

Figure 8.1 Nociceptors of primary afferent fibres (C fibres) use numerous different receptors to detect code and transmit noxious stimuli. The cancer cells invading the bone marrow cavity release a wide variety of factors which act a chemotractants to immune-active cells (macrophages, T cells), and ligands for primary afferent receptors. These include endothelins (ET), which act on endothelin receptors (ET-R), among other actions, prostaglandins (PG) acting on prostaglandin receptor (RG-R) (also released by macrophages) and protons (H$^+$) which act on the vallinoid receptors (VR1), and acid-sensing channels (ASIC), which also detect mechanical deformation of the primary afferent. Extracellular adenosine triphosphate (ATP) binds to purinergic receptors such as P2X3, and nerve growth factor (NGF) binds to the TrKA receptor. Activation of these receptors induces phosphorylation of sodium channels, which in turn decreases the nociceptor activation threshold. (Adapted from Mantyh *et al.* 2002.)

Prostanoids

These derivatives of arachidonic acid can be divided into numerous families among which are PGE, PGD, PGF, prostacyclins and thromboxanes. Their corresponding receptors are coupled to G-proteins to activate secondary messenger pathways. Prostanoids are released by tumour cells and the activated infiltrating immune cells (macrophages and T cells). Prostanoids have been demonstrated to activate prostanoid receptors on primary afferents and induce pain behaviours (Coleman 1997; Murata *et al.* 1997; Bley *et al.* 1998).

Growth factors

One of the most important growth factors, NGF, was characterised over 40 years ago and has been shown to be essential as a trophic factor for small diameter sensory afferents during embryological development, then in the mature animal changing to a regulator of neuronal function in pain, inflammation and synaptic plasticity (Levi-Montalcini *et al.* 1996; Ma & Woolf 1997). NGF is released by tumour and immune cells and interacts with its tyrosine kinase bound receptor (TrkA) on primary afferents (Bonetti *et al.* 1997; Emmett *et al.* 1997).

Cytokines

Cytokines are small soluble proteins that are secreted by one cell, such as immune cells or cancer cells, activate receptors in autocrine and paracrine actions to produce numerous reactions. Cytokines bind to specific receptors which are defined in families: such as the TNF-receptor family or chemokine receptor family. Cytokines are known to be involved in the generation and maintenance of inflammatory and neuropathic pain (Sorkin *et al.* 1997; Arruda *et al.* 1998; Laughlin *et al.* 2000). Numerous cytokines, including TNF, interleukin-1β, interleukin-6 and transforming growth factor, have been shown to be released in *in vitro* studies by tumour and immune-active cells (Basolo *et al.* 1993; Fonsatti *et al.* 1997; Nasu *et al.* 1998).

Endothelin-1

In addition to their vasoconstrictor actions, endothelins (ET) promote pain behaviours when applied to the sciatic nerve, induce nociception through the endothelin receptors in inflammatory pain and are involved in tumour cell signal transduction, mitogenesis, endothelial cell growth and angiogenesis (Asham *et al.* 1998; Davar *et al.* 1998; De-Melo *et al.* 1998). A mouse model in which osteolytic connective tissue carcinoma was injected into and onto the calcaneous bone demonstrated peak pain behaviours on day 10 which correlated with an increase in ET-1 secretion. Further, a blockade of the ET_A receptor reduced nociceptive behaviour (Cain *et al.* 2001). ET microperfusate from tumour sites found increased levels of ET-1 from fibrosarcoma-implanted mice, in which the lesions were hyperalgesic but not melanoma-implanted mice, which demonstrated no hyperalgesia (Wacnik *et al.* 2001).

Other mediators

Numerous other mediators are released by either cancer or immune-active cells that may activate nociceptors of the primary afferents and thus be involved in generating or maintaining pain. These include adenosine triphosphate (ATP) acting at the P2X3 receptor, histamine, serotonin, sympathomimetics, nitric oxide, bradykinin (also implicated in tumour mitogenic behaviour) and proteinase activated receptor (which is cleaved and activated by thrombin and sensitises the primary afferent, evoking neurogenic inflammation through SP and CGRP release) (Millan 1999; Vergnolle *et al.* 2001).

Acidosis

The intracellular and extracellular pH of tumours are lower (pH < 5) than normal tissue. An accumulation of acid metabolites induces the local acidosis, which in turn can directly activate nociceptors (Reeh & Steen 1996; Sutherland *et al.* 2000). Acid-sensing ion channels (ASICs) such as VR1 (senses pH < 6), and the ASIC 3 and others are activated in the presence of low or falling pH (Lingueglia *et al.* 1997). ASICs have been demonstrated to co-localise with CGRP, in small diameter primary afferents, such as those that innervate bone (Olson *et al.* 1998). In addition the release of proteins by infiltrating immune cells as well as the high levels of apoptosis can both contribute to the low pH. As well as primary activation of acid-sensing channels on the primary afferents, the tumour-enhanced low pH allows bone resorption by osteoclasts. Osteoclasts are terminally differentiated multinucleated monocyte-lineage cells, which resorb bone by maintaining a microenvironment of a pH 4–5 at the osteoclast–bone interface.

Primary and secondary sensitisation

As discussed above, there is ample evidence to suggest that tumour invasion of bones causes a primary sensitisation of the primary afferent (Aδ and C fibres) and SNS. The local release of nociceptive agents from the dividing and dying tumour cells as well as from the activated immune infiltrate induces sensitisation and activation of the primary afferents and evokes a corresponding neurogenic inflammatory response through SP/CGRP release. As the tumour invading the bone medulla grows, it compresses and destroys the haematopoietic cells within the marrow as well as compressing, distending and destroying primary afferents within the bone. The direct mechanical injury initially activates ASIC channels (by distension of the neuron) and later directly by proteolysis or ischaemic damage to the primary afferent. The destruction of the primary afferents also leads to primary afferent sensitisation and contributes a neuropathic component to the pain syndrome (Mantyh *et al.* 2002).

In addition, there is evidence for secondary, central sensitisation. Both the mouse and rat models of bone cancer pain have described neurochemical re-organisation of the spinal cord segments that receive nociceptive input from the affected bone. These include an increased expression of the pro-hyperalgesic peptide dynorphin and an astrocyte hypertrophy. SP-NK1 internalisation and an upregulation of *c-fos* gene expression after non-noxious palpation of the affected bone indicate primary afferent sensitisation as seen in other models of inflammation or neuropathy (Honore *et al.* 2000a). Hypertrophy of spinal astrocytes is uncommon in inflammatory models but has been reported after sciatic nerve injury, albeit to a lesser extent than in the bone cancer model where the hypertrophy is up to 300% (Garrison *et al.* 1991; Colburn *et al.* 1997; Coyle 1998; Honore *et al.* 2000a). Whether this massive astrocyte hypertrophy is involved in the generation or maintenance of the pain is as yet unknown, although there is mounting evidence of the involvement of astrocytes in inflammatory and neuropathic hyperalgesia (Watkins *et al.* 1999). In addition the dynorphin and stimulated *c-fos* expression are in the deep laminae in close proximity to the hypertrophied astrocytes (Honore *et al.* 2000a).

Spontaneous C fibre discharge, lowered thermal thresholds and altered epidermal afferent branching have been reported in a mouse model of a connective tissue cancer injected in and around the calcaneal bone (Cain *et al.* 2001). The spontaneous primary afferent activity was confined to unmyelinated fibres, and may contribute to maintaining a central sensitisation consistent with the internalisation of SP (Schwei *et al.* 1999; Cain *et al.* 2001). However, unlike other mouse or rat models of bone cancer pain, no reduction in mechanical threshold was observed (Honore *et al.* 2000a; Cain *et al.* 2001). Up to day 14 post-tumour implantation there was evidence of epidermal nerve fibre increased branching, followed by progressive atrophy. Loss of epidermal innervation accompanying hyperalgesia and pain is seen in several painful neuropathies and may be due to increased activation of second-order sensory neurons (Holland *et al.* 1997; Cain *et al.* 2001).

Osteoclast–osteoblast activation

As the tumour grows the bone is destroyed, improperly remodelled and the pain experienced becomes progressively more severe. In humans the extent of osteoclast activity is related to pain severity. Even in prostate cancer, which is predominately osteosclerotic, there is extensive osteoclast activity and pain (Adami 1997). Osteoclasts descend from the monocyte lineage and are terminally differentiated multinucleated cells, which act to resorb bone from the bone surface. Osteoclast formation requires macrophage colony stimulating factor (M-CSF) and the interaction between the receptor activator for nuclear factor κB (RANK) which is expressed on osteoclast precursors and RANK ligand (RANK-L) expressed on several cell types including osteoblasts (Lacey *et al.* 1998; Yasuda *et al.* 1998).

The normal activation of osteoclast precursors and mature osteoclasts is dependent on the RANK binding to RANK-L on osteoblasts (Hsu *et al.* 1999). To limit the forward feeding cycle, osteoblasts also secrete a cytokine, osteoprotegerin (OPG), which is a member of the soluble TNF receptor family (Lacey *et al.* 1998; Kong *et al.* 1999; Simmonds 1999), OPG acts as a decoy receptor and sequesters RANK-L, preventing RANK activation, and thus is vital to normal bone density and remodelling (Bucay *et al.* 1998) (see Figure 8.2). After the invasion and growth of tumour cells within the bone medulla, an imbalance in osteoclast–osteoblast activation is induced. One mechanism for the ensuing osteolysis is due to the increased secretion of RANK-L by tumour cells and infiltrating activated T cells combined with the sequestration of OGP by tumour cells (Sezer *et al.* 2002; Standal *et al.* 2002) (see Figure 8.2).

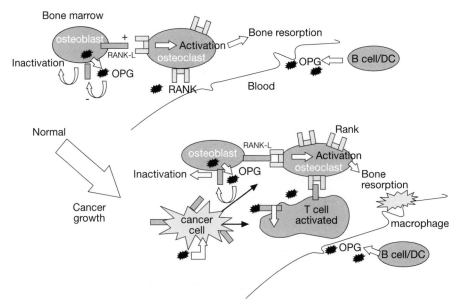

Figure 8.2 A schematic representation of the interaction of RANK-L, RANK and osteoprotegerin (OPG) in the normal bone marrow and after growth of cancer cells. In the normal bone marrow the interaction of RANK-L expressed on activated osteoblasts binds to RANK on osteoclasts and activates the cells to increase bone resorption. A negative feedback loop is present in the autocrine action of secreted OPG also from activated osteoblasts, which binds to and sequesters RANK-L. This is one pathway that maintains a balance between osteoblast and osteoclast activation. After tumour cell invasion and growth, the normal balance is overturned in favour of osteoclast activity. The tumour cells express RANK-L, along with activated T cell, which can bind RANK and activate the osteoclasts. OPG secreted by osteoblasts can be sequestered and degraded by some cancer lines, thus reducing a natural inhibitor. B lymphocytes and dendritic cells (DC) also secrete OPG.

Indeed, in one study, 225 patients with myeloma were shown to have serum OPG levels 18% lower than normal controls, but more than 50% higher in Hodgkin's or non-Hodgkin's lymphoma; the former having extensive painful metastases compared with the latter (Seidel *et al.* 2001; Lipton *et al.* 2002).

However, several cytokines are known to influence osteoclast activation through a RANK-L independent mechanism such as TNF and IL-1, IL-6, IL-11 (Hofbauer *et al.* 2000; Kobayashi *et al.* 2000; Kudo *et al.* 2003). The RANK-L independent pathway for osteoclast formation may be of particular importance in the presence of high levels of cytokines (TNF, IL-1) production such as cancer-induced osteolysis, Pagets disease and rheumatoid arthritis (Roodman *et al.* 1992; Kotake *et al.* 1996; Wierzbowska *et al.* 1999). In addition, as discussed above, there is evidence for a neuronal-based regulation of osteoclast action, and facilitated bone resorption due to the lowered pH in tumour-laden bone.

Modulation of hyperalgesia

Three therapies that modulate bone-cancer-induced pain will be discussed: OPG, cyclo-oxygenase (COX) inhibitors and bisphosphonates, with particular reference to their potential modulation of the mechanisms of hyperalgesia.

Osteoprotegerin

OPG is a potentially an interesting target for analgesia in cancer-induced bone pain. As has been discussed, OPG is a naturally occurring cytokine which sequesters RANK-L and thus prevents activation of osteoclasts through RANK. Cancer growth within the bone alters the osteoclast–osteoblast balance, induces osteolysis and thus pain. Exogenous OPG would theoretically be one way of redressing this balance. In the mouse model of osteosarcoma-induced femoral bone pain and destruction, OPG given subcutaneously from day 5–17 post-sarcoma infusion produced a significant attenuation of bone-cancer-induced pain and virtually eliminated bone destruction (Honore *et al.* 2000b). Of interest, spontaneous flinches of the affected limb were unchanged, but there was a reduction of spinal cord dynorphin expression, stimulated *c-fos* expression, SP-NK1 internalisation and astrocyte hypertrophy (Honore *et al.* 2000b). Several other authors also report the efficacy of OPG, OPG-Fc fusion protein or inhibitory RANK antibodies to treat osteolytic metastases and reduce tumour-associated bone pain (Luger *et al.* 2001; Morony *et al.* 2001; Sezer *et al.* 2002; Zhang *et al.* 2002). In addition, OPG-Fc fusion protein has been administered to humans; post-menopausal women or patients with myeloma, with minimal side effects and a significant reduction in markers of bone turnover equivalent in its effect to intravenous pamidronate (Sezer *et al.* 2002).

Bisphosphonates

Bisphosphonates have been developed over the past 30 years and are primarily used to treat hypercalcaemia (from excess bone resorption) and more recently cancer-induced bone pain (Body 2000). Their exact mode of action is unclear, although there is increasing evidence that bisphosphonates inhibit the recruitment and activation of osteoclasts, in part through an increase in OPG levels (Rogers *et al.* 1997; Viereck *et al.* 2002). In addition they induce osteoclast apoptosis, inhibit cancer cell proliferation, reduce cytokine production and metalloproteinase secretion (Derenne *et al.* 1999; Senaratne *et al.* 2000). Bisphosphonates are pyrophosphate analogues that bind tightly to bone hydroxyapatite and inhibit bone resorption. A Cochrane review of the clinical efficacy of bisphosphonates for pain relief in metastatic bone disease suggested that there was some evidence for their use as analgesics, although the effect was delayed. The number needed to treat to achieve 50% pain relief at 4 weeks was 11, falling to 7 at 12 weeks (Wong *et al.* 2002).

In the rat model of cancer-induced bone pain, infusion of breast carcinoma cells into the tibia produced movement-induced pain and mechanical hyperalgesia from day 14 post cell injection. Chronic treatment with either pamidronate or a new third-generation bisphosphonate, zoledronic acid, revealed little or no attenuation of hyperalgesia by pamidronate, but a significant attenuation by zoledronic acid (Walker *et al.* 2002). In addition, zoledronic acid, but not pamidronate, inhibited cancer cell growth, bone de-mineralisation and preserved trabeculated bone structure (Walker *et al.* 2002). These results are not reflected clinically where clodronate and pamidronate are the most commonly reported bisphosphonates and modest to significant analgesic relief is cited (Body 1997; Mercadante 1997; Wong & Wiffen 2002). The future development of bisphosphonates may be an important area for future reduction of cancer-induced bone pain.

COX inhibitors

Prostaglandins and other pro-inflammatory lipids are formed by the action of COX enzymes cycloxygenase and peroxidase on arachidonic acid and the unstable intermediate prostaglandin (PG) G2, respectively. A series of specific isomerases continue the conversion to a range of PG, thromboxanes and prostacyclins. Two isoforms of COX, COX-1 and COX-2 are expressed. COX-1 is essentially constitutively expressed in most tissues and is responsible for the tonic production of PG for the maintenance of physiological functions. COX-2, in contrast is not detected in normal tissue but is induced by mitogenic or inflammatory stimuli. Oncogenes, cytokines, growth factors and chemotherapy all promote COX-2 transcription (Subbaramaiah *et al.* 2003). The balance between activation of oncogenes and down-regulation of suppressor genes among other factors determine the level of COX-2 in any one tumour type; thus breast, lung and oesophagus cancer, which express mutant p53, have higher levels of COX-2 (Ristimaki *et al.* 2002). COX-2 expression has been implicated in many stages of carcinogenesis: angiogenesis, apoptosis, immune function, invasiveness (Dannenberg *et al.* 2001) and cancer-induced bone pain. Thus COX inhibitors (NSAIDs) and the newer COX-2 inhibitors should be effective in reducing cancer-associated pain and slow cancer progression. Indeed, several studies are now suggesting the use of COX inhibition alongside anti-cancer therapy, such as in colorectal carcinoma (Thun *et al.* 2002; Subbaramaiah *et al.* 2003).

As discussed above, PGs appear to be involved in sensitisation of primary afferents, and centrally through release from activated astrocytes and thus could be central to hyperalgesia. However, clinical data are controversial, with a few studies reporting NSAID efficacy in cancer-induced bone pain, whereas others suggest little benefit (Pace 1995; Mercadante 1997). In the mouse osteosarcoma model of bone pain, a selective COX-2 inhibitor was administered acutely 14 days after tumour infusion or chronically between days 6–14. Both schemes significantly reduced both the ongoing and movement-evoked hyperalgesia, although the chronic administration also reduced tumour burden and bone destruction by more than 50% (Sabino *et al.* 2002). In contrast, the rat model using breast carcinoma to evoke bone pain demonstrated no reduction in mechanical hyperalgesia after chronic (daily) administration of celecoxib (Celebrex) (COX-2 inhibitor), and did not report any attenuation of cancer growth (Walker *et al.* 2002).

Thus although the actions of COX enzymes and the production of prostanoids appear to be involved with tumour growth, primary afferent sensitisation and central sensitisation (through astrocyte release), the current human and animal data do not demonstrate clear anti-hyperalgesic efficacy of COX inhibition. However, with the advent of more selective COX-2 inhibitors and a greater understanding of the mechanisms that PG modulate, more selective and potent analgesics or disease modifiers may be available.

Conclusion

After decades of being ignored, cancer-induced bone pain is coming to the forefront. The development of an animal model whereby the animals remained well, with localised, reproducible pain development that closely parallels the human situation, has allowed elucidation of some of the basic mechanisms that may underlie this pain state.

Bones have been demonstrated to be highly innervated with SNS and primary afferent fibres. The latter consist of noxious coding Aδ and peptidergic C fibres (CRGP, SP-positive). A wide range of nociceptors on the primary afferents are sensitised and activated by invading and growing tumour cells releasing a range of cytokines and prostanoids among others. The tumour cells evoke an extensive inflammatory response, which further sensitises the primary afferents. These mechanisms are well described in inflammatory pain states. However, in addition, there appears to be primary afferent destruction, evidence for spontaneous discharges from damaged C fibres and alteration in the epidermal nerve fibre projection more akin to neuropathic pain models. Although cancer-induced bone pain initially appears to be an intense inflammatory response, evidence both from animal models and clinical observation would suggest that this pain is more complex. Indeed, the dorsal horn response to the primary afferent input does not reflect an inflammatory stimulation, with no increase in CGRP or SP expression. However, nor does it reflect a pure neuropathy, with no alteration in neuropeptide Y or galanin expression. The alterations within the dorsal horn imply a unique set of changes, including a massive astrogliosis and increase dynorphin expression and evidence of secondary, central sensitisation with internalisation of SP.

Clinicians managing cancer-induced bone pain will not be surprised by the results above, suggesting that this is a unique pain state. This type of pain, severe with rapid onset often with movement, has been difficult to effectively treat with common analgesics. The animal models, along with some insight into the unique combination of mechanisms underlying this pain state, have also begun to suggest novel analgesics to treat the pain. One potential analgesic is OPG, which acts by inhibiting osteoclast activation and has been demonstrated to be safe in humans. In addition, third-line bisphosphonates, which have a wide range of actions, may be demonstrated to be powerful analgesics, preventing osteoclastic reaction. Further work on the alterations within the dorsal horn may reveal yet more novel targets to exploit.

However, for the future to be delivered it will require close collaboration between clinicians treating patients with cancer-induced bone pain and research scientists. In such a relatively young field, it is a golden opportunity for palliative care physicians to be at the forefront of developing clinically relevant pain scales and defining the pain terminology, both of which need to be done before accurate assessments of treatments can be made. The essence of bone pain that renders current analgesic therapy ineffective is the inability to adequately control the rapid movement-induced pain (or spontaneous pain) arising from the bone. However, even in animal models, analgesic efficacy is often reported as a composite of background and 'breakthrough' pain (with few definitions of the latter).

References

Adami, S. (1997). Bisphosphonates in prostate carcinoma. *Cancer* **80**, 1674–1679.

Arruda, J. L., Colburn, R. W., Rickman, A. J., Rutkowski, M. D. & DeLeo, J. A. (1998). Increase of interleukin-6 mRNA in the spinal cord following peripheral nerve injury in the rat: potential role of IL-6 in neuropathic pain. *Molecular Brain Research* **62**, 228–235.

Asham, E. H., Loizidou, M. & Taylor, I. (1998). Endothelin-1 and tumour development. *European Journal of Surgical Oncology* **24**, 57–60.

Banning, A., Sjogren, P. & Henriksen, H. (1991). Pain causes in 200 patients referred to a multidisciplinary cancer pain clinic. *Pain* **45**, 45–48.

Basolo, F., Calvo, S., Fiore, L., Serra, C., Conaldi, P. G., Falcone, V., Morganti, M., Squartini, F. & Toniolo, A. (1993). Production of cytokines and response to them in normal and transformed human mammary epithelial cells. *Annals of the New York Academy of Sciences* **698**, 126–130.

Bjurholm, A., Kreicbergs, A., Terenius, L., Goldstein, M. & Schultzberg, M. (1988). Neuropeptide Y-, tyrosine hydroxylase- and vasoactive intestinal polypeptide-immunoreactive nerves in bone and surrounding tissues. *Journal of the Autonomic Nervous System* **25**, 119–125.

Bley, K. R., Hunter, J. C., Eglen, R. M., Smith, J. A. (1998). The role of IP prostanoid receptors in inflammatory pain. *Trends in Pharmacological Science* **19**, 141–147.

Body, J. J. (1997). Clinical research update: zoledronate. *Cancer* **80**, 1699–1701.

Body, J. J. (2000). Current and future directions in medical therapy: hypercalcemia. *Cancer* **88**, 3054–3058.

Bonetti, B., Panzeri, L., Carner, M., Zamboni, G., Rizzuto, N. & Moretto, G. (1997). Human neoplastic Schwann cells: changes in the expression of neurotrophins and their low-affinity receptor p75. *Neuropathology and Applied Neurobiology* **23**, 380–386.

Bruera, E., Schoeller, T., Wenk, R., MacEachern, T., Marcelino, S., Hanson, J. & Suarez-Almozor, M. (1995). A prospective multi-center assessment of the Edmonton staging system for cancer pain. *Journal of Pain and Symptom Management* **10**, 348–355.

Bucay, N., Sarosi, I., Dunstan, C. R., Morony, S., Tarpley, J., Capparelli, C., Scully, S., Tan, H. L., Xu, W., Lacey, D. L., Boyle, W. J. & Simonet, W. S. (1998). Osteoprotegerin-deficient mice develop early onset osteoporosis and arterial calcification. *Genes and Development* **12**, 1260–1268.

Cain, D. M., Wacnik, P. W., Turner, M., Wendelschafer-Crabb, G., Kennedy, W. R., Wilcox, G. L. & Simone, D. A. (2001). Functional interactions between tumor and peripheral nerve: changes in excitability and morphology of primary afferent fibres in a murine model of cancer pain. *Journal of Neuroscience* **21**, 9367–9376.

Chenu, C., Serre, C. M., Raynal, C., Burt-Pichat, B. & Delmas, P. D. (1998). Glutamate receptors are expressed by bone cells and are involved in bone resorption. *Bone* **22**, 295–299.

Colburn, R. W., DeLeo, J. A., Rickman, A. J., Yeager, M. P., Kwon, P. & Hickey, W. F. (1997). Dissociation of microglial activation and neuropathic pain behaviors following peripheral nerve injury in the rat. *Journal of Neuroimmunology* **79**, 163–175.

Coleman, R. E. (1997). Skeletal complications of malignancy. *Cancer* **80**, 1588–1594.

Coyle, D. E. (1998). Partial peripheral nerve injury leads to activation of astroglia and microglia which parallels the development of allodynic behavior. *Glia* **23**, 75–83.

Dannenberg, A. J., Altorki, N. K., Boyle, J. O., Dang, C., Howe, L. R., Weksler, B. B. & Subbaramaiah, K. (2001). Cyclo-oxygenase 2: a pharmacological target for the prevention of cancer. *Lancet Oncology* **2**, 544–551.

Davar, G., Hans, G., Fareed, M.U., Sinnott, C. & Strichartz, G. (1998). Behavioral signs of acute pain produced by application of endothelin-1 to rat sciatic nerve. *Neuroreport* **9**, 2279–2283.

De-Melo, J. D., Tonussi, C. R., D'Orleans-Juste, P. & Rae, G. A. (1998). Articular nociception induced by endothelin-1, carrageenan and LPS in naive and previously inflamed knee-joints in the rat: inhibition by endothelin receptor antagonists. *Pain* **77**, 261–269.

Derenne, S., Amiot, M., Barille, S., Collette, M., Robillard, N., Berthaud, P., Harousseau, J. L. & Bataille, R. (1999). Zoledronate is a potent inhibitor of myeloma cell growth and secretion of IL-6 and MMP-1 by the tumoral environment. *Journal of Bone and Mineral Research* **14**, 2048–2056.

Emmett, C. J., McNeeley, P. A. & Johnson, R. M. (1997). Evaluation of human astrocytoma and glioblastoma cell lines for nerve growth factor release. *Neurochemistry International* **30**, 465–474.

Fonsatti, E., Altomonte, M., Coral, S., Cattarossi, I., Nicotra, M. R., Gasparollo, A., Natali, P.G. & Maio, M. (1997). Tumour-derived interleukin 1alpha (IL-1alpha) up-regulates the release of soluble intercellular adhesion molecule-1 (sICAM-1) by endothelial cells. *British Journal of Cancer* **76**, 1255–1261.

Garrison, C. J., Dougherty, P. M., Kajander, K. C., Carlton, S. M. (1991). Staining of glial fibrillary acidic protein (GFAP) in lumbar spinal cord increases following a sciatic nerve constriction injury. *Brain Research* **565**, 1–7.

Goto, T., Yamaza, T., Kido, M. A. & Tanaka, T. (1998). Light- and electron-microscopic study of the distribution of axons containing substance P and the localization of neurokinin-1 receptor in bone. *Cell and Tissue Research* **293**, 87–93.

Griffiths, J. R. (1991). Are cancer cells acidic? *British Journal of Cancer* **64**, 425–427.

Hill, E. L. & Elde, R. (1991). Distribution of CGRP, VIP, D beta H, SP, and NPY immunoreactive nerves in the periosteum of the rat. *Cell and Tissue Research* **264**, 469–480.

Hill, E. L., Turner, R. & Elde, R. (1991). Effects of neonatal sympathectomy and capsaicin treatment on bone remodeling in rats. *Neuroscience* **44**, 747–755.

Hofbauer, L. C., Khosla, S., Dunstan, C. R., Lacey, D. L., Boyle, W. J. & Riggs, B. L. (2000). The roles of osteoprotegerin and osteoprotegerin ligand in the paracrine regulation of bone resorption. *Journal of Bone and Mineral Research* **15**, 2–12.

Hohmann, E. L., Eldem R. P., Rysavy, J. A., Einzig, S. & Gebhard, R. L. (1986). Innervation of periosteum and bone by sympathetic vasoactive intestinal peptide-containing nerve fibers. *Science* **232**, 868–871.

Holland, N. R., Stocks, A., Hauer, P., Cornblath, D. R., Griffin, J. W. & McArthur, J. C. (1997). Intraepidermal nerve fiber density in patients with painful sensory neuropathy. *Neurology* **48**, 708–711.

Honore, P., Rogers, S. D., Schwei, M. J., Salak-Johnson, J. L., Luger, N. M., Sabino, M. C., Clohisy, D. R. & Mantyh, P. W. (2000a). Murine models of inflammatory, neuropathic and cancer pain each generates a unique set of neurochemical changes in the spinal cord and sensory neurons. *Neuroscience* **98**, 585–598.

Honore, P., Luger, N. M., Sabino, M. A., Schwei, M. J., Rogers, S. D., Mach, D. B., O'Keefe, P. F., Ramnaraine, M. L., Clohisy, D. R. & Mantyh, P. W. (2000b). Osteoprotegerin blocks bone cancer induced skeletal destruction, skeletal pain and pain related neurochemical reorganization of the spinal cord. *Nature Medicine* **6**, 521–528.

Hsu, H., Lacey, D. L., Dunstan, C. R., Solovyev, I., Colombero, A., Timms, E., Tan, H. L., Elliott, G., Kelley, M. J., Sarosi, I. *et al.* (1999). Tumor necrosis factor receptor family member RANK mediates osteoclast differentiation and activation induced by osteoprotegerin ligand. *Proceedings of the National Academy of Sciences of the United States of America* **96**, 3540–3545.

Hukkanen, M., Konttinen, Y. T., Rees, R. G., Gibson, S. J., Santavirta, S. & Polak, J. M. (1992). Innervation of bone from healthy and arthritic rats by substance P and calcitonin gene related peptide containing sensory fibers. *Journal of Rheumatology* **19**, 1252–1259.

Janjan, N. (2001). Bone metastases: approaches to management. *Seminars in Oncology* **28**, 28–34.

Kobayashi, K., Takahashi, N., Jimi, E., Udagawa, N., Takami, M., Kotake, S., Nakagawa, N., Kinosaki, M., Yamaguchi, K., Shima, N. *et al.* (2000). Tumor necrosis factor alpha stimulates osteoclast differentiation by a mechanism independent of the ODF/RANKL-RANK interaction. *Journal of Experimental Medicine* **191**, 275–286.

Kong, Y. Y., Yoshida, H., Sarosi, I., Tan, H. L., Timms, E., Capparelli, C., Morony, S., Oliveira-dos-Santos, A. J., Van, G., Itie, A. *et al.* (1999). OPGL is a key regulator of osteoclastogenesis, lymphocyte development and lymph-node organogenesis. *Nature* **397**, 315–323.

Kotake, S., Sato, K., Kim, K. J., Takahashi, N., Udagawa, N., Nakamura, I., Yamaguchi, A., Kishimoto, T., Suda, T. & Kashiwazaki, S. (1996). Interleukin-6 and soluble interleukin-6 receptors in the synovial fluids from rheumatoid arthritis patients are responsible for osteoclast-like cell formation. *Journal of Bone and Mineral Research* **11**, 88–95.

Kudo, O., Sabokbar, A., Pocock, A., Itonaga, I., Fujikawa, Y. & Athanasou, N. A. (2003). Interleukin-6 and interleukin-11 support human osteoclast formation by a RANKL-independent mechanism. *Bone* **32**, 1–7.

Lacey, D.L., Timms, E., Tan, H.L., Kelley, M.J., Dunstan, C.R., Burgess, T., Elliott, R., Colombero, A., Elliott, G., Scully, S. *et al.* (1998). Osteoprotegerin ligand is a cytokine that regulates osteoclast differentiation and activation. *Cell* **93**, 165–176.

Laughlin, T. M., Bethea, J. R., Yezierski, R. P. & Wilcox, G. L. (2000). Cytokine involvement in dynorphin-induced allodynia. *Pain* **84**, 159–167.

Levi-Montalcini, R., Skaper, S.D., Dal Toso, R., Petrelli, L. & Leon, A. (1996). Nerve growth factor: from neurotrophin to neurokine. *Trends in Neuroscience* **19**, 514–520.

Lingueglia, E., de Weille, J.R., Bassilana, F., Heurteaux, C., Sakai, H., Waldmann, R. & Lazdunski, M. (1997). A modulatory subunit of acid sensing ion channels in brain and dorsal root ganglion cells. *Journal of Biological Chemistry* **272**, 29778–29783.

Lipton, A., Ali, S.M., Leitzel, K., Chinchilli, V., Witters, L., Engle, L., Holloway, D., Bekker, P. & Dunstan, C. R. (2002). Serum osteoprotegerin levels in healthy controls and cancer patients. *Clinical Cancer Research* **8**, 2306–2310.

Luger, N. M., Honore, P., Sabino, M. A., Schwei, M.J. Rogers, S.D., Mach, D.B., Clohisy, D.R. & Mantyh, P.W. (2001). Osteoprotegerin diminishes advanced bone cancer pain. *Cancer Research* **61**, 4038–4047.

Luger, N. M., Sabino, M. A., Schwei, M. J., Mach, D. B., Pomonis, J. D., Keyser, C. P., Rathbun, M., Clohisy, D. R., Honore, P., Yaksh, T. L. & Mantyh, P. W. (2002). Efficacy of systemic morphine suggests a fundamental difference in the mechanisms that generate bone cancer vs. inflammatory pain. *Pain* **99**, 397–406.

Ma, Q. P. & Woolf, C. J. (1997). The progressive tactile hyperalgesia induced by peripheral inflammation is nerve growth factor dependent. *Neuroreport* **8**, 807–810.

Mach, D. B., Rogers, S. D., Sabino, M. C., Luger, N. M., Schwei, M. J., Pomonis, J. D., Keyser, C. P., Clohisy, D. R., Adams, D. J., O'Leary, P. & Mantyh, P. W. (2002). Origins of skeletal pain: sensory and sympathetic innervation of the mouse femur. *Neuroscience* **113**, 155–166.

Mantyh, P. W., Clohisy, D. R., Koltzenburg, M. & Hunt, S. P. (2002). Molecular mechanisms of cancer pain. *Nature Reviews Cancer* **2**, 201–209.

McQuay, H. J., Collins, S. L., Carroll, D. & Moore, R. A. (2000). Radiotherapy for the palliation of painful bone metastases. *Cochrane Database Systematic Reviews*, CD001793.

Medhurst, S. J., Walker, K., Bowes, M., Kidd, B. L., Glatt, M., Muller, M., Hattenberger, M., Vaxelaire, J., O'Reilly, T., Wotherspoon, G. *et al.* (2002). A rat model of bone cancer pain. *Pain* **96**, 129–140.

Mercadante, S. (1997). Malignant bone pain: pathophysiology and treatment. *Pain* **69**, 1–18.

Mercadante, S. & Arcuri, E. (1998). Breakthrough pain in cancer patients: pathophysiology and treatment. *Cancer Treatment Reviews* **24**, 425–432.

Mercadante, S., Maddaloni, S., Roccella, S. & Salvaggio, L. (1992). Predictive factors in advanced cancer pain. *Pain* **50**, 151–155.

Mercadante, S., Radbruch, L., Caraceni, A., Cherny, N., Kaasa, S., Nauck, F., Ripamonti, C. & De Conno, F. (2002). Episodic (breakthrough) pain: consensus conference of an expert working group of the European Association for Palliative Care. *Cancer* **94**, 832–839.

Millan, M. J. (1999). The induction of pain: an integrative review. *Progress in Neurobiology* **57**, 1–164.

Morony, S., Capparelli, C., Sarosi, I., Lacey, D. L., Dunstan, C. R., Kostenuik, P. J. (2001). Osteoprotegerin inhibits osteolysis and decreases skeletal tumor burden in syngeneic and nude mouse models of experimental bone metastasis. *Cancer Research* **61**, 4432–4436.

Murata, T., Ushikubi, F., Matsuoka, T, Hirata, M., Yamasaki, A., Sugimoto, Y., Ichikawa, A., Aze, Y., Tanaka, T., Yoshida, N. *et al.* (1997). Altered pain perception and inflammatory response in mice lacking prostacyclin receptor. *Nature* **388**, 678–682.

Nasu, K., Matsui, N., Narahara, H., Tanaka, Y. & Miyakawa, I. (1998). Effects of interferon-gamma on cytokine production by endometrial stromal cells. *Human Reproduction* **13**, 2598–2601.

Olson, T.H., Riedl, M.S., Vulchanova, L., Ortiz-Gonzalez, X.R. & Elde, R. (1998). An acid sensing ion channel (ASIC) localizes to small primary afferent neurons in rats. *Neuroreport* **9**, 1109–1113.

Pace, V. (1995). Use of nonsteroidal anti-inflammatory drugs in cancer. *Palliative Medicine* **9**, 273–286

Portenoy, R. K. & Hagen, N. A. (1990). Breakthrough pain: definition, prevalence and characteristics. *Pain* **41**, 273–281.

Portenoy, R. K., Payne, D. & Jacobsen, P. (1999). Breakthrough pain: characteristics and impact in patients with cancer pain. *Pain* **81**, 129–134.

Reeh, P. W. & Steen, K. H. (1996). Tissue acidosis in nociception and pain. *Progress in Brain Research* **113**, 143–151.

Ristimaki, A., Sivula, A., Lundin, J., Lundin, M., Salminen, T., Haglund, C., Joensuu, H. & Isola, J. (2002). Prognostic significance of elevated cyclooxygenase-2 expression in breast cancer. *Cancer Research* **62**, 632–635.

Rogers, M. J., Watts, D. J. & Russell, R. G. (1997). Overview of bisphosphonates. *Cancer* **80**, 1652–1660.

Roodman, G. D., Kurihara, N., Ohsaki, Y., Kukita, A., Hosking, D., Demulder, A., Smith, J. F. & Singer, F. R. (1992). Interleukin 6. A potential autocrine/paracrine factor in Paget's disease of bone. *Journal of Clinical Investigation* **89**, 46–52.

Sabino, M. A., Ghilardi, J. R., Jongen, J. L., Keyser, C. P., Luger, N. M., Mach, D. B., Peters, C. M., Rogers, S. D., Schwei, M. J., de Felipe, C. & Mantyh, P. W. (2002). Simultaneous reduction in cancer pain, bone destruction, and tumor growth by selective inhibition of cyclooxygenase-2. *Cancer Research* **62**, 7343–7349.

Safieh-Garabedian, B., Poole, S., Allchorne, A., Winter, J. & Woolf, C. J. (1995). Contribution of interleukin-1 beta to the inflammation induced increase in nerve growth factor levels and inflammatory hyperalgesia. *British Journal of Pharmacology* **115**, 1265–1275.

Schwei, M. J., Honore, P., Rogers, S. D., Salak-Johnson, J. L., Finke, M. P., Ramnaraine, M. L., Clohisy, D. R. & Mantyh, P. W. (1999). Neurochemical and cellular reorganization of the spinal cord in a murine model of bone cancer pain. *Joural of Neuroscience* **19**, 10886–10897.

Seidel, C., Hjertner, O., Abildgaard, N., Heickendorff, L., Hjorth, M., Westin, J., Nielsen, J. L., Hjorth-Hansen, H., Waage, A., Sundan, A. & Borset, M. (2001). Serum osteoprotegerin levels are reduced in patients with multiple myeloma with lytic bone disease. *Blood* **98**, 2269–2271.

Senaratne, S. G., Pirianov, G., Mansi, J. L., Arnett, T. R. & Colston, K. W. (2000). Bisphosphonates induce apoptosis in human breast cancer cell lines. *British Journal of Cancer* **82**, 1459–1468.

Serafini, A. N. (2001). Therapy of metastatic bone pain. *Journal of Nuclear Medicine* **42**, 895–906.

Serre, C. M., Farlay, D., Delmas, P. D. & Chenu, C. (1999). Evidence for a dense and intimate innervation of the bone tissue, including glutamate-containing fibers. *Bone* **25**, 623–629.

Sezer, O., Heider, U., Zavrski, I., Kuehne, C. A. & Hofbauer, L. C. (2002). RANK ligand and osteoprotegerin in myeloma bone disease. *Blood* **7**, 7.

Simmonds, M. A. (1999). Management of breakthrough pain due to cancer. *Oncology (Huntington)* **13**, 1103–1108.

Sorkin, L. S., Xiao, W. H., Wagner, R. & Myers, R. R. (1997). Tumour necrosis factor alpha induces ectopic activity in nociceptive primary afferent fibres. *Neuroscience* **81**, 255–262.

Standal, T., Seidel, C., Hjertner, O., Plesner, T., Sanderson, R. D., Waage, A., Borset, M. & Sundan, A. (2002). Osteoprotegerin is bound, internalized, and degraded by multiple myeloma cells. *Blood* **100**, 3002–3007.

Subbaramaiah, K. & Dannenberg, A. J. (2003). Cyclooxygenase 2: a molecular target for cancer prevention and treatment. *Trends in Pharmacological Science* **24**, 96–102.

Sutherland, S. P., Cook, S. P. & McCleskey E. W. (2000). Chemical mediators of pain due to tissue damage and ischemia. *Progress in Brain Research* **129**, 21–38.

Suzuki, K. & Yamada, S. (1994). Ascites sarcoma 180, a tumor associated with hypercalcemia, secretes potent bone resorbing factors including transforming growth factor alpha, interleukin-1 alpha and interleukin 6. *Bone and Mineral* **27**, 219–233.

Swanwick, M., Haworth, M. & Lennard, R. F. (2001). The prevalence of episodic pain in cancer: a survey of hospice patients on admission. *Palliative Medicine* **15**, 9–18.

Thun, M. J., Henley, S. J. & Patrono, C. (2002). Nonsteroidal anti-inflammatory drugs as anticancer agents: mechanistic, pharmacologic, and clinical issues. *Journal of the National Cancer Institute* **94**, 252–266.

Vergnolle, N., Bunnett, N. W., Sharkey, K. A., Brussee, V., Compton, S. J., Grady, E. F., Cirino, G., Gerard, N., Basbaum, A. I., Andrade-Gordon, P. *et al.* (2001). Proteinase-activated receptor-2 and hyperalgesia: a novel pain pathway. *Nature Medicine* **7**, 821–826.

Viereck, V., Emons, G., Lauck, V., Frosch, K. H., Blaschke, S., Grundker, C. & Hofbauer, L. C. (2002). Bisphosphonates pamidronate and zoledronic acid stimulate osteoprotegerin production by primary human osteoblasts. *Biochemical and Biophysical Research Communications* **291**, 680–686.

Wacnik, P. W., Eikmeier, L. J., Ruggles, T. R., Beitz, A. J. & Wilcox, G. L. (2000). Cancer pain mechanisms and animal models of cancer pain. In *Proceedings of the 9th World Congress on Pain* (ed. M. R. M. Devor & Z. Wiesenfeld-Hallin), pp. 615–637. Seattle: IASP Press.

Wacnik, P. W., Kehl, L. J., Trempe, T. M., Ramnaraine, M. L., Beitz, A. J. & Wilcox, G. L. (2003). Tumor implantation in mouse humerus evokes movement-related hyperalgesia exceeding that evoked by intramuscular carrageenan. *Pain* **101**, 175–186.

Wacnik, P. W., Eikmeier, L. J., Ruggles, T. R., Ramnaraine, M. L., Walcheck, B. K., Beitz, A. J. & Wilcox, G. L. (2001). Functional interactions between tumor and peripheral nerve: morphology, algogen identification, and behavioral characterization of a new murine model of cancer pain. *Journal of Neuroscience* **21**, 9355–9366.

Walker, K., Medhurst, S. J., Kidd, B. L., Glatt, M., Bowes, M., Patel, S., McNair, K., Kesingland, A., Green, J. & Chan, O. *et al.* (2002). Disease modifying and anti-nociceptive effects of the bisphosphonate, zoledronic acid in a model of bone cancer pain. *Pain* **100**, 219–229.

Watkins, L. R., Wiertelak, E. P., Furness, L. E. & Maier, S. F. (1994). Illness-induced hyperalgesia is mediated by spinal neuropeptides and excitatory amino acids. *Brain Research* **664**, 17–24.

Watkins, L. R., Hansen, M. K., Nguyen, K. T., Lee, J. E. & Maier, S. F. (1999). Dynamic regulation of the proinflammatory cytokine, interleukin-1beta: molecular biology for non-molecular biologists. *Life Sciences* **65**, 449–481.

Wierzbowska, A., Urbanska-Rys, H. & Robak, T. (1999). Circulating IL-6-type cytokines and sIL-6R in patients with multiple myeloma. *British Journal of Haematology* **105**, 412–419.

Wong, R. & Wiffen, P. J. (2002). Bisphosphonates for the relief of pain secondary to bone metastases. *Cochrane Database Systematic Reviews*, CD002068.

Woolf, C. J., Allchorne, A., Safieh-Garabedian, B. & Poole, S. (1997). Cytokines, nerve growth factor and inflammatory hyperalgesia: the contribution of tumour necrosis factor alpha. *British Journal of Pharmacology* **121**, 417–424.

Yasuda, H., Shima, N., Nakagawa, N., Mochizuki, S. I., Yano, K., Fujise, N., Sato, Y., Goto, M., Yamaguchi, K., Kuriyama M. *et al.* (1998). Identity of osteoclastogenesis inhibitory factor (OCIF) and osteoprotegerin (OPG): a mechanism by which OPG/OCIF inhibits osteoclastogenesis in vitro. *Endocrinology* **139**, 1329–1337.

Zhang, J., Dai, J., Lin, D. L., Habib, P., Smith, P., Murtha, J., Fu, Z., Yao, Z., Qi, Y. & Keller, E. T. (2002). Osteoprotegerin abrogates chronic alcohol ingestion-induced bone loss in mice. *Journal of Bone and Mineral Research* **17**, 1256–1263.

Chapter 9

Neuropathic pain: evidence-base and clinical effectiveness of novel interventions

Marie T. Fallon and John D. Walley

Introduction

Despite advances in pain management, relieving cancer pain associated with damage to the peripheral or central nervous system can still prove to be a difficult therapeutic challenge. Although the presence of neuropathic pain may confer a poor prognosis for pain control, there is pre-clinical and clinic research evidence to suggest that certain treatment modalities can be effective in managing pain produced by this mechanism. However, even for investigators with access to sophisticated diagnostic tools, the ability to infer pain mechanisms in individual patients remains relatively primitive. In addition, a proven mechanism-based, pain therapy algorithm is not yet a reality and mechanistic inferences have not been rigorously tested to determine if they can help improve treatment outcomes for heterogeneous cancer pain populations (Woolf & Decosterd 1999; Woolf *et al.* 1998).

The pathophysiology of neuropathic pain can be summarised as a composite of a series of reactions involving combinations of the following: chemical, mechanical, thermal and anatomical changes. Reactions can occur at any point from the periphery to the central nervous system. Typically, this pain mechanism is associated with changes in gene expression in the cell bodies of sensory neurons and marked alterations in the central processing of sensory information, particularly within the dorsal horn of the spinal cord.

Although neuropathic pain produces changes in pain pathways that are extremely complex, most patients can be treated with standard drugs in a predictable way. The general approach to neuropathic pain follows the principles of the World Health Organization analgesic ladder, using a combination of a standard and an adjuvant analgesic (World Health Organization 1996). This approach has been shown to provide meaningful pain relief for most patients with neuropathic cancer pain (Ventafridda *et al.* 1987; Zech *et al.* 1995; Grond *et al.* 1999). The strength of the standard analgesic chosen will depend on the severity of the pain. The choice of adjuvant will depend on the individual patient's analgesic history, tolerance to drugs previously tried and the presence of co-morbidities that may be adversely affected by particular adjuvant agents.

It is a common misconception that neuropathic pain is resistant to opioid analgesia. This is in fact untrue. However, it can be said that the opioid responsiveness of neuropathic pain is generally less than that of non-neuropathic pain, as higher dosages of opioids are often required to control the former (Dellemijn 1997, 1999; Kupers *et al.* 1991). It is often the onset of side effects that limits opioid responsiveness, not inherent resistance (Fallon & Hanks 1993; Hanks & Forbes 1997; Portenoy *et al.* 1990). Clearly, larger doses of opioids will be more commonly associated with unacceptable side effects. This is why it is particularly important in the management of neuropathic pain to have the early and appropriate introduction of a suitable adjuvant analgesic (Moore 1999).

Accepting that a trial of an opioid with appropriate dose titration remains fundamental in the management of neuropathic cancer pain, five other medication categories are often employed to treat this pain mechanism. These can be grouped as follows:

1. Antidepressants.
2. Anticonvulsants.
3. Topical agents.
4. TENS.
5. Spinal analgesia with local anaesthetic with or without clonidine.

Acupuncture is mentioned in Chapter 14, and should not be discounted.

Antidepressants

Although some patients find drugs labelled for use in depression to be unpalatable, it has to be acknowledged that no medication in any category has been proven to be unequivocally superior to tricyclic antidepressants for the management of neuropathic pain. Pain relief and relief of depression are independent factors (Sindrup *et al.* 1992a). Essentially, every blinded clinical trial with tricyclic antidepressants has found them to be efficacious (McQuay *et al.* 1996).

Non-tricyclic antidepressants are also widely used for the management of pain. They include selective serotonin reuptake inhibitors (SSRIs), antidepressants that alter both serotonergic (5-HT) and noradrenergic (NA) neurotransmission and NA-selective antidepressants. Although evidence for the analgesic activity of the newer antidepressants continues to accrue, so far there have only been a few controlled studies conducted in neuropathic pain disorders (McQuay & Moore 1998). Comparisons of tricyclic antidepressants with non-tricyclics have rarely been performed. The most instructive of these was a cross-over trial comparing the tricyclic antidepressant imipramine and the SSRI paroxetine for the treatment of pain caused by diabetic neuropathy. Paroxetine was equal to imipramine in most subjects, inferior in 30–40% and essentially never superior. A recent review of published work on the analgesic role of SSRIs, which included all types of pain and all types of literature report, identified 19 publications regarding fluoxetine, three with sertraline, six with paroxetine, three with fluvoxamine, three with citalopram and nine with trazodone. Except for paroxetine, controlled studies have not shown SSRIs to be superior to placebo for neuropathic pain (Rowbotham 2002).

Antidepressants that are either noradrenalin selective (maprotiline, bupropion) or that affect both 5-HT and noradrenalin (venlafaxine) may be more effective analgesics than SSRIs. Bupropion, almost completely selective for noradrenalin, was found effective for mixed neuropathic pain in a small placebo controlled cross-over trial. Maprotiline has also been found to be effective in the treatment of post-herpetic neuralgia, but less so when compared with a tricyclic antidepressant. Although reports of controlled clinical trials for neuropathic pain have not yet appeared for venlafaxine, anecdotal reports and abstract presentations are very favourable (Schrieber *et al.* 1999; Taylor & Rowbotham 1996; Pernia *et al.* 2000; Boyd 1998).

The presumed mechanisms underlying antidepressant analgesia involve the facilitation of descending serotonergic and noradrenergic pain modulatory pathways. However, this may not be their only mechanism of action. Tricyclic antidepressants, in addition to blocking serotonin and noradrenalin reuptake, are relatively potent sodium channel blockers and may act as *N*-methyl-D-aspartate (NMDA) receptor antagonists. Also, some have significant sympatholytic effects.

Whereas in general the non tricyclic antidepressants are safer and have a better side-effect profile than the tricyclic antidepressants, this cannot be assumed to be the case in every individual, and side effects and withdrawal reactions are still a potential issue for all these drugs. On balance, the choice of an adjuvant analgesic depends on several factors, including co-existing depression. In this situation, when a true antidepressant dose is required, it is probably safer and more practical in the cancer pain population to use a non-tricyclic antidepressant such as venlafaxine.

Anticonvulsants

Anticonvulsants are only tied together by their ability to suppress epileptic seizures. Other than trigeminal neuralgia, where carbamazepine has been shown to have an excellent effect, comparisons between anticonvulsants are rare, even in pre-clinical literature (Backonja *et al.* 1998).

Anticonvulsants differ in their mechanisms of action. Many drugs have a common ability to block sodium channels in a use-dependent manner. However, some anticonvulsants may also exert their effect through non-sodium-channel mechanisms which are thought to involve actions on sensitised central neurons. Examples include direct or indirect inhibition of the release of excitatory amino acids, blockade of neuronal calcium channels and augmentation of the CNS inhibitory pathways by increasing GABAergic transmission.

The tricyclic antidepressants and the anticonvulsants have been examined in systematic reviews, and analysis has shown that the number needed to treat to gain significant analgesia is three (NNT = 3) (McQuay & Moore 1998). Gabapentin was not included in this systematic review but it would seem from the literature that it is likely that the number needed to treat is also three. However, gabapentin has the potential benefit of a more favourable side effect profile when compared with most other anticonvulsants (Backonja et al.1998; McQuay et al. 1995; Mellegers et al. 2001; Rice et al. 2001; Rosenberg et al. 1997; Rowbotham et al. 1998a). In effect, this means that more patients can tolerate this treatment, which is probably more valuable clinically than numbers needed to treat.

As with antidepressants, the choice of anticonvulsant depends very much on the individual patient, the past history of adjuvant use and any co-morbidities that would influence the choice for or against a particular drug. As with the other drugs mentioned, randomised controlled trials of gabapentin have not been conducted in cancer pain. However, they have been performed in other neuropathic pain syndromes, the mechanisms of which can be extrapolated to the common neuropathic cancer pain mechanisms.

The key to the use of an adjuvant analgesic, whether antidepressant or anticonvulsant, is to choose a drug for the individual patient and titrate its dose to achieve analgesia without unacceptable side effects. It is common to prescribe an adjuvant and to fail to be sufficiently aggressive when titrating its dose.

Antidepressant and anticonvulsant drug combinations are difficult to use in cancer pain because of the number of potential drug interactions. Combinations should be avoided where possible and used with great care when needed.

Topical agents

Morphine

Topical agents such as morphine are of increasing interest in the management of neuropathic pain. We know that there are peripheral opioid receptors and there are anecdotal reports of the efficacy of topical opioids in a variety of skin problems, the mechanisms of which are partly neuropathic. Morphine can be prepared in instilagel at a dose of 20 mg in 10 ml and applied topically to the skin. The morphine dose can be titrated up if required. Clearly the evidence for this route and appropriateness in different pain syndromes needs further evaluation.

Capsaicin

When used topically, this is effective for some patients with cutaneous neuropathic pain (Petersen et al. 2000; Watson 1994; Watson et al. 1993). This acts through vanilloid receptors and it can be useful when applied after local anaesthetic cream for scar pain, e.g. thoracotomy, mastectomy.

Lignocaine

Topical lignocaine patches, licensed in North America for the management of post-herpetic neuralgia, have a purely cutaneous mechanism of action with no significant systemic absorption (Galer *et al.* 1999, Rowbotham & Fields 1989a; Rowbotham *et al.* 1996a). These can be useful in cancer pain that has a cutaneous neuropathic element.

Others

Other topical agents are in development and are in fact available in other countries, such as topical ketamine, clonidine and gabapentin (Byas-Smith *et al.* 1995). Cream containing the tricyclic antidepressant doxepin is now available commercially.

TENS

Trans-cutaneous electrical nerve stimulation (TENS) has been shown to be effective in some patients with neuropathic pain. TENS is much underused in cancer pain. Also, when it is used, it is often in a sub-optimal way. Advice from someone properly trained in the use of TENS can be useful for patients with neuropathic pain and a helpful adjunct to other treatments (McQuay & Moore 1998).

Spinal analgesia

Spinal analgesia is sometimes necessary for patients with difficult neuropathic pain. We know from randomised controlled studies that it is not usually spinal opioids that make the difference in neuropathic pain but rather the addition of such drugs as local anaesthetic or clonidine. Evidence for the latter is largely based on case series and anecdotal reports and no robust clinic trial has been conducted to provide good evidence for the use of spinal analgesia in difficult neuropathic pain. There is one randomised controlled trial of best pharmacological management versus implanted intrathecal pumps, published in the *Journal of Clinical Oncology* (Smith *et al.* 2002). This study looks more at difficult cancer pain in general rather than neuropathic pain *per se*. Also, there would seem to be some methodological problems with this study, as there is insufficient clarity about the pharmacological management, adjuvants and other methods used in their patient population.

Acupuncture

Acupuncture, in particular, paravertebral points, can be particularly useful for some forms of neuropathic pain from anecdotal experience. This should not be forgotten for those who have this expertise and its use and evidence base is covered more fully in another chapter.

NMDA Antagonists

Finally, it would be appropriate to mention drugs such as ketamine that act as NMDA receptor antagonists. At a pre-clinical level there is no doubt that they are exceedingly impressive analgesics in neuropathic pain (Chapman & Dickenson 1992; Bennett 1994). In addition, a variety of clinical studies have demonstrated efficacy in non-malignant neuropathic pain (Mitchell & Fallon 2002; Nikolajsen *et al.* 1997; Graven-Nielsen *et al.* 2000). Case series in cancer pain have been reported (Fallon & Welsh 1996). These drugs seem to be exceptionally effective for a group of patients. However, definition of this group remains difficult clinically and high-level evidence in cancer pain is lacking. The side effects of ketamine can be a problem for some patients and a search for a more selective NMDA antagonist is required.

In summary, there are several approaches in the management of difficult neuropathic pain. Effective analgesic management is based on sound clinical assessment, the use of basic drugs such as opioids, and an adjuvant to suit the patient's clinical situation. All strategies to minimise opioid side-effects and therefore increase opioid responsiveness should be used. Appropriate titration of adjuvants is always necessary and other treatments such as TENS should not be forgotten. Spinal analgesia may be necessary in a few patients predominantly, because of the role of local anaesthetic and/or clonidine. NMDA antagonists can be effective in selective patients; however, clarity about their use in malignant neuropathic pain is lacking.

As with all types of cancer pain the general distress that many of our patients experience should not be forgotten and assessment of distress, anxiety and depression with the most appropriate management is fundamental to helping to raise the pain threshold in this pain syndrome, as in others.

References

Backonja, M., Beydoun, A., Edwards, K. R., Schwarz, S., Fonesca, M., Hes, L., LaMoreaux, L., Garofalo, E. (1998). Gabapentin for the symptomatic treatment of painful neuropathy in patients with diabetes mellitus: a randomised controlled trial. *Journal of the American Medical Association* **280**, 1831–1836.

Bennett, G. J. (1994). Animal models of neuropathic pain. In *Proceedings of the 7th World Congress on Pain, Progress in Pain Research and Management*, vol. 2. (ed. G. F. Gebhart, D. L. Hammond & T. Jensen), pp. 495–510. Seattle, WA: IASP Press.

Boyd, I. W. (1998). Venlafaxine withdrawal reactions. *Medical Journal of Australia* **169**, 91–92.

Byas-Smith, M. G., Max, M. B., Muir, J., Kingman, A. (1995). Transdermal clonidine compared to placebo in painful diabetic neuropathy using a two-stage "enriched enrolment" design. *Pain* **60**, 267–274.

Chapman, V. & Dickenson, A. H. (1992). The combination of NMDA antagonism and morphine produces profound antinociception in the rat dorsal horn. *Brain Research* **573**, 321–323.

Dellemijn, P. (1997). Randomised double-blind active-placebo-controlled crossover trial of intravenous fentanyl in neuropathic pain. *The Lancet* **349**, 753–758.

Dellemijn, P. (1999). Are opioids effective in relieving neuropathic pain? *Pain* **80**, 453–462.

Fallon, M. & Hanks, G. W. (1993). Opioid responsiveness – sense or nonsense? *Pain Clinic* **6**, 205–206.

Fallon, M. T. & Welsh, J. (1996). The role of ketamine in pain control. *European Journal of Palliative Care* **3**, 143–146.

Galer, B. S., Rowbotham, M. C., Perander, J., Friedman, E. (1999). Topical lidocaine patch relieves postherpetic neuralgia more effectively than a vehicle topical patch: results of an enriched enrolment study. *Pain* **80**, 533–538.

Graven-Nielsen, T., Aspegren Kendall, S., Hennksson, K. G., Bengtsson, M., Sorenson, J., Johnson, A., Gerde, B., Arendt-Nielson, L. (2000). Ketamine reduced muscle pain, temporal summation and referred pain in fibromyalgia patients. *Pain* **85**, 483–491.

Grond, S., Radbruch, L., Meuser, T., Sabatokowski, R., Loick, G., Lehmann, K. A. (1999). Assessment and treatment of neuropathic cancer pain following WHO guidelines. *Pain* **79**, 15–20.

Hanks, G. W. & Forbes, K. (1997). Opioid responsiveness. *Acta Anaesthesiologica Scandinavica* **41**, 151–158.

Kupers, R. C., Konings, H., Adriaensen, H., Gybels, J. M. (1991). Morphine differentially affects the sensory and affective pain ratings in neurogenic and idiopathic forms of pain. *Pain* **45**, 5–12.

McQuay, H., Carroll, D., Jadad, A. R., Wiffen, P., Moore, A. (1995). Anticonvulsant drugs for management of pain: a systematic review. *British Medical Journal* **311**, 1047–1052.

McQuay, H. J., Tramer, M., Nye, B. A., Carroll, D., Wiffen, P., Moore, R. A. (1996). A systematic review of antidepressants in neuropathic pain. *Pain* **68**, 217–227.

McQuay, H. & Moore, A. (1998). An evidence-based resource for pain relief. Oxford: Oxford Medical Publications.

Mellegers, M. A., Furlan, A. D., Mailis, A. (2001). Gabapentin for neuropathic pain: systematic review of controlled and uncontrolled literature. *Clinical Journal of Pain* **17**, 284–295.

Mitchell, A. C. & Fallon, M. T. (2002). A single infusion of intravenous ketamine improves pain relief in patients with critical limb ischaemia: results of a double blind randomised controlled trial. *Pain* **97**, 275–281.

Moore, R. A. (1999). New developments in evidence-based decision-making: relevance to pain treatment and research. In *Pain 1999 – an updated review: refresher course syllabus* (ed. M. Max), pp. 423–430. Seattle, WA: IASP Press.

Nikolajsen, L., Ilkhaer, S., Kroner, K., Christensen, J. H., Jensen, T. S. (1997). The influence of preamputation pain on post amputation stump and phantom pain. *Pain* **72**, 393–405.

Pernia, A., Mico, J. A, Calderon, E., Torres, L. M. (2000). Venlafaxine for the treatment of neuropathic pain. *Journal of Pain and Symptom Management* **19**, 408–410.

Petersen, K. L., Fields, H. L., Brennum, J., Sandroni, P., Rowbotham, M. C. (2000). Capsaicin activation of "irritable" nociceptors in post-herpetic neuralgia. *Pain* **88**, 125–133.

Portenoy, R. K., Foley, K. M. & Inturrisi, C. E. (1990). The nature of opioid responsiveness and its implications for neuropathic pain: new hypotheses derived from studies of opioid infusions. *Pain* **43**, 273–286.

Rice, A. S. & Maton, S. (2001). Gabapentin in postherpetic neuralgia: a randomised, double blind, placebo controlled study. *Pain* **94**, 215–224.

Rosenberg, J. M., Harrell, C., Ristic, H., Werner, R. A., de Rosays, A. M. (1997). The effect of gabapentin on neuropathic pain. *Clinical Journal of Pain* **13**, 251–255.

Rowbotham, M. C. & Fields, H. L. (1989). Topical lidocaine reduces pain in post-herpetic neuralgia. *Pain* **38**, 297–301.

Rowbotham, M. C., Davies, P. S., Verkempinck, C., Galer, B. S. (1996). Lidocaine patch: double-blind controlled study of a new treatment method for post herpetic neuralgia. *Pain* **65**, 39–44.

Rowbotham, M., Harden, N., Stacey, B., Bernstein, P., Magnus-Miller, L. (1998). Gabapentin for the treatment of post herpetic neuralgia: a randomised controlled trial. *Journal of the American Medical Association* **280**, 1837–1842.

Rowbotham, M. C. (2002). Neuropathic pain: from basic science to evidence-based treatment. In *Pain 2002 – an updated review* (ed. M.A. Giamberardino), pp. 165–173. Seattle, WA: IASP Press.

Schrieber, S., Backer, M. M. & Pick, C. G. (1999). The antinociceptive effect of venlafaxine in mice is mediated through opioid and adrenergic mechanisms. *Neuroscience Letters* **273**, 85–88.

Sindrup, S. H., Brosen, K. & Gram, L. F. (1992a) Antidepressants in pain treatment: antidepressant or analgesic effect? *Clinical Neuropharmacology* **15**, 636A–637A.

Smith, T. J., Staats, P. S., Deer, T., Stearns, L. J., Rauck, R. L., Boortz-Marx, R. L., Buchser, E., Catala, E., Bryce, D. A., Coyne, P., Pool, G. E. (2002). Randomised clinical trial of an implantable drug delivery system compared with comprehensive medical management for refractory cancer pain: impact on pain, drug-related toxicity and survival. *Journal of Clinical Oncology* **20**, 4040–4049.

Taylor, K. & Rowbotham, M. C. (1996). Venlafaxine hydrochloride and chronic pain. *Western Journal of Medicine* **165**, 147–148.

Watson, C. P. N. (1994). Topical capsaicin as an adjuvant analgesic. *Journal of Pain and Symptom Management* **9**, 425–433.

Watson, C. P., Tyler, K. L., Bickers, D. R., Millikan, L. E., Smith, S., Coleman, E. (1993). A randomised vehicle-controlled trial of topical capsaicin in the treatment of postherpetic neuralgia. *Clinical Therapy* **15**, 510–526.

Woolf, C. J. & Decosterd, I. (1999). Implications of recent advances in the understanding of pain pathophysiology for the assessment of pain in patients. *Pain* (Aug.) (Suppl. 6), S141–S147.

Woolf, C. J., Bennett, G. J., Doherty, M., Dubner, R., Kidd, B., Koltzenberg, M., Lipton, R., Loeser, J. D., Payne, R., Torebjork, E. (1998). Towards a mechanism-based classification of pain? *Pain* **77**, 227–229.

World Health Organization (1996). *Cancer pain relief*, 2nd edn. Geneva: World Health Organization.

Ventafridda, V., Tamburini, M., Caraceni, A., De Conno, F., Naldi, F. (1987). A validation study of the WHO method for cancer pain relief. *Cancer* **59**, 850–856.

Zech, D. F., Grond, S., Lynch, J., Hertel, D., Lehmann, K. A. (1995). Validation of World Health Organization guidelines for cancer pain relief: a 10 year prospective study. *Pain* **63**, 65–76.

Chapter 10

Non-physical pain: suffering in action

Rob George and Jonathan Martin

> '*To be, or not to be: that is the question: whether 'tis nobler in the mind to suffer the slings and arrows of outrageous fortune or to take arms against a sea of troubles, and by opposing end them?*'

> '*To die: to sleep; no more; and, by a sleep to say we end the heart-ache and the thousand natural shocks that flesh is heir to, 'tis a consummation devoutly to be wished.*'

> '*To die, to sleep; to sleep: perchance to dream: ay, there's the rub; for in that sleep of death what dreams may come when we have shuffled off this mortal coil, must give us pause. There's the respect that makes calamity of so long life…*'

> Hamlet, William Shakespeare

The context

Shakespeare touched on the fundamental issues that face us all as illness and death finally take hold. The battle to overcome or to 'beat this' disease; the overwhelming disappointment of the battle being lost; conflicts with the desire that pretty well all our patients have, at some time, to call it a day, and yet the worry that there may be something out there beyond death '*…that makes calamity of so long life*'. The struggle to find meaning or make sense from physical deterioration and discomfort; the 'pain of passing' that is felt between the leaver and those being left, coupled with the review of a life led, is a process through which we all must go. The term 'pain' applies rightly to much of this struggle. Indeed, anguish, sadness and other emotions may be felt physically with knots in the stomach, difficulty in getting warm, breathlessness, etc. Clearly these physical descriptions or phenomena do not have a *prima facie* basis in the physical, but the patient feels pain all the same.

It is this symptomatology that we address briefly in this chapter. This manifestation of psychological and spiritual, ontological or existential crises, which accompanies the dying process, entitles those of us specialising in palliative care to emphasise the interdisciplinary and complex nature of diagnosing and managing symptoms in the face of a person's uncertain future and the suffering that can entail. Notwithstanding the need for technical expertise and a firm grounding in pharmacology and evidence-based prescribing, the challenge and kernel of the specialty is the management of suffering and uncertainty that goes beyond the nosology (science) of medicine and rather is in the wisdom and art of its practice.

Whereas the concept of emotional, spiritual and 'total' pain are familiar to the speciality and defined in all the textbooks, placing this with other symptoms susceptible to the intangible effects of the mind, soul and spirit under the rubric of suffering, to our knowledge, is not.

Our premise is that suffering is a function of the conflicts within a person, and that our endeavour, therefore, should be to promote the environment for the patient and family for choices and changes to be made that resolve these tensions. In this modelling, Hope becomes the notion that the future can be different and better, not that disease can be cured and morality conquered. The chapter concludes with mechanisms that can assist this.

Before looking specifically at suffering and an accessible way in which to approach it, we shall begin by discussing two basic concepts that unify our approach to symptoms and form the foundation of our model of suffering: the idea of a symptom threshold, and the relationship and distinction between the pathological *mechanism* underlying a symptom, that is its *pathology*, and the *meaning* of the symptom to the patient as a *person*.

The concepts

Pain thresholds

Figure 10.1 is a pictorial representation of the relationship between a linear stimulus (dotted line) given in a controlled environment, such as the measurable pressure of a pin or temperature of a probe on the skin (ordinate 1), compared with the reported sensation (solid line). Sensation (ordinate 2) will move from awareness through discomfort to overwhelming distress. This is some form of exponent. The point at which the subject reports the symptom – in this case as pain – is called the threshold. Both the form of the curve and the threshold depend upon factors that are summarised in Figure 10.2. However, the dotted line is a function of the pathology and mechanism leading to the symptom, such as the degree of trauma and neuropharmacology of pain pathways.

In short, pain can be exacerbated every bit as much, if not more, by the psychological, social and ontological consequences of a disease as its pathology. These in turn are the sources of conflict in the person when the meaning of an illness leads to the emergence of hidden fears, memories and perceptions. This brings us to the issue of meaning.

Interpretation: the link between mechanism & meaning

Biomedicine

> '... 'tis nobler in the mind to suffer the slings and arrows of outrageous fortune or to take arms against a sea of troubles, and by opposing end them?'

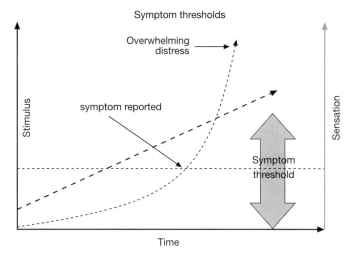

Figure 10.1 The relation between a noxious stimulus (e.g. pain) and the reported symptom is exponential. Once past its threshold, without adequate treatment or a reduction in the process, the symptom will soon become intolerable. If the patient's threshold falls, the symptom will escalate, even when the underlying disease is stable.

Symptom thresholds and what can change them

? adequate technical
  symptom control
? explanation
? exploration
? strategies

disease stable

increased
threshold

symptom
reduced

Nausea
pain
dyspnoea

Increase

Thresholds

Decrease

reduced
disease

symptom
reduced

threshold stable

? inadequate
  curative option
? ignorance
? denial
? secrecy
? psychol. distress
? spiritual distress

disease stable

decreased
threshold

symptom
worse

Figure 10.2 This figure shows three clinical situations. In the top panel, the symptom is reduced by increasing the threshold in the face of stable disease, e.g. by giving adequate pain control, explaining the situation and what it means for the patient, and developing strategies that will ensure that they learn to use adequate analgesia when necessary and develop other coping mechanisms. In the middle panel, the disease is reduced by, say, palliative radiotherapy, chemotherapy or surgery in the face of a stable pain threshold. Hence the pain is reduced. In the lower panel, whilst the disease is stable, factors such as those in the accompanying panel on the left have reduced the pain threshold and led to a worsening clinical picture despite stable disease. The cases below illustrate this clearly.

We now come to the personal rather than the pathological. Once a symptom is experienced, it is evaluated and interpreted, the negative and extreme experience being suffering. Cassel (1982) defines suffering as '...the state of severe distress associated with events that threaten the intactness of the person'. He notes that suffering, as distinct from physical distress, is experienced by persons, not merely by bodies.

For most people, perhaps for all, the *experience* of 'dis-ease' is always a source of some distress: 'Is this something to worry about? I can't afford time off work. Who will pay the mortgage? What have I done to cause this?', etc. This is the seedbed of suffering as the person enters the surgery wanting a simple and remediable diagnosis. He wants an answer. The doctor's job in the first instance then is to investigate and treat. If the patient's cough and chest discomfort is a straightforward problem like a chest infection, the remedy is simple and the problem resolved. In this sense the pre-emptive 'management' of suffering lies clearly within the biomedical domain (Figure 10.3, left-hand side).

However, the reverse is clearly not true: not all suffering is disease. Say the doctor spots the R Horner's Syndrome and refers the patient for a chest X-ray and an urgent thoracic opinion. The odds are that the patient will now become much more anxious and symptomatic as he begins to worry about lung cancer and what that may mean to him and his family. Nothing has changed, except the patient's perception, as he explores the implications of his symptoms. The doctor's cycle is looking for a *mechanism*; the patient though is now asking very different *meaning* questions (Figure 10.3, right-hand side).

The apical small-cell cancer initially remits well with chemotherapy and the patient resolves to beat it. Later in this disease journey, he develops metastases. Even though the consultant knows they will be futile, she offers the patient more cycles of chemotherapy, which are taken up. The patient wants cure to be free of the accumulating pressures. The doctor is trained to do this and approaches him with the only biomedical option she can: more of the same. Ultimately she will feel a failure and he will feel let down and abandoned unless he begins to understand that the strategy is ultimately futile and another must be adopted. Cynically, perhaps, we refer to this as the 'Dance of denial' (Figure 10.4).

Later, local painful bony lesions require single shots of radiotherapy. By now he is very symptomatic, miserable and is referred for a palliative care opinion as there is nothing more that oncology can do.

Palliative care: transitions to a balance

'*To die: to sleep; no more; and, by a sleep to say we end the heart-ache and the thousand natural shocks that flesh is heir to, 'tis a consummation devoutly to be wished.*'

It emerges that his home life had fallen apart when his latest girlfriend was discovered by his wife on his first hospital admission and he is now alone in a bed-sit. His family

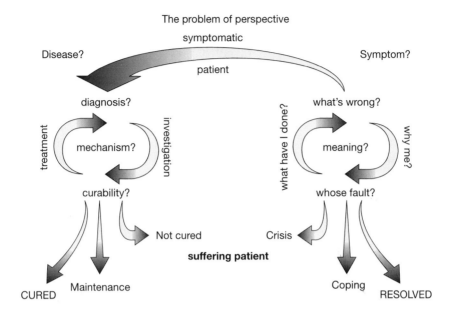

Figure 10.3 The difference between a biomedical view and that of the patient leads to key issues being missed.

has disowned him and say he deserves the cancer for what he has done. He feels like turning his face to the wall.

Worse still, his elderly mother plans to come and collect him: 'You'd better come home—I said it would catch up with you in the end'. He had left home under a cloud 20 years earlier having decided not to enter the priesthood. He'd not entered a church since.

The sources of this suffering are now palpable and nothing to do with the cancer *per se*: the pain of broken relationships and of aloneness complicated probably by an understandable depression. Guilt and remorse is weighing heavy; and maybe mum is right that there is a God in Heaven. If there is, the worry is finding a way back.

> '*To die, to sleep; to sleep: perchance to dream: ay, there's the rub; for in that sleep of death what dreams may come when we have shuffled off this mortal coil, must give us pause. There's the respect that makes calamity of so long life...*'

As far as palliative care is concerned, there is a great deal more to be done, but it requires a shift to a different epistemology* and approach. Although it is generally accepted that the relief of suffering is a function of the intrinsic aim of medicine (that

---

*This means a knowledge base and approach that is different and more appropriate to the problem in hand. It is seen in research, for example, as the move from quantitative methods in evidence-based therapeutics about diseases to qualitative ones in social and anthropologically based evidence about people.

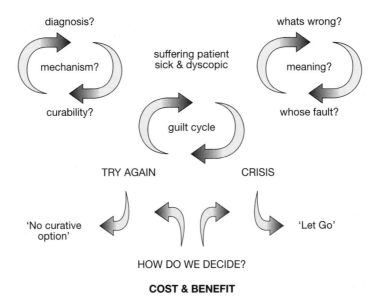

Figure 10.4 lead-in caption title: Contracts of conflict: The dance of denial

Figure 10.4 The natural and understandable tendency when disease recurs is for acute physicians to continue doing what they do well: to investigate and treat disease. However, the cost is that it is difficult often to face the incurability of disease. It is less 'painful' to have one more go with therapy than to confront the need to change course and face the reality of the patient's suffering, especially when there is no simple strategy to adopt.

of promoting a 'medical good') (Randall & Downie 1999), this idea is usually conceived of entirely in relation to physical symptoms (including mental illness). To what extent all healthcare professionals should attempt to help a patient's non-physical suffering is therefore better phrased as: to what extent should we promote a patient's 'total good'? In palliative care, and similarly in general practice, we believe that helping a patient to address non-physical suffering is a legitimate and necessary, if extrinsic, aim of what we do.

Physical pain, and other symptoms such as breathlessness and nausea, is experienced as suffering in a direct and obvious way. But the intensity and meaning of these symptoms will be deeply personal:

- Has a similar pain been experienced before, and what was the outcome?
- Has someone known to the patient experienced an apparently similar symptom, and what did it mean for him or her?

- What could a new symptom signify? For example, could increasing pain signal a new bone metastasis or an escalation of disease, the symptoms of which were previously well controlled?
- What memories, fears, regrets, etc. are allowed conscious space when facing the uncertain meaning of a symptom?
- And ultimately, does this symptom signify the approach of death?

In other words, the neurogenic signal generated by, say, bone pain is modulated and transformed as it passes through a patient's conscious and subconscious filters to be interpreted and reported as a symptom with meaning (Figure 10.5).

What these questions illustrate is that physical suffering, while happening in the present, has both past and future associations: our past experiences may inform our understanding (correctly or incorrectly) of the meaning of a present symptom; and the present symptom, correctly or incorrectly evaluated, may give rise to fears about what the future is likely to hold. It is therefore impossible to predict which symptoms may give rise to how much suffering, although it is probably true to say that certain forms of injury almost invariably cause suffering.

Symptoms thus have both universal and individual aspects (Ira Byock: www.dyingwell.com).

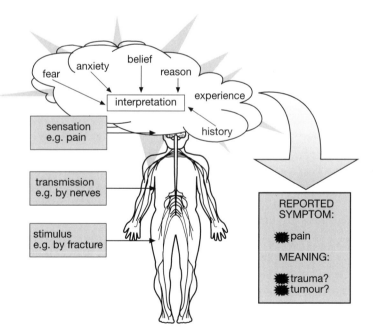

Figure 10.5 Here we refer to the sentient characteristics and functions of the brain as the 'Black box'.

The wide-ranging nature of this kind of suffering, however, is such that traditional medical and nursing training, including basic counselling and communication skills, does not equip the healthcare professional for this work. Rather, a practical wisdom borne of experience of life, reflective practice, mentorship and a humanitarian approach is most likely to be helpful, and as such may be the purview of non-healthcare professionals as much as that of doctors, nurses, psychologists and so on (Randall & Downie 1999). In this sense we are keen not to 'medicalise' non-physical suffering.

For the clinician, the significances of such meanings perceived by patients lie in two areas:

- *Ideas, concerns and expectations (ICE)*. The clinician may not attach the same set of implications to the presentation of physical symptoms as does the patient. Hence we need to ask the patient about these. This is encapsulated in general practice teaching as the need to ask about *ICE*.
- *Creating 'decision space'*. One key objective in controlling symptoms, aside from an end in itself, is to understand the need for adequate treatment as a means of creating 'space' in which the individual may start to address the underlying meanings and conflicts and to resolve them.

Why then is a patient more likely to present with physical symptoms, than with existential questions? Whereas many believe, and we share this view, that medicine now occupies the priestly role in our 'post-religious' society, one obvious reason is the expediency and legitimacy that physical symptoms bring to a person's need for attention: they are tangible and demand exploration and action, or as Autton (1986) puts it: 'It is easier to say you have a pain in the stomach than that your heart is hurting'. However, there are other ways of looking at this:

- The socially sanctioned process of gaining attention from symptoms results in a partial change of responsibility: the patient 'hands over' a degree of control to the clinician and may assume a 'sick role'. This in turn can bestow certain privileges upon the patient, such as the freedom to be absent from work for a 'physical' illness.
- Allied to this new position is the hope that the symptom, and whatever its underlying cause, is resolvable by others (this may represent a defence against the fear of death and the idea that the patient will be rescued by an external 'hero' (Ira Byock: www.dyingwell.com)).
- Presenting to the medical profession in this way with a 'medical' problem is considered legitimate for another reason: doctors are most comfortable in the biomedical domain.
- Physical symptoms are in some ways a 'protective' buffer or barrier to the patient, in that they focus attention on the surface of things, allowing the deeper 'internal landscapes' to remain unexamined.

An understanding of factors such as these is useful when considering suffering in a more general sense, and in particular when defining it in a practical sense as a sign of conflict.

It is difficult, of course, to know whether such deeper ontological corollaries of physical symptoms are always present in an individual—in our experience they usually are. What is clearer is that these meanings often do not reside within the conscious awareness of the patient. However, it is our common experience that looking for and addressing them often results in a lessening of overall suffering. The problem is that such meanings are more difficult to uncover or address while the patient is experiencing significant physical distress. In this sense, taking clinical steps to relieve the physical symptoms must be our initial concern.

In summary, by treating physical symptoms appropriately – i.e. a satisfactory balance between control and side effects of drugs or other interventions – the clinician is not only relieving the suffering arising as a direct result of the symptoms, but is also creating the 'decision space' within which the patient may choose to begin addressing non-physical suffering.

We believe it is the central role and purposes of specialist palliative care to help create the environment and circumstances in which the patient is free to address the roots of their suffering, should they wish. The following case serves as an example.

Suffering in action: the case of Nina

This young woman was at the end of her breast cancer journey with severe lymphoedema of the arm and cutaneous metastases. She developed pain as her disease progressed. However, this was extremely brittle and fluctuated even during periods of remitting or quiescent disease. We attempted unsuccessfully to explore any emotional or spiritual need as she refused categorically at all stages to face the possibility of deterioration or death; instead she continued her pursuit of a cure and many opinions on her treatment. At one stage, the instability of her pain necessitated admission for observation.

Investigation confirmed that there was no clinical basis for this. However, combining the nursing and medical notes revealed the full story. Figure 10.6 shows two traces. The upper bar chart details her breakthrough analgesia. This logs her requests for additional morphine for periods of intensifying pain. Because these requests were made in the face of clinically stable disease, they reflect fluctuations in the pain threshold. The lower line, therefore, is a simple inversion of these doses to show by proxy the variations in the pain threshold directly. The correlation with mood and emotionally stressful events is striking and suggests that her pain threshold has a psychological or possibly spiritual component, or both. She was from a religious, Jewish, family, but had taken a different path: she was an atheist and a feminist working as an academic on the suffering of women in the 20th century. Her whole professional life was therefore influenced by unconscious cultural and societal drivers.

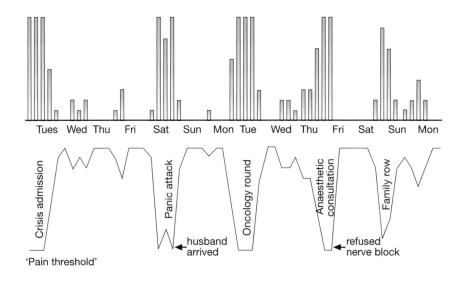

Figure 10.6 Case study of Nina (for explanation see text on page 115).

We revisited these areas with her, but sadly and ironically she was unable to see or engage them for herself. Predictably, she needed significant sedation to manage her terminal restlessness.

A practical model of suffering†

A relevant model of person

Having considered how a mechanistic view cannot answer meaning questions and how this may present clinically, we now simplify the puzzling array of potential sources of suffering as a visual model, and then apply this model to a process that can take a patient from suffering and conflict to hope and change.

This model is very simple and is intended to offer a further element to a framework through which to work. It is in two parts. First, we present a schematic view into our world through its layers to the core (Figure 10.7). Secondly, we can then apply this in the individual case as the ingredients of suffering become known, to address them systematically and explore what is remediable.

---

†First, the model is based within contemporary Western culture. The needs of those from other cultures may be quite different and require different sensitivities. Secondly, the focus is on the needs of patient who is suffering. However, those close to the patient may also suffer greatly as a result of the patient's distress.

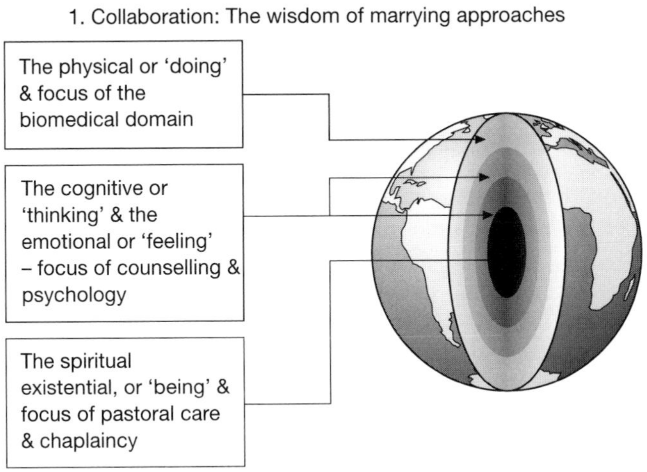

1. Collaboration: The wisdom of marrying approaches

| The physical or 'doing' & focus of the biomedical domain |
| The cognitive or 'thinking' & the emotional or 'feeling' – focus of counselling & psychology |
| The spiritual existential, or 'being' & focus of pastoral care & chaplaincy |

Figure 10.7 The schematic layers within our world relevant to suffering. See text on page 116.

The physical or 'doing' domain

General points

These are the 'surface' or immediately consuming issues through which we interact initially with the outside. They include:

1. Symptoms such as physical pain and, importantly, undiagnosed depression (which, of course, crosses all domains).
2. Uncertainties that influence the tasks the patient might want to do such as:

   (*a*) An idea of the remaining useful time.
   (*b*) The *Aspiration:Achievement Gap* that is the principal determinant of quality of life. The actual physical restrictions of the disease, symptoms and abilities, and what can be done, versus what hopes the patient carries about physical functioning, and what they want to do.
   (*c*) Actual disability and its impact.

Apart from being very practical problems, discussing them openly in the context of the patient's *real* life is the entrée through which one may begin to expose the deeper meanings and fears that will surface with disability, deterioration or dying.

Helplessness

The cardinal expression of this is helplessness, or more accurately, the feeling of loss of control. The patient feels denuded of their independence, prestige and privacy—classical 'hiding places for the insecurities of our soul'. Any illness does this, but irreversible disability and dependence does this ultimately, as we can no longer dictate our own boundaries and find solace in being a *human doing* rather than a *human being.*

The psychological, emotional or 'feeling' domain

Psychological suffering moves us deeper into the person and may expose the underlying meanings about thoughts, emotions and behaviours. Although there can be overlap between the two, we consider this source of suffering to be distinct from defined mental illness, which is, for the time being at least, a biomedical diagnosis. In this area of feeling:

(*a*) Some will relate to the common experiences of living and the emotional impact and strain of practical concerns or financial pressure.

(*b*) Mood varies and it is important to understand what the patient is feeling as distinct from how they want to feel, what influences this and how it manifests. More explicitly, for example:

   (i)   How are symptoms affecting the patient and those around them, and how in turn does that feed itself back to the patient?

   (ii) Does the patient trust the healthcare staff to deal effectively with these symptoms, now and in the future?

   (iii) If a patient's mood is flat, is it appropriate sadness, or is there a depressive element? Although suicidal or euthanastic ideation lies well below 5% and falls as disease progresses, diagnosing depression is notoriously difficult (Kissane & Kelly 2000).

Finally,

(*c*) What is the state of important emotional relationships? This last area deserves closer attention.

   (i)   Almost all, and even the healthiest, will need attention or facilitation.

   (ii) Broken relationships may be those close to the patient, i.e. within the patient's immediate family or friends, or may be more distant, in both space and time.

   (iii) 'Dead' relationships are an essential and frequently neglected area to explore. By dead we mean those where the person concerned has deceased: parental relationships are the most obvious. More difficult are relationships that have failed, yet the person is still around. Examples are divorces or family estrangements.

(iv) Finally, those who have lived through human conflict will have wounds deeply buried. Among the elderly, the World War II is still casting its shadow. In this day, the refugees and survivors of wars are increasingly presenting with disease and suffering, though their needs are very specialised.

All these areas of psychological and emotional suffering can be resolved given the right expertise and approach, and motivation by the patient. However, the work may be time consuming and may need specialist help. Nevertheless, if you do not look, you will not uncover these remediable areas.

The spiritual/existential domain

'To die, to sleep; to sleep: perchance to dream: ay, there's the rub; for in that sleep of death what dreams may come when we have shuffled off this mortal coil, must give us pause. There's the respect that makes calamity of so long life...'

The spiritual and existential domain, or more completely the ontological‡, encompasses the fundamental questions of life and death. It is worth remembering that although some patients may not wish to address these questions explicitly, they may still underlie the intensity of the suffering arising in the psychological and biomedical domains. For those who have a strong religious or atheist conviction, some of the following questions are still relevant, particularly when the patient is facing the reality of impending death. Without prejudice, this is quite simply because all beliefs are based in faith rather than fact, and when death approaches, the robustness of most people's beliefs are stretched to the full. The questions are common in theme, but vary according to age, background, etc.

1. The inevitability and irreversibility of death crowds everyone at some stage, as patients (and ourselves) are usually able to avoid it throughout life and even a disease journey if one has paid into the biomedical model. This fends off the conscious implications, responsibilities, pursuant consequences and fears until they can no longer wait. For example,

(*a*) How we, or others, have used our freedom. Although freedom is usually valued when we can ignore the consequences, the responsibilities it brings for our decisions and actions may find final focus when '*...we have shuffled off this mortal coil*'. Although Britain is now post-religious, its Judeo-Christian beliefs of judgement still affect all of us to some extent, if only as a shadow. Patients and families from other cultures bring particular spins to this eternal question.

---

‡Our ontology is the way in which we see the nature of our being, which for some extends beyond death, and therefore is beyond the existential, which in modern parlance limits itself to this time and space.

(*b*) The consequent guilt and bitterness of a mixed past may erupt with frightening clarity and detail, or fill a soul with amorphous but destructive anger and fear when chains of regrets and recriminations have polluted our sense of worth or dignity yet have origins lost in our history.

(*c*) The ultimate aloneness in dying, on the one hand that we worry that the buck stops here, yet on the other that we can never have all the facts: we can never know someone else fully, nor fully be known.

2. Resolving and integrating our personal meaning into the universal. This is the 'existential paradox': is there meaning and order in the universe, or do we seek meaning and certainty in a universe with neither? Whatever the answer is, have we done our bit?

The need for the giving and receiving of forgiveness mentioned above is the area of overlap with the psychological domain. The way that patients frequently voice these issues is through questions such as:

(*a*) What does my life mean now?
(*b*) What has it meant, to me and to others (did I matter or make a difference)?
(*c*) What is the meaning of my illness and death (why me, why now)?
(*d*) What happens next?

For some, answers may be found in spiritual beliefs. For others there are no answers, although these questions may be made less significant through the perceived importance of 'meaningful' achievements and relationships with others, including healthcare professionals (Ira Byock: www.dyingwell.com).

Those who continue to repress these beliefs will report dreams and may be vulnerable to 'hallucinations' when given any psychoactive drug, including opiates. Dreams and hallucinations should be dealt with as such and explored as means to bring the unconscious forward in symbolic ways. This may need help from someone trained in work with the unconscious and imagination.

Collaboration: the wisdom of marrying approaches

We emphasise that our approach in no sense commits a biomedical approach to the bin; rather, that it must be balanced with the individual's construction of meaning around the three matched areas of tasks (biomedicine, etc.), relationships (the psychological) and resolution (the spiritual and ontological) as summarised in Figure 10.8. Above all, it is interdisciplinary.

Suffering: a simple algorithm

Finally, we may draw all the threads together to develop a simple and effective algorithm that gives the key elements in our analysis (Figure 10.9). The figure should

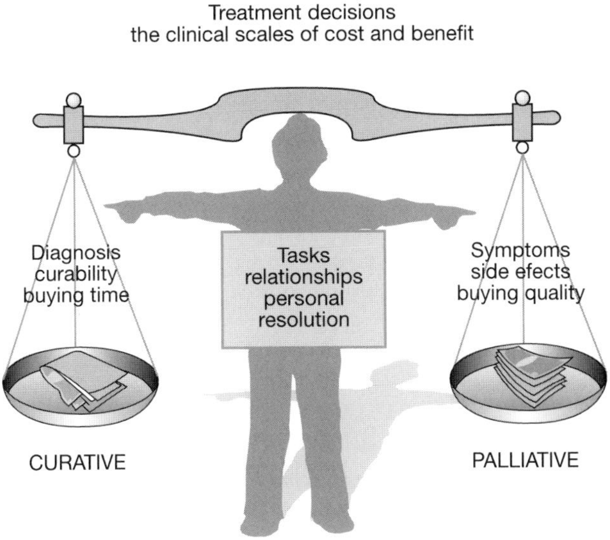

Treatment decisions
the clinical scales of cost and benefit

Diagnosis
curability
buying time

Tasks
relationships
personal
resolution

Symptoms
side efects
buying quality

CURATIVE

PALLIATIVE

Figure 10.8 However expressed, biomedical versus ontological or curative and palliative medicine, the approaches are not mutually exclusive. They must be balanced around the needs and agenda of the patient as s/he seeks to resolve their suffering.

be read from the left and offers the four main roots of conflict that we see in specialist palliative care. These at least should be looked at, ideally before a patient is in distress, to map areas of likely internal conflict. The team's responsibility is then to work at clearing a 'space' for the individual to have the time, energy, tools and motivation to examine relevant areas in a productive and calm way. In essence this involves:

- Review of the areas in question.
- Re-evaluation to discriminate between the facts of a problem and the perceived truth of what it means.
- Response to the problem. For example, the remorse or guilt of a past indiscretion when examined again may reveal to the individual that it is a paper tiger, or else that there is genuinely something that must be done. This may involve contact with a person, a letter written, a confession, etc. The help of a cleric may be necessary here.

The outcomes aimed for are:

- Resolution of the problem if it is a misperception.

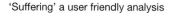

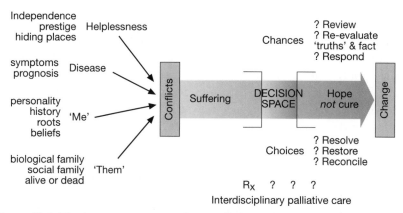

Figure 10.9 The keys to movement from suffering to hope is to offer manageable and achievable opportunities and approaches for patient and family to engage and transform conflicts into the vehicles for change. These challenges are complex and although they must be understood by physicians, they are the collective task of the interdisciplinary team. The areas are represented by the following symbols: R_x, technical symptom control; φ, psychological care; θ, spiritual care; ς, social care.

- Restoration of a belief if a patient has misunderstood some element of their faith. Or
- Reconciliation of a broken relationship if the person is alive, perhaps through a written letter, confession with an appropriate witness or the use of imagery, or of problems with people who are either dead or uncontactable may release a burden from a person's mind. Patients who have lived through wars or who have issues with dead relatives can gain enormous benefit from some ceremonial way of dealing with a problem that has life, reality and meaning for them.

These approaches are the elements of change within the person that may restore some sense of control or the freedom from images, thoughts or memories that have terrorised them up until then. They may appear false or banal to the fit and healthy. However, for the dying, in whom thoughts and the transcendent are far more real than the temporal, simple measures such as these can change their view of themselves, their intrinsic value and therefore their sense of being to astonishing degrees.

Conclusions

Although these models of the person and their symptoms may help professionals address uncertainties surrounding the suffering of their patients, by providing a framework within which to understand some of the relevant issues, it offers the bare bones of how to diagnose and begin to help patients access and address the meanings of their sufferings.

As we have stated above, the cardinal virtue for success in this is a practical wisdom. It is true that colleagues in other disciplines, such as psychologists, social workers and pastoral carers, have skills that are relevant to some of the issues raised. However, having said that, it behoves us all to strive to help our patients through their difficulties. In some, such as Nina, we will fail, but provided that we approach their troubles in a respectful manner, being aware of the great vulnerabilities that they bring to us and the vulnerabilities that we bring to them, it is better to have tried and failed than not to have tried at all. This is the essence of being human and helping each other to find water.

References

Autton, N. (1986). *Pain: an exploration*. London: Darton, Longman & Todd.

Byock, I. www.dyingwell.com

Cassel, E. J. (1982). The nature of suffering and the goals of medicine. *New England Journal of Medicine* **306**, 639–645.

Kissane, D. W. & Kelly, B. J. (2000). Demoralisation, depression and desire for death: problems with the Dutch guidelines for euthanasia of the mentally ill. *Australian and New Zealand Journal of Psychiatry* **34**, 325–333.

Randall, F. & Downie, R. S. (1999). *Palliative care ethics – a companion for all specialties*, 2nd edition. Oxford: Oxford University Press.

PART 3

The prevention and control of therapy-related nausea and vomiting

Chapter 11

Nausea and vomiting associated with chemotherapy: physiological mechanisms and pharmacological perspectives

Robin L. Jones and Paul L. R. Andrews

The biological context of nausea and vomiting

Both nausea and vomiting are elements of the physiological mechanism used by the body to protect against the accidental ingestion of toxins. However, for many cancer patients they are the most feared and troublesome side effects of cytotoxic chemotherapy and radiotherapy, and hence require anti-emetic treatment.

Chemotherapy-associated nausea and vomiting

Nausea and vomiting secondary to chemotherapy can reduce the quality of life of cancer patients (Morrow & Dobkin 1988; Stewart 1990) as well as leading to further complications, such as dehydration, anorexia, metabolic imbalances, psychological problems and anticipatory nausea and vomiting (Bilgrami & Fallon 1993). This can lead to treatment delays and reduce compliance with therapy. For highly emetic chemotherapy regimes (e.g. cisplatin greater than 70 mg/m^2), acute, delayed and anticipatory phases of nausea and vomiting can be identified (see below). Several studies have suggested that patients typically regard the control of nausea as more important than that of vomiting, whereas medical staff tend to have the opposite view.

Nausea can be described as the unpleasant sensation associated with the urge to vomit, which is frequently accompanied by autonomic nervous system activity, particularly the parasympathetic. Likewise, vomiting can be defined as the forceful oral expulsion of gastric contents.

Mechanisms

The sensation of nausea may be accompanied by indications of autonomic activation (tachycardia, cutaneous vasoconstriction, sweating, salivation). Large increases in plasma vasopressin (antidiuretic hormone: ADH) and disturbed gastric motility (e.g., tachyantria associated with decreased motility, proximal gastric relaxation) are consistently associated with nausea but a causal link has not been established (for references see Andrews (1999)). The precise brain pathways by which this sensation is generated are not known but imaging has implicated the inferior frontal gyrus. Understanding nausea is still a major challenge, particularly as this is often perceived by the patient (but not necessarily the doctor) as more troublesome than vomiting and because of its protracted nature. Most anti-emetics show efficacy against nausea but this is usually lower than the efficacy against vomiting.

Before the onset of vomiting the proximal stomach relaxes under the influence of the inhibitory neurotransmitters nitric oxide and vasoactive intestinal peptide, and a retrograde contraction (transmitter acetylcholine) of the small intestine occurs, both of which are under vagal efferent control (for references see Andrews (1999)). These changes are not the cause of the sensation of nausea. Forceful compression of the stomach by the diaphragm (innervated by the phrenic nerve) and anterior abdominal muscles results in the forceful oral expulsion of gastric contents. Coordination of the autonomic and somatic motor components occurs in the brainstem, which receives inputs from four main sources capable of inducing nausea, retching and vomiting: (i) vestibular system (motion sickness); (ii) 'higher regions' of the brain (e.g. amygdala); (iii) area postrema: this is one of the circumventricular organs, a region of the brainstem where the blood–brain barrier is relatively permeable and agents in the circulation may act to induce vomiting, e.g. morphine; (iv) abdominal vagal afferents (involved in vomiting evoked by gut distension, mucosal irritation and some systemic agents).

Treatment (including surgery and concomitant medication such as morphine), the physical effects of the malignancy itself (e.g. obstructing the gut or pressing on the brainstem) and tumour products could activate one or more of the above pathways to induce nausea and vomiting or to sensitise the pathway to other stimuli.

Acute and delayed nausea and vomiting

In the treatment of chemotherapy patients, it is important to distinguish between acute and delayed nausea and vomiting, which typically occurs after high doses of highly emetogenic agents such as cisplatin (greater than 50 mg/m^2) (Martin 1996). The acute phase is usually regarded as the first 24 h after administration of the chemotherapeutic agent, with emesis usually being most intense in the first 12 h (Hesketh *et al.* 2003). In the absence of anti-emetic prophylaxis, almost all patients treated with cisplatin greater than 50 mg/m^2 will experience acute emesis. In the acute phase, experimental studies have suggested that chemotherapy and radiation induce the formation of free radicals in the 5-hydroxytryptamine (5-HT) containing enterochromaffin (EC) cells in the small intestine, leading to local exocytotic release of 5-HT which activates the ligand-gated ion channel 5-HT$_3$ receptors located on the terminals of the abdominal vagal afferents projecting to the brainstem. The efficacy of 5-HT$_3$ receptor antagonists such as ondansetron (Zofran), granisetron (Kytril) and dolasetron (Anzemet) in the acute phase of chemotherapy-induced emesis supports this mechanism and it is proposed that the predominant site of the anti-emetic effect of this class of agent is peripheral, but this does not exclude a contribution from a central site probably in the nucleus tractus solitarius where the receptors are present in high density (Andrews 1995).

Delayed emesis after chemotherapy persists for 5–7 days with the peak being between days 2 and 3. In patients treated with cisplatin greater than 50 mg/m^2 the incidence is between 57% and 89% (Kris *et al.* 1994). The relative lack of efficacy of 5-HT$_3$ receptor antagonists in this phase implicates a different mechanism from the acute phase. It probably involves multiple mechanisms including the products of cell breakdown (perhaps acting on the area postrema), inflammation (local mediators such as substance P could act on vagal afferents) and disrupted gastrointestinal motility (detected by mechanosensitive vagal afferents); the limited efficacy of dexamethasone and metoclopramide supports this proposal but additional mechanistic studies are still required. Even with best current anti-emetic prophylaxis (a 5-HT$_3$ receptor antagonist or metoclopramide and dexamethasone), up to 50% of patients still experience delayed emesis although this may change with the introduction of the neurokinin$_1$ (NK$_1$) receptor antagonists that act on the preferred receptor for substance P (see below) (Hesketh 2001).

Anticipatory nausea and vomiting

Patients who experience symptoms with their initial cycles of chemotherapy can develop nausea and vomiting in expectation of their subsequent cycles of therapy. Anticipatory nausea and vomiting develops in approximately 30% of patients by their fourth cycle of chemotherapy. In addition, certain patient characteristics are associated with anticipatory nausea and vomiting: (i) age younger than 50; (ii) nausea and vomiting after last chemotherapy; (iii) susceptibility to motion sickness; (iv) expectations of post-therapy nausea; (v) anxiety; (vi) hostility or depression; (vii) generalized weakness, sweating or 'feeling warm all over' after the last chemotherapy session (Morrow 1993). It has been suggested that the development of anticipatory nausea and vomiting involves classical conditioning (Montgomery & Bovbjerg 1997). Once this problem has become apparent it is virtually impossible to treat with drug intervention but behavioural treatment can be used to alleviate it.

However, a patient who experiences no post-therapy nausea or vomiting is very unlikely to develop anticipatory symptoms so the emphasis should be on optimal anti-emetic therapy from the first course of chemotherapy.

Predictive factors

The variation in the severity and frequency of nausea and vomiting associated with chemotherapy has led to the suggestion that there are endogenous factors that make patients more or less sensitive to these side effects of chemotherapy. Several of the factors identified above as risk factors for anticipatory nausea and vomiting are also factors that influence the responses in the acute and delayed phases. The patients most at risk are young females who do not drink alcohol. In addition in both sexes previous emetic history (e.g. sensitivity to motion, pregnancy sickness) is also a risk factor. In post-operative nausea and vomiting (PONV) tobacco smoking is protective (Apfel *et al.* 1999) but it is not clear if this is also the case in chemotherapy-induced emesis. Racial factors have been little studied but it is well established that Orientals are more sensitive to motion sickness than are Westerners (Xu *et al.* 1993). Understanding these factors is of considerable interest so that anti-emetic treatment algorithms incorporating patient characteristics and chemotherapy emetogenicity can be produced to improve patient care. Such algorithms are well established in PONV (see, for example, Apfel *et al.* 2002) and could provide a model for their development in chemotherapy-induced nausea and vomiting. There has been considerable interest in identifying 'physiological' predictive factors so that patients at most risk could be identified and their anti-emetic regime tailored or dose schedules modified to coincide with when the onset of nausea or emesis is expected. The autonomic nervous system and hypothalamic pituitary axis have been most studied and are outlined briefly

Autonomic nervous system

Several studies have shown that changes in the autonomic nervous system may predict the response of individual patients to chemotherapy (see, for example, Fredrikson *et al.* 1993; Bellg *et al.* 1995). In patients with ovarian cancer treated with cisplatin, Morrow *et al.* (2000) showed that the onset of the first report of nausea occurred consistently after the standard deviation of successive differences (SDSD; a measure of cardiac parasympathetic nerve activity used as marker for more general parasympathetic changes) began to decline after reaching a peak. It could be possible to use this peak to time administration of an anti-emetic agent.

Hypothalamic–pituitary–adrenal axis

Many of the side effects associated with chemotherapy (nausea, vomiting and fatigue), are also characteristic of adrenal insufficiency. It is thus possible that cytotoxic drugs may directly or indirectly influence the activity of the hypothalamic–pituitary–adrenal axis. Dexamethasone (and other steroids including methylprednisolone) is widely used as an anti-emetic in oncology, and as a consequence investigators have studied the role of cortisol in chemotherapy-induced emesis. Hursti *et al.* (1993) have shown a relation between nocturnal urinary cortisol and the intensity of nausea on the day of treatment and for 2 days afterwards. Cortisol production follows a circadian rhythm, the level being at its lowest in late evening and highest between 05.00 and 09.00; this has been linked to the observation that emesis after platinum is lowest when the cytotoxic is given at 18.00 compared with when it is given at 06.00 (Seymour *et al.* 1993).

A pharmacogenetic study of 5-HT_{3B} receptor gene polymorphisms in cancer patients undergoing chemotherapy and given a 5-HT_3 receptor antagonist to treat the emesis revealed that patients homozygous for the -100_-102delAAG deletion variant of the promoter region had more episodes of vomiting in the acute phase of emesis than patients who were not homozygous for this deletion (Tremblay *et al.* 2003). The authors comment that only a small part of the therapeutic failure of the 5-HT_3 receptor antagonist could be ascribed to the deletion variant. Similar studies in PONV patients would be of considerable interest especially if combined with assessment of more conventional risk factors.

A study of 23 women with ovarian cancer was performed for serial cortisol levels before and after platinum-based chemotherapy over two cycles. Samples were also taken on a comparison day when no chemotherapy was given, but patients underwent all the procedures experienced apart from the administration of cytotoxic therapy (Morrow *et al.* 2002). After administration of the platinum-based therapy an acute fall in serum cortisol was found. No progressive fall in basal cortisol levels was observed over the two treatment cycles.

Despite these studies a conclusive causal relation has not been demonstrated. However, if a causal relation were shown, then cortisol levels could possibly be used as a means of identifying patients at risk of nausea and vomiting, along with other predictive parameters.

5-Hydroxytryptamine$_3$ receptor antagonists

5-HT$_3$ receptors are one of at least 14 different types or subtypes of 5-HT receptor. The 5-HT$_3$ receptor belongs to the ligand-gated ion channel family of receptors so that when 5-HT binds to the receptor it opens an ion channel leading to cell depolarisation. They are widely distributed in the nervous system and those of most relevance to emesis are located on vagal afferent fibres, in the nucleus tractus solitarius (high density) and on EC cells in the gut. These drugs have a predominately peripheral site anti-emetic action blocking the effect of 5-HT released from the EC cells on the 5-HT$_3$ receptors located on the abdominal vagal afferent terminals, but a contribution from the 5-HT$_3$ receptors in the brainstem cannot be excluded. The role (if any) of these central 5-HT$_3$ receptors in emesis is unclear as 5-HT$_3$ receptor antagonists do not appear to have anti-emetic effects against motion or opioid-induced emesis (Shoji *et al.* 1999) although their efficacy in PONV is difficult to explain without invoking at least a contribution from central receptors (Andrews 2003). It must be noted that a lack of efficacy of a 5-HT$_3$ receptor antagonist in emesis does not exclude the involvement of 5-HT in emesis as the 5-HT could be acting upon one or more of the many other types of receptor.

The past 15 years have seen a dramatic improvement in the treatment of acute phase nausea and vomiting associated with chemotherapy because of the introduction of 5-HT$_3$ receptor antagonists (e.g. ondansetron, granisetron, dolasetron, tropisetron). They are clinically better at controlling vomiting compared with earlier anti-emetic drugs, but may become less effective with repeated chemotherapy cycles (De Wit *et al.* 1996). Unfortunately, they do not appear to be more effective than previous drugs at controlling nausea (Morrow *et al.* 1998).

The anti-emetic effects of the 5-HT$_3$ receptor antagonists can be potentiated if they are used in combination with the glucocorticoid dexamethasone. In a study reported by Roila *et al.* (1993) emesis on day 1 (acute phase) was completely controlled in 79% of patients who received this combination, compared with 59% in those who received high dose metoclopramide, dexamethasone and diphenhydramine ($p < 0.002$).

On days 2–4 (delayed phase) patients in both arms received metoclopramide and dexamethasone. It was found that significantly fewer patients who received ondansetron on day 1 developed delayed emesis (84–86% and 68–71%, respectively; $p < 0.006$) (Roila et al. 1993). Other investigators have found that the efficacy of this combination of a 5-HT$_3$ receptor antagonist and dexamethasone is not maintained with successive cycles of chemotherapy. De Wit et al. (1996) report an initial complete control rate of 71% decreasing to 43% with the sixth cycle of chemotherapy. This apparent reduction in efficacy is a problem that needs to be addressed in the development of any novel approaches to anti-emesis.

Cannabinoids

Anecdotal reports that smoking marijuana had a beneficial effect against cytotoxic-induced emesis, lead to 9-tetra-hydrocannabinol being investigated as an anti-emetic (Sallan et al. 1980). Over the past few years, requests have been made for the legalisation of this class of drug for use in various medical conditions. Side effects associated with these drugs can include sedation, dizziness, dysphoria, hallucinations and paranoia. A combination of nabilone and prochlorperazine was found to have a significant reduction in the incidence of adverse effects on the central nervous system; the exact mechanism of this finding has not been explained (Cunningham et al. 1985). A recent systemic review evaluated the efficacy and adverse effects associated with this class of compound in the treatment of chemotherapy-induced emesis (Tramer et al. 2001). In this review oral nabilone and dronabinol and intramuscular levonantradol displayed slightly superior activity compared with conventional anti-emetics after chemotherapy. Despite the potentially serious side-effect profile, patients expressed a preference for these agents. However, adverse effects are likely to limit the widespread use of this class of drug, although they may still have a role in a selected group of patients as mood-enhancing adjuncts in the control of chemotherapy-induced emesis.

Recently there appears to have been a resurgence of interest in cannabinoid pharmacology. Two pre-clinical studies have demonstrated that agonists at the cannabinoid$_1$ receptor (CB$_1$) were anti-emetic when tested against emesis induced by morphine or morphine-6-glucuronide (Simoneau et al. 2001; Van Sickle et al. 2001). Advances in pharmacology may mean that the development of selective cannabinoid agonists devoid of unacceptable side effects may be possible. One of the studies also showed that the emetic threshold could be reduced by treatment with a CB$_1$ receptor antagonist, providing evidence that endogenous cannabinoids may be involved in modulating emetic sensitivity. Such endogenous modulatory systems are likely to be involved in determining an individual patient's emetic response to treatment.

Neurokinin-1 receptor antagonists

Substance P is an 11 amino acid neuropeptide of the tachykinin family of peptides and is the preferred endogenous ligand for the neurokinin-1 (NK$_1$) receptor. It is a neurotransmitter in both the central and the autonomic divisions of the nervous system and is also found in high concentrations in the intestinal mucosal EC cells (i.e. the same location as 5-HT, see above). The development of small molecular mass, brain penetrant, non-peptide, selective antagonists allowed the functions of the NK_1 receptor and substance P to be explored. Pre-clinical studies have shown that in contrast to $5-HT_3$ receptor antagonists, NK_1 receptor antagonists are able to antagonize a much broader spectrum of emetic stimuli (see Watson *et al.* 1995; Andrews & Rudd 2004). Their action requires entry into the central nervous system and it is proposed that their site of action is in the brainstem, most likely in the nucleus tractus solitarius (see above). In the ferret and piglet, NK_1 receptor antagonists have displayed activity in both acute and delayed emesis (Rudd *et al.* 1996; Grelot *et al.* 1998). These observations prompted clinical trials in chemotherapy-induced nausea and vomiting, with a particular emphasis on the delayed phase. In the absence of anti-emetic prophylaxis, almost 90% of patients receiving highly emetogenic regimes (e.g. cisplatin not less than 80 mg/m^2) will have nausea and vomiting in the delayed phase, and even with current standard anti-emetic prophylaxis approximately 50% of patients will develop delayed emesis (Kris *et al.* 1994; Tavorath *et al.* 1996).

The first reported phase I/II trial used the NK_1 receptor antagonist CP-122, 721 in combination with a $5-HT_3$ receptor antagonist and dexamethasone. Kris *et al.* (1997) found that 17% of patients who received the NK_1 receptor antagonist in combination with the other two standard drugs developed delayed emesis. This compared favourably with 83% developing delayed emesis in the group that received dexamethasone and a $5-HT_3$ antagonist.

Studies comparing regimes including an NK_1 receptor antagonist or ondansetron were done by Cocquyt *et al.* (2001) and Van Belle *et al.* (2002). The former compared the effect of either L-758, 298 (the pro-drug for L-754-030 / MK-806) or ondansetron administration to patients receiving cisplatin in the absence of dexamethasone. In the acute phase there was no significant difference between the two treatments in the number of patients who were emesis free, but in the delayed phase significantly more patients were emesis free in the L-758, 298 group (72%) compared with the ondansetron group (30%). In this study anti-emetics were only given on day 1, and this provides some evidence for a 'carry-over' effect of the NK_1 receptor antagonist into the delayed phase. In the Van Belle *et al.* (2002) study, the MK-869 pro-drug L-758, 298 was investigated. The first group received 100 mg intravenously of L-758, 298, then dexamethasone followed by cisplatin on day 1. A dose of 300 mg of MK-869 was given orally on days 2–5. The second group received the same regimen on day 1 followed by placebo on days 2–5. The final group were given ondansetron and dexamethasone followed by cisplatin on the first day. It was found that the dexamethasone and ondansetron combination was significantly ($p < 0.05$) better at controlling acute emesis. However, the group that received continued dosing with MK-869 experienced better control of delayed emesis, although there was no statistically significant difference between the three regimens.

Hesketh *et al.* (1999) randomised patients between granisetron and dexamethasone with or without the NK_1 receptor antagonist CJ-11,974 before cisplatin chemotherapy. The primary end-point of this study was the frequency of delayed emesis. In the CJ-11, 974 arm, 67.8% of patients had no delayed emesis compared with 36.6% in the other arm ($p = 0.0425$). The patients who received the NK_1 receptor antagonist also had less delayed nausea, but this difference was not statistically significant.

The largest trial investigating the use of NK_1 receptor antagonists was published by Campos *et al.* (2001). Patients receiving platinum-based therapy were randomised into four groups. All received dexamethasone before cisplatin. The first group were treated with granisetron before chemotherapy and then placebo on days 2–5. Group two received granisetron and MK-869 on the first day and placebo on days 2–5. The third arm received two doses of MK-869, 12 h apart on day 1. Subsequently, they were given MK-869 on days 2–5. The last group were randomised to MK-869 before cisplatin, followed by MK-869 on days 2–5. The combination of an NK_1 antagonist and dexamethasone was less effective than granisetron and dexamethasone. Delayed emesis was better controlled in arms that received MK-869 compared with the arm that was treated with granisetron and dexamethasone. However, the best overall results were observed with an NK_1 receptor antagonist combined with dexamethasone and granisetron. These results are supported by two other earlier studies by Hesketh *et al.* (1999) and Navari *et al.* (1999).

Clearly, additional randomised controlled trials are required to elucidate the exact role of these agents in the treatment and prevention of nausea and vomiting associated with chemotherapy. At the doses used in the above studies no dose limiting toxicities have been reported and their adverse event profile has been very encouraging. Their efficacy, combined with dexamethasone, in preventing acute cisplatin-induced emesis is inferior to that of a $5\text{-}HT_3$ receptor antagonist and dexamethasone. However, when the three drug classes are combined, control of acute emesis is improved by 20–30% over a two-drug regimen consisting of dexamethasone and a $5\text{-}HT_3$ antagonist. These agents improve control of delayed cisplatin-induced emesis by 30–40% compared with a placebo. There is also some evidence that their efficacy is maintained over repeated cycles (up to six) of chemotherapy.

The first member of this class of agent (Emend®, Aprepitant/MK–869) was approved by the US Food and Drug Administration (FDA) in April 2003 for use in combination with other anti-emetic agents for the prevention of acute and delayed nausea and vomiting associated with highly emetogenic cancer chemotherapy. This agent has also been licensed for a similar indication by the European Medicine Evaluation Agency in July 2003.

Conclusion

Chemotherapy-induced nausea and vomiting are among the most common and significant side effects of cytotoxic treatment. The use of $5\text{-}HT_3$ receptor antagonists has revolutionised the treatment of acute emesis associated with chemotherapy. These agents, in combination with dexamethasone, are now used extensively as prophylaxis for the treatment of acute and delayed emesis (Gralla *et al.* 2000). Many patients continue to experience delayed emesis. NK_1 receptor antagonists (with other drugs) are promising candidates for achieving better control of delayed emesis but further randomised controlled trials are required to elucidate their exact role. Such studies will also improve our understanding of the neuropharmacology of chemotherapy-induced nausea and vomiting in humans.

References

Andrews, P. L. R. (1995). 5-HT_3 receptor antagonists and anti-emesis.. In *5-HT-3 receptor antagonists* (ed. F. D. King, B. J. Jones, G. J. Sanger), pp. 255–317. Boca Raton, Florida: CRC Press.

Andrews, P. L. R. (2003). Approaching an understanding of the mechanism of post-operative nausea and vomiting. In *The effective prevention and management of post-operative nausea and vomiting. 2nd Edition.* (ed. L. Strunin, D. Rowbotham & A. Miles), pp. 3–28. London: Aesculapius Medical Press, London.

Andrews, P. L. R. (1999). Nausea, vomiting and the autonomic nervous system. In *Autonomic failure: a textbook of clinical disorders of the autonomic nervous system*, 4th edition (ed. C. J. Mathias & R. Bannister), pp. 126–135. Oxford: Oxford University Press.

Andrews, P. L. R. and Rudd, J. G. (2004). Neurokinin$_1$ receptors and emesis. In *Handbook of experimental pharmacology* (ed. P. Holzer). Berlin and Heidelberg: Springer. (In the press.)

Apfel, C. C., Katz, M. H., Kranke, P., Goepfert, C., Papenfuss, T., Rauch, S., Heineck, R., Greim, C.-A. & Roewer, N. (2002). Volatile anaesthetics may be the main cause of early but not delayed postoperative vomiting: a random controlled trial of factorial design. *British Journal of Anaesthesia* **88**, 1–10.

Apfel, C. C., Laara, E., Koivuranta, M., Greim, C. A. & Roewer, N. (1999). A simplified risk score for predicting postoperative nausea and vomiting: conclusions form cross-validations between two centres. *Anesthesiology* **91**, 693–700.

Bilgrami, S. & Fallon, B. G. (1993). Chemotherapy-induced nausea and vomiting. Easing patients' fears and discomfort with effective antiemetic regimens. *Postgraduate Medicine* **94**, 55–58.

Campos, D., Rodrigues-Pereira, J., Reinhardt, R. R., Carracedo, C., Ploi, S., Vogel, C., Martinez-Cedillo, J., Erazo A, Wittreich J, Eriksson L.-O. *et al.* (2001). Prevention of cisplatin-induced emesis by the oral neurokinin-1 antagonist, MK-869, in combination with granisetron and dexamethasone or with dexamethasone alone. *Journal of Clinical Oncology* **19**, 1759–1767.

Cocquyt, V., Van Belle, S., Reinhardt, R.R., Decramer, M.L.A., O'Brien, M., Schellens, J.H.M., Borms, M., Verbeke, L., Van Aelst, F., De Smet, M. *et al.* (2001). Comparison of L-758, 298, a prodrug for the selective neurokinin-1 antagonist, L-754-030, with ondansetron for the prevention of cisplatin-induced emesis. *European Journal of Cancer* **37**, 835–842.

Cunningham, D., Forrest, G. J., Soukop, M. *et al.* (1985). Nabilone and prochlorperazine: a useful combination for emesis-induced by cytotoxic drugs. *British Medical Journal* **291**, 864–865.

De Wit, R., Schmitz, P. I., Verweij, J., de Boer-Dennert, M., de Mulder, P. H., Planting, A. S., van der Burg, M. E. & Stoter, G. 1996. Analysis of cumulative probabilities shows the efficacy of 5HT_3 antagonist prophylaxis is not maintained. *Journal of Clinical Oncology* **14**, 644–651.

Fredrikson, M., Hursti, T., Sami, P., Borjeson, S., Furst, C. J., Peterson, C. & Steineck, G. (1993). Conditioned nausea after cancer chemotherapy and autonomic nervous system conditionability. *Scandinavian Journal of Psychology* **34**, 318–327.

Gralla, R. J., Osoba, D., Kris, M. G., Kirkbride, P., Hesketh, P. J., Chinnery, L. W., Clark-Snow, R., Gill, D.P., Grosheen, S., Grunberg S. *et al.* (2000). Recommendations for the use of antiemetics: evidence-based, clinical practice guidelines. *Journal of Clinical Oncology* **17**, 2971–2994.

Grelot, L., Dapzol, J., Estève, E., Frugiere, A., Bianchi, A. L., Sheldrick, R. L., Gardner, C. J. & Ward, P. (1998). Potent inhibition of both the acute and delayed emetic responses to cisplatin in piglets treated with GR205171, a novel highly selective tachykinin NK1 receptor antagonist. *British Journal of Pharmacology* **124**, 1643–1650.

Hesketh, P. J. (2001). Potential role of the NK1 receptor antagonists in chemotherapy-induced nausea and vomiting. *Supplementary Care in Cancer* **9**, 350–354.

Hesketh, P. J., Gralla, R. J., Webb, R. T., Ueno, W., Del Prete, S., Bachinsky, M. E., Dirlam, N. L., Stack, C. B. & Silberman, S. L. (1999). Randomised phase II study of the neurokinin-1 receptor antagonist CJ-11, 974 in the control of cisplatin-induced emesis. *Journal of Clinical Oncology* **17**, 338–343.

Hesketh, P. J., Van Belle, S., Aapro, M., Tattersall, F. D., Naylor, R. J., Hargreaves, R., Carides, A. D., Evans, J. K. & Horgan, K. J. (2003). Differential involvement of neurotransmitters through the time course of cisplatin-induced emesis as revealed by therapy with specific receptor antagonists. *European Journal of Cancer* **39**, 1074–1080.

Hursti, T., Fredrikson, M., Steineck, G., Borjeson, S. & Peterson, C. (1993). Endogenous cortisol exerts antiemetic effect similar to that of exogenous corticosteroids. *British Journal of Cancer* **68**, 112–114.

Kris, M.G., Pisters, K. M. W. & Hinkley, L. (1994). Delayed emesis following anti-cancer chemotherapy. *Supplementary Care in Cancer* **2**, 297–300.

Kris, M. G., Radford, J., Pizzo, B. A., Inabinet, R., Hesketh, A. G. & Hesketh, P. (1997). Control of emesis following cisplatin by CP-122,721, a selective NK1 receptor antagonist. *Journal of the National Cancer Institute* **89**, 817–818.

Martin, M. (1996). The severity and pattern of emesis following different cytotoxic agents. *Oncology* **53**, 26–31.

Montgomery, G. H. & Bovbjerg, D. H. (1997). The development of anticipatory nausea in patients receiving adjuvant chemotherapy for breast cancer. *Physiology and Behavior* **61**, 737–741.

Morrow, G. R. (1993). Psychological aspects of nausea and vomiting: Anticipation of chemotherapy. In *The Handbook of Nausea and Vomiting* (ed. M. H. Sleisenger), pp. 11–25. New York: Parthenon Publishing.

Morrow, G. R., Andrews, P. L., Hickok, J. T. & Stern, R. (2000). Vagal changes following cancer chemotherapy: implications for the development of nausea. *Psychophysiology* **37**, 378–384.

Morrow, G. R. & Dobkin, P. L. (1988). Anticipatory nausea and vomiting in cancer patients undergoing chemotherapy treatment: prevalence, etiology and behavioural interventions. *Clinical Psychology Review* **8**, 517–556.

Morrow, G. R., Roscoe, J. A., Hynes, H. E., Flynn, P. J., Pierce, H. I. & Burish, T. (1998). Progress in reducing anticipatory nausea and vomiting: a study of community practice. *Supportive Care in Cancer* **6**, 46–50.

Morrow, G. R., Hickok, J. T., Andrews, P. L. R. & Stern, R. M. (2002). Reduction in serum cortisol after platinum based chemotherapy for cancer: a role for the HPA axis in treatment-related nausea? *Psychophysiology* **39**, 491–495.

Navari, R. M., Reinhardt, R. R., Gralla, R. J., Kris, M. G., Hesketh, P. J., Khojasteh, A., Kindler, H., Grote, T. H., Pendergrass, K., Grunberg, S. M. *et al.* (1999). Reduction of cisplatin-induced emesis by a selective neurokinin receptor antagonist. *New England Journal of Medicine* **340**, 190–195.

Roila, F. and the Italian Group for Antiemetic Research (1992). Ondansetron+dexamethasone vs. metoclopramide +dexamethasone+diphenhydramine in prevention of cisplatin-induced emesis. *The Lancet* **340**, 96–99.

Roscoe, J. A., Hickok, J. T & Morrow, G. R. (2000). Patient expectations as predictor of chemotherapy-induced nausea. *Annals of Behavioural Medicine* **22**, 121–126.

Rudd, J. A., Jordan, C. C. & Naylor, R. J. (1996). The action of an NK1 tachykinin receptor antagonist, CP99,994, in antagonizing the acute and delayed emesis induced by cisplatin in the ferret. *British Journal of Pharmacology* **119**, 931–936.

Sallan, S. E., Zinberg, N. E. & Frei, E. (1980). Antiemetic effect of delta-9-tetrahydrocannabinol and prochlorperazine. *New England Journal of Medicine* **302**, 135–138.

Seymour, M. T. (1993). The pharmacokinetics and pharmacodynamics of chemotherapeutic agent. In *Emesis in anti-cancer therapy, mechanisms and treatment* (ed. P. L. R. Andrews & G. J. Sanger), pp. 9–44. London: Chapman and Hall.

Shoji, A., Toda, M., Suzuki, K., Takahashi, K., Yoshiike, Y., Ogura, T., Watanuki, Y., Nishiyama, H. & Odagiri, S. (1999). Insufficient effectiveness of 5-hydroxytryptamine-2 receptor antagonisms due to oral morphine administration in patients with cisplatin-induced emesis. *Journal of Clinical Oncology* **17**, 1926–1930.

Simoneau, I. I., Hamza, M. S., Mata, H. P., Siegel, E. M., Vanderah, T. W., Porreca, F., Makriyannis, A. & Malan, T. P. (2001). The cannabinoid agonist WIN55, 212-2 suppresses opioid-induced emesis in ferrets. *Anesthesiology* **94**, 882–887.

Stewart, D. J. (1990). Cancer therapy, vomiting and antiemetics. *Canadian Journal of Physiology and Pharmacology* **68**, 304–313.

Tavorath, R. & Hesketh, P. J. (1996). Drug treatment of chemotherapy-induced delayed emesis. *Drugs* **52**, 639–648.

Tramer, M. R., Carroll, D., Campbell, F. A., Reynolds, D. J. M., Moore, R. A. & McQuay, H. J. (2001). Cannabinoids for control of chemotherapy induced nausea and vomiting: quantitative systemic review. *British Medical Journal* **323**, 1–8.

Tremblay, P. B., Kaiser, R., Sezer, O., Roler, N., Schelenz, C., Possinger, K., Roots, I. & Brockmoller, J. (2003). Variations in the 5-HT_{3B} receptor gene as predictors of the efficacy of anti-emetic treatment in cancer patients. *Journal of Clinical Oncology* **21**, 2147–2155.

Van Belle, S., Lichinitser, M. R., Navari, R. M., Garin, A. M., Decramer, M. L. A., Riviere, A., Thant, M., Brestan, E., Bui, B., Eldridge, K. *et al.* (2002). Prevention of cisplatin-induced acute and delayed emesis by the selective neurokinin-1 antagonists, L-758, 298 and MK-869. *Cancer* **94**, 3032–3041.

Van Sickle, M. D., Oland, L. D., Ho, W., Hillard, C. J., Mackie, K., Davison, J. S. & Sharkey, K. A. (2001). Cannabinoids inhibit emesis through CB1 receptors in the brainstem of the ferret. *Gastroenterology* **121**, 767–774.

Watson, J. W., Gonsalves, S. F., Fossa, A. A., McLean, S., Seeger, T., Obach, S. & Andrews, P. L. R. (1995). The anti-emetic effects of CP-99, 994 in the ferret and the dog: role of the NK_1 receptor. *British Journal of Pharmacology* **115**, 84–94.

Xu, L. H., Koch, K. L., Summy-Long, J., Stern, R. M., Seaton, J. F., Harrison, T. S., Demers, L. M. & Bingaman, S. (1993). Hypothalamic and gastric myoelectrical responses during circular vection-induced nausea in healthy Chinese subjects. *American Journal of Physiology, Endocrinology and Metabolism* **265**, E578–E583.

Chapter 12

Therapy-induced nausea and vomiting: assessment of severity and indications for treatment

Nicola S. Stoner

Introduction

The prevention and control of nausea and vomiting are paramount in the treatment of cancer patients. The goal of anti-emetic therapy is to prevent nausea and vomiting completely (Gralla *et al.* 1999). This has been achieved for many patients by the improved control of emesis over the past 20 years. However, nausea and vomiting remain two of the more distressing and feared side effects to cancer patients and their families (Gralla *et al.* 1999; Grunberg *et al.* 2002). Nausea and vomiting can also result in serious metabolic derangements, nutritional depletion and anorexia, deterioration of patients' physical and mental status, oesophageal tears, fractures, withdrawal from potentially useful and curative chemotherapy treatment, and degeneration of self-care and functional ability (National Cancer Institute website 2002). Further research is required to ensure the reduction in this side effect continues (Gralla *et al.* 1999).

Assessment of nausea and vomiting

Vomiting is usually measured by counting the number of vomiting episodes, and it is the most important end point. Complete control (no vomiting) is achievable in most patients in the first 24 h, and in approximately 45% of patients during the first 5–7 days of chemotherapy. It is a highly accurate and reliable measure. Complete control of vomiting correlates highly with patients' perception of emesis, and their satisfaction with treatment, which demonstrates the validity of this measure. Lesser control rates, such as major control (zero to two or one to two emetic episodes) or minor control (three to five emetic episodes), have been useful in the past and may still have some value in particularly difficult emetic situations (Gralla *et al.* 1999).

The mechanisms responsible for mediating nausea are less well explained. Nausea, or the perception that emesis may occur, can only be judged by the patient. The incidence of nausea correlates well with the incidence of vomiting. However, chemotherapy-induced nausea occurs at a greater frequency than vomiting. Questionnaires using either visual analogue or categorical scales are widely used to assess nausea (Gralla *et al.* 1999). Nausea can be classified as mild, moderate and severe (Gralla *et al.* 1999; National Cancer Institute website 2002).

Total control (no vomiting or nausea) is essentially identical to the complete nausea control rate, so this category does not provide further useful information. Nausea and vomiting should be assessed separately (Gralla *et al.* 1999).

Classification of nausea and vomiting

Commonly used classifications of nausea and vomiting are anticipatory nausea and vomiting (ANV), acute nausea and vomiting (or emesis), delayed nausea and vomiting (or emesis), and chronic nausea and vomiting.

ANV is a classical conditioning response, which occurs days to hours before a new cycle of chemotherapy, in response to conditioned stimuli such as the smells, sights and sounds of the treatment room. It is a classically conditioned response that typically occurs after three or four prior chemotherapy treatments, usually following which the person experiences acute or delayed nausea and vomiting. Anticipatory nausea occurs in 29% and anticipatory vomiting in 11% of patients receiving chemotherapy. The introduction of the serotonin receptor antagonists does not seem to have reduced the incidence of anticipatory nausea and vomiting (National Cancer Institute website 2002).

Acute nausea and vomiting occurs in the initial 24 h after therapy. Its incidence and severity varies according to the drug or field of radiation, dose, schedule of administration and individual patient variables (Feyer *et al.* 1998).

Delayed nausea and vomiting occurs more than 24 h after chemotherapy administration. It is associated with cisplatin, cyclophosphamide, doxorubicin, ifosfamide when given at high doses or on more than two consecutive days. Patients who experience acute emesis with chemotherapy are significantly more likely to have delayed emesis (National Cancer Institute website 2002).

Chronic nausea and vomiting occurs in patients with advanced cancer. It is associated with a variety of potential aetiologies, such as physical complications of cancer like brain metastases or bowel obstruction, or metabolic complications like hypercalcaemia, or unrelated factors like gastric ulcers or gastroenteritis (National Cancer Institute website 2002). Any underlying emesis needs to be considered before giving therapy, when deciding on an anti-emetic regimen.

Patient risk factors

The frequency, severity and onset of emesis are related to the emetic potential of the therapy and to the emetic risk profile of the patient for both chemotherapy- and radiotherapy-induced nausea and vomiting (Feyer *et al.* 1998; Gralla 1999). Several patient factors have been shown to predict poor anti-emetic control. These factors include female sex, younger age, a history of sickness (pregnancy, motion), poor control with prior chemotherapy, underlying nausea and vomiting, or a low chronic alcohol intake or history (Gralla *et al.* 1999). A history of high alcohol use is considered to be greater than 100 g of alcohol per day for a period of several years.

Generally the higher the alcohol intake history, the lower the emetic risk with chemotherapy (Gralla *et al.* 1999). Patients with a history of motion sickness and poor control with previous chemotherapy are predisposed to anticipatory emesis (Gralla *et al.* 1999).

Emetic risk of chemotherapy

Chemotherapy agents are classified by emetic potential, which helps select appropriate anti-emetics (Table 12.1). The American Society of Clinical Oncology (ASCO) (Gralla *et al.* 1999) and European Society for Medical Oncology (ESMO) (Fauser *et al.* 1999; Herrstedt 2000) guidelines place all these agents in the same category for anti-emetic treatment recommendations. Prospective documentation of the potential of a chemotherapy drug to cause emesis has only been rigorously established for a few agents. There is no clear evidence of the emetic potential for most chemotherapy agents and combinations. General categories are based on experience rather than on specific data. Combination treatment increases the emetic potential.

However, for the highly emetic chemotherapy, the literature clearly documents the incidence of emesis with cisplatin. Cisplatin causes acute emesis in all patients without active anti-emetics, and delayed emesis in 60–90% of patients. The risk of acute emesis with dacarbazine and mustine is greater than 90%. The risk of emesis with cyclophosphamide is also well established. The risk of emesis with the other agents in this group is greater than 30% (Gralla *et al.* 1999).

The risk of acute emesis in the intermediate emetic group is 10–30%. The emesis induced in this group is easier to control than that found in the higher-risk category. The incidence of delayed emesis is 20–30%. Irinotecan could be considered on the border of the higher category, and some of the other agents could be considered on the border of the lower category, e.g. mitomycin (Fauser *et al.* 1999; Gralla *et al.* 1999; Herrstedt 2000). The risk of emesis with low emetic risk agents is less than 10% (Gralla *et al.* 1999).

Radiotherapy-induced emesis

Radiotherapy-induced nausea and vomiting is generally less severe than that induced by chemotherapy. The latent period preceding the onset of nausea and vomiting is shorter after radiotherapy than that seen after chemotherapy. The pattern of emesis is easier to determine with single-fraction radiotherapy than with fractionated treatment. Fractionated treatment can comprise up to 40 sessions given over a period of 6–8 weeks. Nausea and vomiting during that length of period can be particularly distressing for patients (Feyer *et al.* 1998).

Acute emesis is seen most frequently with radiotherapy. The latent period ranges from 30 min to 4 h in single fraction studies, and is shorter with higher doses of radiation (Feyer *et al.* 1998). Acute emesis lasts 6–8 h, followed by a recovery period (Tramer *et al.* 1998). Delayed emesis is not seen with radiotherapy like that seen with

Table 12.1 Emetic risk of chemotherapy (Fauser *et al.* 1999; Gralla *et al.* 1999; Herrstedt 2000)

1. High emetic risk
cisplatin
dacarbazine
actinomycin-D
mustine
carmustine
carboplatin
oxaliplatin
daunorubicin
doxorubicin ≥60 mg/m^2
epirubicin ≥90 mg/m^2
idarubicin
cytarabine
ifosfamide
cyclophosphamide

2. Intermediate emetic risk
irinotecan
topotecan
mitoxantrone
paclitaxel
docetaxel
gemcitabine
etoposide
teniposide
mitomycin
methotrexate 50–250 mg/m^2

3. Low emetic risk
busulfan (low dose)
chlorambucil
fludarabine
hydroxyurea
methotrexate ≤50 mg/m^2
vinca alkaloids
5-fluorouracil
bleomycin

cisplatin, and anticipatory emesis is extremely rare. However, prolonged emesis lasting 2–3 days is reported by up to 40% of patients (Feyer *et al.* 1998).

The most important factors influencing radiation-induced emesis are shown in Table 12.2 (Feyer *et al.* 1998). Fractionated irradiation may have a lower risk of nausea and vomiting. There is a direct relationship between the cumulative dose of irradiation and the severity of radiation-induced sickness (Tramer *et al.* 1998). Treatment field is one of the major determinants of emetic risk, as well as dose of radiotherapy administered per fraction and the fractionation pattern (Gralla *et al.* 1999).

Table 12.2 Factors influencing radiation-induced emesis (Feyer *et al.* 1998)

Single and total dose, dose rate
Fractionation
Field size
    Irradiated volume
Site of irradiation
    Organs included in the radiation field
Patient positioning
Radiation technique
Energy, beam quality
Previous or simultaneous influencing therapy
General health status of the patient

Total body irradiation and irradiation of the upper part of the abdomen or whole abdomen are the most emetic radiotherapy regimens and are associated with nausea, vomiting, anorexia and diarrhoea (Table 12.3). Emesis can occur 2–3 weeks after the onset of treatment in approximately 50% of patients receiving conventionally fractionated radiation to the upper abdomen (1.8–2.0 Gy) or to the whole abdomen. Emesis occurs in over 80% of patients when single treatments are given to the abdominal area. Radiotherapy to the pelvic region causes emesis in only 40% of patients if no anti-emetic treatment is administered. More attention needs to be given to the selection of patients requiring anti-emetic therapy (Feyer *et al.* 1998).

Table 12.3 Emetic risk of radiotherapy (Feyer *et al.* 1998)

High risk:
Total body irradiation
Upper half body irradiation
Total nodal irradiation

Moderate risk:
Lower thorax region
Upper abdominal region
Pelvis
Craniospinal

Low risk:
Head and neck
Extremities

Considerations for anti-emetic therapy and indications for treatment

Factors that need to be considered when choosing an anti-emetic regimen include the therapy being administered and its emetic risk. The emetic risk is affected by the therapy dose and schedule, and radiotherapy field. The patient risk factors of emesis also need to be considered.

Other considerations include the mechanisms of action of the anti-emetics being prescribed, their adverse effects, the response to anti-emetics already given if patients are on subsequent cycles of chemotherapy or if they have other causes of nausea, and the type of emesis (anticipatory, acute or delayed) being treated. The effects of anti-emetics on gastro-intestinal motility should be considered to ensure that prokinetics (e.g. metoclopramide or domperidone) and anti-kinetics (anticholinergics) are not prescribed simultaneously. The final common pathway for prokinetic drugs is cholinergic; antimuscarinic (anticholinergic) drugs (including cyclizine) block their prokinetic action.

Combination therapy is more effective than single agents, so this is usually always necessary for chemotherapy and highly emetic radiotherapy. Anti-emetics should be given regularly and prophylactically. It is much harder to stop vomiting once it has started. The role of non-drug treatments also needs to be considered. Clinical practice guidelines should be used to ensure that anti-emetics are prescribed cost effectively.

References

Fauser, A. A., Fellhauer, M., Hoffmann, M., Link, H., Schlimok, G., Gralla, R. J. (1999). Guidelines for anti-emetic therapy: acute emesis. *European Journal of Cancer* **35**, 361–370.

Feyer, P. C., Stewart, A. L., Titlbach, O. J. (1998). Aetiology and prevention of emesis induced by radiotherapy. *Supportive Care in Cancer* **6**, 253–260.

Gralla, R. J., Osaba, D., Kris, M. G., Kirkbride, P., Hesketh, P. J., Chinnery, L. W., Clark-Snow, R., Gill, D. P., Groshen, S. *et al.* (1999). Recommendations for the use of anti-emetics: evidence-based, clinical practice guidelines. *Journal of Clinical Oncology* **17**, 2971–2994.

Grunberg, S. M., Hansen, M., Deuson, R., Mavros, P. (2002). Incidence and impact of nausea/vomiting with modern anti-emetics: perception vs. reality. *Proceedings of the American Society of Clinical Oncology*, abstract no. 996.

Herrstedt, J. (2000). European Society for Medical Oncology (ESMO) Recommendations for prophylaxis of chemotherapy-induced nausea and vomiting (NV). www.esmo.org/reference/anti_emetics.htm.

National Cancer Institute (2002). Nausea and vomiting (PDQ). www.nci.nih.gov/cancer.

Tramer, M. R., Reynolds, D. J. M., Stoner, N. S., Moore, R. A., McQuay, H. J. (1998). Efficacy of 5-HT$_3$ receptor antagonists in radiotherapy-induced nausea and vomiting: a quantitative systematic review. *European Journal of Cancer* **34**, 1836–1844.

Chapter 13

Evidence for selection and use of anti-emetic agents and regimens: therapy-induced nausea and vomiting

Nicola S. Stoner

Introduction

The goal of anti-emetic therapy is to prevent emesis completely. Despite improvements in the control of emesis over the past 20 years, a significant number of patients still experience emesis (Gralla *et al.* 1999; Grunberg *et al.* 2002). Newer anti-emetics have fewer side effects than older regimens, and are more convenient to use for both patients and healthcare professionals (Gralla *et al.* 1999).

Factors that need to be considered when choosing an anti-emetic regimen include the emetic risk of therapy, its dose, and schedule; the anti-emetic mechanism of action and routes of administration; the type of emesis being treated (anticipatory, acute, delayed); the patient risk of emesis; and the adverse effects of the drugs. Anti-emetics should be given regularly and prophylactically. Combinations are significantly more effective than single agents. Goals related to the complete control of emesis include providing care that is convenient for the patient, reducing hospitalisation, and enhancing patient quality of life. Practitioners need to be aware of reducing costs of treatment while achieving these goals (Gralla *et al.* 1999). The use of clinical practice guidelines ensures appropriate and cost-effective anti-emetic use (Gralla *et al.* 1999; Herrstedt 2002; National Cancer Institute 2002).

5-Hydroxytryptamine$_3$ receptor antagonists

The introduction of 5-hydroxytryptamine$_3$ (5-HT$_3$: serotonin) receptor antagonists has dramatically improved the management of chemotherapy-induced emesis (Roila *et al.* 1997). Ondansetron, granisetron, dolasetron and tropisetron are the commercially available 5-HT$_3$ receptor antagonists (Fauser *et al.* 1999, Gralla *et al.* 1999).

5-HT$_3$ receptor antagonist anti-emetics and corticosteroids are two of the most effective classes of anti-emetics, with the fewest side effects and are convenient to use. They are recommended in combination for highly and moderately–highly emetogenic chemotherapy regimes. When possible, these agents should be given orally in single doses. (Roila *et al.* 1997; Fauser *et al.* 1999; Gralla *et al.* 1999). The combination of a 5-HT$_3$ receptor antagonist plus dexamethasone is able to completely prevent chemotherapy-induced vomiting in approximately 80% of patients receiving cisplatin, and in approximately 90% of patients receiving moderately emetogenic chemotherapy (Roila *et al.* 1997; Gralla *et al.* 1999; Licitra *et al.* 2002).

The anti-emetic activity and tolerability of ondansetron, granisetron, dolasetron and tropisetron is almost identical in the prevention of cisplatin-induced emesis, so there is no reason to prefer one over the others (Roila *et al.* 1997; Fauser *et al.* 1999; Gralla *et al.* 1999). There is excellent evidence available for ondansetron, granisetron, and dolasetron; however, the studies with tropisetron are less rigorous. There is, however, adequate evidence available to support their equivalence (Fauser *et al.* 1999; Gralla *et al.* 1999). There is scant information available on the use of 5-HT$_3$ receptor antagonists in moderately emetic chemotherapy, and more studies should be carried out in this group of patients (Roila *et al.* 1997). All four agents have the same side effect profile, which includes mild headache, constipation, and transient asymptomatic transaminase elevations most commonly (Roila *et al.* 1997; Gralla *et al.* 1999).

The practical issues of choosing a 5-HT$_3$ receptor antagonist anti-emetic include the available formulations, the frequency of administration, its licensed indications and cost. Consideration has to be made as to whether it will be administered orally or intravenously, and the frequency of administration of each of these routes. Most hospitals would prefer to stock a single 5-HT$_3$ receptor antagonist, so it would be preferable for that antagonist to be licensed for all indications including chemotherapy, radiotherapy, post-operatively and in children. Some of the 5-HT$_3$ receptor antagonists are available in several formulations including tablets, syrups, suppositories, intravenous injections or dispersible tablets. Consideration needs to be given to the emetic risk that will be covered with a single 5-HT$_3$ receptor antagonist: will it be used for both highly and moderately emetic therapy? Economically, differences may exist and are related to the dose and schedule of administration of each agent.

Established proven doses of the 5-HT$_3$ receptor antagonists are shown in Table 13.1. There is a threshold effect for these agents, so once all relevant receptors are saturated, higher doses do not enhance any aspect of activity. Single oral doses are preferred for convenience and cost. Excellent absorption is found with all agents: reports indicate 50–80% bioavailability. Because 5-HT$_3$ receptors are found in the enterochromaffin cells in the gut, with vagal afferent fibres in this area, it has been suggested that oral administration may be particularly appropriate for these agents. Single-dose administration is the most cost-effective and minimises the side effects experienced (Gralla *et al.* 1999; National Cancer Institute 2002).

Table 13.1 Recommended oral daily doses of 5-HT$_3$ receptor antagonists (Gralla *et al.* 1999).

ondansetron	16–24 mg
granisetron	2 mg
dolasetron	100 mg
tropisetron	5 mg

Corticosteroids

Dexamethasone was one of the first agents to be introduced, and is the corticosteroid used most extensively in combination with other anti-emetics. Very few data are available on its efficacy against placebo, and most efficacy data were established as adjunctive treatment to 5-HT$_3$ receptor antagonists (Fauser *et al.* 1999; Gralla *et al.* 1999; Loannidis *et al.* 2000). A meta-analysis of randomised evidence on the efficacy of dexamethasone for patients receiving highly and moderately emetogenic chemotherapy was published in 2000 (Loannidis *et al.* 2000). Dexamethasone was shown to be effective in protecting both acute and delayed emesis. Emesis is avoided in one patient out of six treated (15 out of 100 patients vomit free in the first 24 h). Dexamethasone increases the chance of not vomiting by 25–30% in the first 24 h (Loannidis *et al.* 2000).

Dexamethasone is one of the most effective treatments for delayed emesis. Dexamethasone increases the chance of not vomiting by 25–30% in the delayed phase, and offers an additional 15 out of 100 patients a vomit-free rate (Loannidis *et al.* 2000). There is no randomised evidence from trials in which dexamethasone has been administered only in the delayed phase, so it is difficult to establish how much of its efficacy of preventing delayed emesis is due to its effect in acute emesis.

There is not a strong dose–response relation for either acute or delayed vomiting, as shown in cumulative meta-analyses of studies ordered by increasing dexamethasone dosages (Loannidis *et al.* 2000). However, the authors suggested that a subtle dose–response relation could not be ruled out for total doses less than 20 mg, with saturation of dexamethasone receptors at higher doses. Nevertheless, even low doses showed clear efficacy (Gralla *et al.* 1999; Loannidis *et al.* 2000). Single doses are recommended, and although there are no formal trials comparing oral and intravenous formulations, acceptable oral bioavailability encourages oral use of dexamethasone (Gralla *et al.* 1999). Side effects of single doses of dexamethasone include sleep disturbances and raised serum glucose levels, but these are rare (Gralla *et al.* 1999). Acutely doses of 20 mg daily are recommended, whereas doses of 4–8 mg are used in the delayed phase to provide efficacy for 2–4 days (Gralla *et al.* 1999; Loannidis *et al.* 2000; National Cancer Institute 2002).

Other anti-emetic agents

There are several classes of agents with anti-emetic activity that are less efficacious than the serotonin receptor antagonists or corticosteroids. These agents have more side effects, usually because they are less selective than 5-HT$_3$ receptor antagonists (Table 13.2).

The first three groups are primarily dopamine type 2 receptor antagonists. Metoclopramide is generally more effective than phenothiazines or butyrophenones. Side effects include dystonic reactions, akathisia, and sedation. In doses of 20–40 mg given two to four times per day for 3–4 days, metoclopramide has efficacy for delayed emesis (Gralla *et al.* 1999).

Table 13.2 Anti-emetic agents: lower therapeutic index (Gralla *et al.* 1999)

dopamine antagonists (e.g. metoclopramide)
butyrophenones (e.g. haloperidol)
phenothiazines (e.g. prochlorperazine, levomepromazine)
cannabinoids (nabilone)
benzodiazepines (e.g. lorazepam)
antihistamines (e.g. cyclizine)

Cannabinoids have an anti-emetic effect alone or in combination with other agents (Gralla *et al.* 1999).

Benzodiazepines and antihistamines are useful adjuncts to anti-emetic drugs, but are not recommended as single agents. Lorazepam has limited anti-emetic activity, but because of its potent anti-anxiety effects it is useful added to combination anti-emetics. It is also effective for anticipatory nausea and vomiting (Gralla *et al.* 1999).

Antihistamines can be administered as anti-emetics and as adjunctive agents to prevent dystonic reactions with dopamine antagonists. However, because dopamine receptor antagonist agents are no longer first-choice drugs, the role for antihistamines is limited (Gralla *et al.* 1999).

These agents should be used for patients who are refractory to serotonin receptor antagonists and corticosteroids (Gralla *et al.* 1999). If patients fail first-line treatment, consideration should be given to the use of phenothiazines (prochlorperazine or levomepromazine), lorazepam, or nabilone in addition to a serotonin receptor antagonist and dexamethasone (National Cancer Institute 2002).

Combinations of anti-emetics

Extensive research has shown that combinations of anti-emetics are significantly more effective than single agents when used with chemotherapy to prevent acute and delayed emesis. When combination chemotherapy is given, the patient should be treated for the agent in the combination with the highest emetic risk (Tables 13.3 and 13.4). If multiple day chemotherapy is administered, anti-emetics appropriate for the risk class of the chemotherapy should be administered for each day of the chemotherapy (Fauser *et al.* 1999; Gralla *et al.* 1999).

Chemotherapy of high emetic risk should be treated with a serotonin receptor antagonist and corticosteroid before chemotherapy. Corticosteroids are the most consistently useful drugs for the prevention of delayed emesis, and can be used for 2–4 days after chemotherapy to minimise side effects. Doses of dexamethasone are usually 8 mg for 2–3 days, occasionally tapering to 4 mg for one to two additional days. Metoclopramide is efficacious when given in combination with corticosteroids in doses of 20–40 mg two to four times daily for 3–4 days, and is generally well tolerated. Akathisia (restlessness) may occur in some patients, and occasionally

Table 13.3 Emetic risk of chemotherapy (Fauser *et al.* 1999; Gralla *et al.* 1999; Herrstedt 2000)

---

1. High emetic risk
cisplatin
dacarbazine
actinomycin-D
mustine
carmustine
carboplatin
oxaliplatin
daunorubicin
doxorubicin $\geq$60 mg/m^2
epirubicin $\geq$90 mg/m^2
idarubicin
cytarabine
ifosfamide
cyclophosphamide

2. Intermediate emetic risk
irinotecan
topotecan
mitoxantrone
paclitaxel
docetaxel
gemcitabine
etoposide
teniposide
mitomycin
methotrexate 50–250 mg/m^2

3. Low emetic risk
busulfan (low dose)
chlorambucil
fludarabine
hydroxyurea
methotrexate $\leq$50 mg/m^2
vinca alkaloids
5-fluorouracil
bleomycin

---

dystonic reactions. There are conflicting results in studies of the use of serotonin antagonists for delayed emesis (Gralla *et al.* 1999; Herrstedt 2002).

A corticosteroid is suggested for patients treated with agents of intermediate emetic risk. The complete control rate should exceed 90% with the use of a single

Table 13.4 Combinations of anti-emetics to prevent chemotherapy-induced nausea and vomiting (Gralla *et al.* 1999; Herrstedt 2002)

High emetic risk	
Acutely:	serotonin receptor antagonist
	corticosteroid, e.g. dexamethasone 20 mg stat. or 8 mg b.d.
Delayed phase:	corticosteroid, e.g. dexamethasone 8 mg daily for 2–3 days, can be reduced to 4 mg daily for one to two additional days
	metoclopramide 20–40 mg two to four times daily for 3–4 days
Intermediate emetic risk	
Acutely	corticosteroid, e.g. dexamethasone 4–8 mg orally once before chemotherapy
Delayed Phase	no regular preventative use of anti-emetic
	metoclopramide as needed
Low emetic risk	
	no regular preventative use of anti-emetics
	Metoclopramide as needed

dose of a corticosteroid. There is no formal documentation of efficacy with anti-emetic treatments for these lower-risk chemotherapy agents.

Patients treated with agents of low emetic risk do not routinely need to be administered with anti-emetics before chemotherapy (National Cancer Institute 2002).

Treatment of anticipatory nausea and vomiting

Prevention of chemotherapy-induced emesis is the best strategy for preventing anticipatory emesis. Behavioural therapy with systematic desensitisation is effective and suggested for the treatment of anticipatory emesis (Gralla *et al.* 1999). However, this treatment is not widely available in this country.

Lorazepam can be a useful drug in this situation, used in doses of up to 1mg three times daily.

Neurokinin-1 (substance P) antagonists

Efforts to improve anti-emetic control further are ongoing. The most interesting new class of anti-emetics under development are the neurokinin-1 (or substance P) antagonists. Substance P is a neuropeptide of the tachykinin family of peptides, comprising 11 amino acids, and has been found to mediate an emetic response. It is located mainly within the gastrointestinal tract and the central nervous system. Substance P exerts its effects by binding to the tachykinin neurokinin NK_1 receptor (Hesketh 2001).

NK_1 receptor antagonists differ from the $5\text{-}HT_3$ receptor antagonist in several ways. They are able to antagonise a broader spectrum of emetic stimuli than the $5\text{-}HT_3$ receptor antagonists, including those to morphine, motion and anaesthetics (Hesketh 2001). NK_1 receptor antagonists require entry into the central nervous system to exert their anti-emetic effect, whereas $5\text{-}HT_3$ receptor antagonists appear to work peripherally (Hesketh 2001).

Clinical trials done so far indicate that these agents are less effective than $5\text{-}HT_3$ antagonists in acute chemotherapy-induced nausea and vomiting, but have superior efficacy to available agents in delayed emesis (Campos *et al.* 2001; Hesketh 2001; de Wit *et al.* 2002; Hesketh *et al.* 2002; Loewen 2002; Van Belle *et al.* 2002). When an NK_1 receptor antagonist is combined with a $5\text{-}HT_3$ receptor antagonist and dexamethasone, control of acute cisplatin-induced emesis is improved by 20–30% over that obtained with the two-drug combination of a $5\text{-}HT_3$ receptor antagonist and dexamethasone. Complete control of cisplatin-induced delayed emesis is better by 30–40% with the use of these agents than with placebo (Campos *et al.* 2001; Hesketh 2001; de Wit *et al.* 2002; Hesketh *et al.* 2002; Loewen 2002; Van Belle *et al.* 2002).

All of the agents tested so far have a favourable safety profile (Hesketh 2001). Aprepitant (Emend®) was approved by the US FDA in April 2003 and by the European Medicine Evaluation Agency in July 2003. Additional clinical trials are required to compare the activity of these agents with dexamethasone or metoclopramide, and to clarify their role in moderately emetogenic chemotherapy. Further clinical experience will clarify the optimal doses and full toxicity profile of these agents (Hesketh 2001).

Other new agents in the future

There clearly remains a need to identify additional effective anti-emetic approaches. In addition to the NK_1 antagonists, other pharmacological strategies in development focus on other serotonin-related targets and agonising CB_1 (cannabinoid) receptors. Serotonin-related targets include additional antagonists of the type 3 receptor and agonists of the type 1A and 2A/2C receptors (Hesketh 2001; Loewen 2002).

$5\text{-}HT_3$ receptor antagonists in radiotherapy-induced emesis

The introduction of the $5\text{-}HT_3$ receptor antagonists has resulted in a dramatic improvement in the control of emesis precipitated by radiotherapy. There are only few published studies with radiotherapy, but the benefits are clear, especially in highly emetogenic regimens (Feyer *et al.* 1998). Radiotherapy with high risk of inducing emesis (Table 13.5) should be treated with serotonin-receptor antagonists with or without dexamethasone (Table 13.6) before each fraction (Feyer *et al.* 1998; Gralla *et al.* 1999; Tramer *et al.* 1998). Total body irradiation should be treated with a serotonin receptor antagonist and for at least 24 h after, with response rates of 50–90% (Feyer *et al.* 1998).

Table 13.5 Emetic risk of radiotherapy (Feyer *et al.* 1998).

High risk
Total body irradiation
Upper half body irradiation
Total nodal irradiation
Moderate risk
Lower thorax region
Upper abdominal region
Pelvis
Craniospinal
Low risk
Head and neck
Extremities

Table 13.6 Treatment of radiotherapy-induced emesis

High risk	serotonin-receptor antagonists with or without dexamethasone before each fraction
Moderate risk	serotonin or dopamine receptor antagonists prophylactic use
Low risk	dopamine receptor antagonists as-needed basis

Single-fraction radiotherapy to the upper abdomen treated with 5-HT$_3$ receptor antagonists controls acute emesis completely in 75% of patients, compared with 50% with metoclopramide. Complete or major control of vomiting is seen in 77–91% of patients and mild or no nausea in 72–77% of patients after single treatments to the upper abdomen (Feyer *et al.* 1998).

Hemibody irradiation-induced emesis is completely controlled in 86% of patients receiving 5-HT$_3$ receptor antagonist and dexamethasone (Feyer *et al.* 1998).

Conventional daily fractionated radiotherapy to the abdominal region has complete control with 5-HT$_3$ receptor antagonist in 61% of patients compared with 35% if patients received prochlorperazine (Feyer *et al.* 1998).

The role of corticosteroids in combination with 5-HT$_3$ receptor antagonists has not been widely studied, but these are recommended because of findings in preliminary reports (Gralla *et al.* 1999). The National Cancer Institute in Canada has, however, published a trial showing that dexamethasone is effective in preventing radiation-induced emesis. In this study, 70% of 75 patients receiving 2 mg dexamethasone three times a day versus 49% of 75 patients receiving placebo for fractionated radiotherapy to fields involving the upper abdomen had complete protection from vomiting (Kirkbride *et al.* 2000).

Radiotherapy of intermediate risk (Table 13.5) should be treated with a serotonin or dopamine antagonist (Table 13.6) before each fraction. There may be smaller differences between these agents, and therefore dopamine receptor antagonists may be more appropriate, particularly in patients receiving craniospinal or lower-half-body radiotherapy, where there is somewhat less risk of emesis (Tramer et al. 1998).

The efficacy of 5-HT$_3$ receptor antagonists may decrease after the first week of treatment, making it difficult to suggest what the optimal duration of prophylactic treatment should be (Gralla et al. 1999).

Low emetic risk radiotherapy (Table 13.5) should be treated only on an as-needed basis (Table 13.6). The incidence of emesis in this group is low (0–30%). Dopamine receptor antagonists are advised. Anti-emetics should be continued prophylactically for each remaining radiation treatment day. Serotonin receptor antagonists should be reserved for rescue treatment (Gralla et al. 1999).

Clinical practice guidelines

The use of evidence-based clinical practice guidelines for anti-emetics ensures appropriate and cost-effective prescribing, particularly for 5-HT$_3$ receptor antagonists (Fauser et al. 1999; Gralla et al. 1999; Dranitsaris et al. 2001). Practice guidelines are systematically developed statements to assist the practitioner and patient in making decisions about appropriate healthcare for specific clinical circumstance. Good clinical guidelines include considerations of validity, reliability, reproducibility, clinical applicability, clinical flexibility, clarity, multidisciplinary process, review of evidence and documentation. Guidelines cannot always account for individual variation among patients, and are not intended to replace clinician judgement for particular patients or special clinical situations (Fauser et al. 1999; Gralla et al. 1999). Evidence can differ in level and grade, and practice guidelines can rate it according to specific criteria (Fauser et al. 1999; Gralla et al. 1999). Evidence-based clinical practice guidelines have been produced by the American Society of Clinical Oncology (Gralla et al. 1999) and the European Society of Medical Oncology (Herrstedt 2002), which can be adapted to local needs. Anti-emetic clinical trials have not answered all the questions related to emesis in cancer, and additional research into the prevention and treatment of emesis is still required (Gralla et al. 1999).

References

Campos D., Pereira, J. R., Reinhardt, R. R., Carracedo, C., Poli, S., Vogel, C., Martinez-Cedillo, J., Erazo, A., Wittreich, J., Eriksson, L. O. et al. (2001). Prevention of Cisplatin-Induced Emesis by Oral Neurokinin-1 Antagonist, MK-869, in combination with granisetron and dexamethasone or with dexamethasone alone. *Journal of Clinical Oncology* **19**(6), 1759–1767.

de Wit, R., Herrstedt, J., Rapoport, B. L., Elmer, M. E., Schmidt, C., Carides, A., Horgan, K. J. (2002). Maintenance of protection against chemotherapy induced nausea and vomiting in multiple cycles with the oral NK$_1$ antagonist MK-0869. *Proceedings of the American Society of Clinical Oncology*, Abstract no. 1467.

Dranitsaris G., Leung, P., Warr, D. (2001). Implementing evidence based anti-emetic guidelines in setting: results of a 4-month prospective intervention. *Supportive Care in Cancer* **9**(8), 611–8.

Fauser A. A., Fellhauer, M., Hoffmann, M., Link, H., Schlimok, G., Gralla, R. J. (1999). Guidelines for anti-emetic therapy: acute emesis. *European Journal of Cancer* **35**(3), 361–370.

Feyer P. C., Stewart, A. L., Titlbach, O. J. (1998). Aetiology and prevention of emesis induced by radiotherapy. *Supportive Care in Cancer* **6**, 253–260.

Gralla R. J., Osoba, D., Kris, M. G., Kirkbride, P., Hesketh, P. J., Chinnery, L. W., Clark-Snow, R., Gill, D. P., Groshen, S., Grunberg, S. *et al.* (1999). Recommendations for the Use of Antiemetics: Evidence-Based, Clinical Practice Guidelines. *Journal of Clinical Oncology* **17**(9), 2971–2994.

Grunberg S. M., Hansen, M., Deuson, R., Mavros, P. (2002). Incidence and impact of nausea/vomiting with modern antiemetics: perception vs. reality. *Proceedings of the American Society of Clinical Oncology*, Abstract no. 996.

Herrstedt J. (2000). European Society for Medical Oncology (ESMO) Recommendations for Prophylaxis of Chemotherapy-Induced Nausea and Vomiting (NV), www.esmo.org/reference/anti_emetics.htm.

Hesketh P. J. (2001). Potential role of the NK_1 receptor antagonists in chemotherapy-induced nausea and vomiting. *Supportive Care in Cancer* **9**, 350–354.

Hesketh P. J., Carides, A., Horgan, K. J. (2002). Differential time course of cisplatin induced emesis with a $5HT_3$ antagonist or an NK antagonist: rationale for combination therapy. *Proceedings of the American Society of Clinical Oncology*, Abstract no. 1476.

Kirkbridge P., Bezjak, A., Pater, J., Zee, B., Palmer, M. J., Wong, R., Cross, P., Gulavita, S., Blood, P., Sun, A. *et al.* (2000). Dexamethasone for the prophylaxis of radiation-induced emesis: a National Cancer Institute of Canada Clinical Trials Group phase III study. *Journal of Clinical Oncology* **18**(9), 1960–6.

Licitra L., Spinazze, S., Roila, F. (2002). Anti-emetic therapy. *Critical Reviews in Oncology and Hematology* **43**(1), 93–101.

Loannidis, J. P. A., Jesketh, P. J. & Lau, J. (2000). Contribution of Dexamethasone to Control Chemotherapy-Induced Nausea and Vomiting: A Meta-Analysis of Randomized Evidence. *Journal of Clinical Oncology* **18**, 3409–3422.

Loewen P. S. (2002). Anti-emetics in development. *Expert Opinion in Investigational Drugs* **11**(6), 801–5.

National Cancer Institute (NCI) (2002). Nausea and Vomiting (PDQ). www.nci.nih.gov/cancer.

Roila F., Ballatori, E., Tonato, M., Del Favero, A. (1997). $5\text{-}HT_3$ Receptor Antagonists: Differences and Similarities. *European Journal of Cancer* **33**(9), 1364–1370.

Tramer M. R., Reynolds, D. J. M., Stoner, N. S., Moore, R. A., McQuay, H. J. (1998). Efficacy of $5\text{-}HT_3$ Receptor Antagonists in Radiotherapy-induced Nausea and Vomiting: A Quantitative Systematic Review. *European Journal of Cancer* **34**(12), 1836–1844.

Van Belle S., Lichinitser, M. R., Navari, R. M., Garin, A. M., Decramer, M. L. A., Riviere, A., Thant, M., Brestan, E., Bui, B., Eldridge, K. *et al.* (2002). Prevention of Cisplatin-Induced Acute and Delayed Emesis by the Selective Neurokinin-1 Antagonists, L-758,298 and MK-869. *Cancer* **94**(11), 3032–3041.

Chapter 14

Non-pharmacological intervention for nausea and vomiting

Jacqueline Filshie and Albert Koomson

Introduction

The problem of nausea and vomiting during treatment of cancer remains a challenge despite better knowledge of the mechanisms by which it is caused. Management of cancer may involve surgery, chemotherapy, radiotherapy, hormonal manipulation, novel or immunological therapy. Treatment is usually given by multidisciplinary teams, and in many cases is multimodal. All of the methods of treatment can potentially induce nausea and vomiting, making an already stressful situation unbearable. In advanced disease, treatment might be essentially palliative, with emphasis on symptom control such as pain relief, and relief of other mechanical problems such as intermittent or acute bowel obstruction which can cause vomiting.

There are limitations to the control of nausea and vomiting, despite the wide range of anti-emetic drugs available to the clinician. As a result, the impact of uncontrolled nausea and vomiting may be significant enough for patients to consider abandoning potentially curative or palliative anticancer treatment. Anti-emetics may lack efficacy in certain clinical situations, and be more effective for early – rather than late – onset post-operative nausea and vomiting (PONV). Treatment with anti-emetic agents can be both costly and associated with unwanted side effects, such as extrapyramidal effects or drowsiness (Bateman 1991; Cunningham 1990). Non-pharmacological interventions such as acupuncture are gaining increasing importance in alleviating symptoms such as nausea and vomiting (Bender *et al.* 2002), pain and dyspnoea, unrelieved by conventional medication (Filshie & Thompson 2003).

Acupuncture is the first-line treatment for many pain and non-pain conditions for therapeutic and preventative purposes, and has been used in China for over 2,000 years. The National Institutes of Health consensus statement in 1996 (National Institutes of Health Technology Assessment Panel on Integration of Behavioral and Relaxation Approaches into the Treatment of Chronic Pain and Insomnia 1996) recommended the use of acupuncture as a useful clinical modality of treatment. This was based partly on the systematic review by Vickers (1996) on acupuncture for nausea and vomiting. This chapter includes an overview of the use of acupuncture for nausea and vomiting in cancer patients.

Hypnosis is the induction of a deeply relaxed state, with increased suggestibility and suspension of critical faculties (Vickers & Zollman 1999). Trance experiences have been used since the time of the ancient Greeks. There is an accumulating evidence base that shows the efficacy of hypnosis for nausea and vomiting: this will be presented. Hypnotised subjects become absorbed in the hypnotic experience, with distortion of awareness of time, and are curiously receptive to suggestions implanted at the time. In addition to reduction of symptoms of procedure-related pain, hypnosis has been found to be helpful for alleviation of anticipatory chemotherapy-related nausea and vomiting, as well as anxiety and stress. The use of hypnosis and other forms of non-drug treatment for nausea and vomiting in cancer patients are also briefly discussed.

Acupuncture

The exact origins of acupuncture in China are somewhat uncertain, though stone needles 'bian shi' were used in the Stone Age, and bone needles have been found dated 21st–16th centuries BC (Ma 1992). Ötzi, the Tyrolean Ice Man, found in 1991 and dated as approximately 5,200 years old, had numerous tattoos, which suggested an acupuncture-like technique (Dorfer *et al.* 1999). Acupuncture is a therapeutic technique, which involves the insertion of fine needles through the skin for therapeutic or preventative purposes. Traditional Chinese acupuncturists use an alternative diagnostic system based on the detection of an 'imbalance' of 'Qi' (vital energy) in the circulation, which is thought to flow through a continuous network of channels or 'meridians' around the body. The balancing of 'Yin and Yang' (opposing forces) is thought to be crucial for normal health. The concepts of 'Qi' and 'Yin and Yang' predate the discoveries of the circulation of blood, normalisation of autonomic function and the concept of homeostasis.

In contrast, many Western medical acupuncturists employ a pragmatic approach to treatment, following an orthodox medical diagnosis, and use a mixture of segmental points, appropriate to the disordered structure; trigger points – mainly for control of myofascial pain; and strong traditional points, some of which have a sound evidence base and many of which have stood the test of time (Filshie & Cummings 1999).

Mechanisms of action

Acupuncture works through Aδ nerve stimulation to release multiple endogenous analgesic substances. Its actions can be blocked by pre-treatment with local anaesthetic injections. It releases β-endorphin, enkephalins and dynorphins. A course of acupuncture 'up-regulates' analgesic gene production, and this explains why 'top-ups' are required to maintain the gene expression in a 'switched on' mode, and why a course of treatment, for example six weekly acupuncture sessions, are necessary for chronic pain states. It also has widespread autonomic effects and releases endogenous steroids. Table 14.1 outlines some of these mechanisms. It is interesting to note that some of the mechanisms overlap mechanisms of action of anti-emetics in current use.

Table 14.1 Some of the mechanisms involved in the action of acupuncture (adapted from Filshie & Thompson (2003))

Primary action is to stimulate $A\delta$ nerve endings. Local anaesthetics block the action of acupuncture.	Bowsher 1998 Chiang *et al.* 1973 Dundee & Ghaly 1991

Neurotransmitter system involved	Neurotransmitter released and clinical effect(s)	
Endogenous opioids released:		
β-endorphin	μ opioid (MOR) agonist: analgesia	Han & Sun 1990 Han *et al.* 1991
Metenkephalin	δ opioid (DOR) agonist: analgesia	Han & Sun 1990 Han *et al.* 1991
Dynorphins A and B	κ opioid (KOR) agonist: analgesia	Han & Sun 1990 Han *et al.* 1991
Pre-prometenkephalin Pre-prodynorphin	Up-regulation of analgesic gene expression. Increases amount and distribution of opioid peptides.	Guo *et al.* 1996
Orphanin (OFQ, nociceptin)	Role unclear, but may modulate opioid systems and thereby antagonise opioid effects of acupuncture.	Tian *et al.* 1997
Cholecystokinin Serotonin (5-HT)	Opioid antagonist: antagonises analgesia. 5-HT is released in the descending inhibitory pathways of the spinal cord to produce analgesia and mood elevation	Zhou *et al.* 1993 Han & Terenius 1982
Autonomic nervous system	Noradrenaline (norepinephrine) is released (a) in the descending inhibitory pathways of the spinal cord to produce analgesia and (b) in the hypothalamus to activate the efferent sympathetic pathways to produce circulatory and metabolic effects.	Han & Terenius 1982 Lundeberg 1999
Adrenocorticotrophic hormone (ACTH)	ACTH (co-released with β-endorphin) through steroid release produces anti-inflammatory effect.	Roth *et al.* 1997
Oxytocin	Analgesic and sedative.	Uvnäs Moberg 1993
Substance P, VIP, glutamate and aspartate	Actions blocked by acupuncture-induced release of opioids. Some have indirect effects on NK_1 receptors.	Dickenson 1996

Evidence base

Based on systematic reviews and meta-analyses, acupuncture has been found to be of benefit for experimental pain (White 1999), dental pain (Ernst & Pittler 1998), headache (Melchart *et al.* 2001), fibromyalgia (Berman *et al.* 1999) and osteoarthritis of the knee (Ezzo *et al.* 2001). Some of the strongest evidence for treatment of nausea and vomiting has been for PONV, chemotherapy-induced nausea and vomiting and nausea and vomiting in pregnancy (Vickers 1996). A further meta-analysis of acupuncture for PONV showed acupuncture to be effective for these symptoms (Lee & Done 1999). There are mixed results for stroke (Park *et al.* 2001), asthma (Linde *et al.* 2000) and back pain (Ernst & White 1998; Smith *et al.* 2000; van Tulder *et al.* 1999) and the reasons for this have been explored (Cummings 2000).

The use of acupuncture for nausea and vomiting

The late Professor John Dundee, having been impressed by the effects of acupressure at the traditional acupuncture point PC6 on the forearm – as used in China for nausea and vomiting in pregnancy – undertook several exploratory studies to show its efficacy on nausea and vomiting from a variety of causes (Dundee *et al.* 1987; Dundee and Yang 1990; McMillan *et al.* 1991). The point PC6 is approximately 5 cm up from the medial surface of the wrist, and lies between the tendons flexor carpi radialis and palmaris longus. Stimulation of this point with a fine acupuncture needle can cause a sensation of numbness, heaviness and parasthesia – 'De Qi' or 'needling sensation'. The needle can be either manually or electrically stimulated. Christine McMillan has summarised many of the original studies on PC6 anti-emesis and gives additional insight into some of the pitfalls when undertaking acupuncture research in this area (McMillan 1998).

Methods of stimulation

Stimulation of an acupuncture point can be invasive or non-invasive. When needles are used, the acupuncture point is stimulated either manually or electrically. Pressure over the acupuncture site could be applied manually, 'acupressure', or by an elasticised band with a large plastic stud positioned directly over the point. These bands (Choy bands), which were specifically devised by Daniel Choy for the stimulation of PC6 are now available commercially under the name of 'Sea bands'. In electro-acupuncture (EA) and transcutaneous electrical nerve stimulation (TENS) the electrical apparatus used is a battery operated, direct current, rectangular wave stimulator, which has the capability for the current and frequency of output to be varied. A variety of other stimuli include semi-permanent needles (studs), which are minute, short acupuncture needles held in place with some form of plaster dressing. Laser therapy and magnetic disc treatment over PC6 are other forms of non-invasive stimulation. The use of acupuncture for treating nausea and vomiting resulting from a variety of causes, including PONV, chemotherapy-induced nausea and vomiting, and nausea and vomiting in palliative care, will be considered separately.

Acupuncture for post-operative nausea and vomiting

Most patients with early or potentially curable cancer undergo some form of surgical procedure. Patients with advanced cancer, needing chemotherapy, might require placement of central venous lines under general anaesthesia or sedation, whereas others might undergo debulking procedures of the tumour or surgery to relieve symptoms and signs caused by the cancer.

The factors influencing the incidence of PONV after cancer surgery are essentially similar to those impacting on other surgical procedures or surgery performed for a different reason. However, additional factors like recent or ongoing chemotherapy and/or radiotherapy might make patients with cancer more susceptible to PONV.

Nausea and vomiting can be profoundly unpleasant and distressing to patients and, if prolonged, can cause dehydration and metabolic and electrolyte disturbances. The consequences could be delayed discharge and increased numbers of unplanned hospital admissions, and may thus affect health costs. Vomiting and retching have also been known to cause or potentiate wound dehiscence, bleeding from flaps, increased intracranial pressure, aspiration pneumonia and, rarely, oesophageal rupture (Kenny 1994). Prolonged nausea and vomiting is associated with absence from work, with its attendant cost implications.

Peri-operative features that increase the risk of PONV include patient, anaesthetic, surgical and post-operative factors. In one study, when 16,000 patients were interviewed, PONV was found to affect between 22% and 38% in four different hospitals (Cohen *et al.* 1994).

The experience of the anaesthetist influences the way an anaesthetic technique is delivered (Belville & Bross 1960). Minor airway mismanagement can lead to a raised intra-gastric pressure after injudicious insufflation of the stomach with gas. An elevated intra-gastric pressure is a recipe for nausea and vomiting. Experienced anaesthetists understand the demands of various types of surgical procedures and how they affect the gastro-intestinal system, and endeavour to use anaesthetic techniques that are less likely to cause PONV.

The choice of anaesthetic agents (Smith 1996) is important in reducing the incidence of PONV, and propofol, especially used as total intravenous anaesthesia (TIVA), is associated with a reduced risk of early PONV (Hannallah *et al.* 1994). Local anaesthetic (LA) blocks, used alone or as adjuncts to general anaesthesia, tend to be opioid-sparing and reduce the amount of inhalational agents necessary to achieve the three basic tenets of anaesthesia, namely: unconsciousness, muscle relaxation and pain relief.

Children are twice as likely as adults to experience PONV (Korttila 1992). Females have a two- to fourfold greater likelihood of having PONV than males (Cookson 1986). A previous history of PONV, motion sickness and any condition associated with a delay in gastric emptying are risk factors for PONV. Excessive anxiety can increase levels of endogenous catecholamines, which reduce gastric emptying and potentially cause sickness (Palazzo & Strunin 1984). Patients who smoke are less likely to vomit (Cohen *et al.* 1986).

Certain types of surgery, cancer and non-cancer, increase the risk of PONV. These include major intra-abdominal (Dupeyron *et al.* 1993), gynaecological (Madej & Simpson 1986), laparoscopic (Hovorka *et al.* 1989), plastics and reconstructive, orthopaedic (Korttila *et al.* 1979), ear, nose and throat (Grunwald *et al.* 1993), and ophthalmic, especially operations to correct strabismus (Abramowitz *et al.* 1983). Pain causes anxiety and increases the risk of PONV. Mobilisation, sudden movements, trolley rides and early intake of fluids and food in the early post-operative period could cause sickness. Hypotension and hypoxaemia can complicate the post-operative period, and they too increase the risk of PONV. Ear, nose and throat operations are frequently associated with swallowing of blood, which is a gastric irritant. Opioids given intra-operatively and post-operatively are a powerful cause of PONV.

Apfel *et al.* (1999) outlined a simplified risk scoring system designed to identify high-risk patients pre-operatively. Often, more than one anti-emetic approach would be given to these patients to try to pre-empt PONV.

In the West, acupuncture is gaining popularity in the treatment of PONV. The PC6 point has been studied extensively, compared with other acupuncture anti-emetic points. Dundee and colleagues compared non-invasive with invasive stimulation of PC6, and assessed the optimal treatment parameters and frequency needed if electrical stimulation was added in the form of EA or TENS to achieve the best anti-emetic effect. They recommended that acupuncture be given before an opioid or emetic stimulus, and noted that the frequency of stimulation in both EA and TENS was more effective at 10–15 Hz (Dundee & McMillan 1991; McMillan & Dundee 1991*a*). They also noted that acupuncture was more effective for nausea than vomiting whereas prochlorperazine was more helpful in dealing with vomiting than nausea (Dundee 1990). Nausea is often a more distressing symptom than vomiting.

In 1996 Andrew Vickers published a systematic review of acupuncture anti-emesis trials. The review included PC6 stimulation, invasively and non-invasively, and its efficacy in preventing nausea and vomiting due to PONV, chemotherapy, and morning sickness due to pregnancy. He included 33 trials, of which 21 were for PONV. Sixteen out of the 21 PONV trials showed efficacy of PC6 stimulation in preventing or treating PONV. They compared different forms of PC6 stimulation, including invasive needling and non-invasive pressure, electrical stimulation, etc. with a variety of controls, such as injection of local anaesthetic before stimulation, 'wrong point', no treatment, etc. The results strengthened the case for PC6 anti-emesis. However, he observed that when acupuncture was administered under general anaesthesia there was less efficacy of PC6 stimulation.

Lee & Done (1999) performed a meta-analysis on acupuncture for PONV. Nineteen studies met their inclusion criteria. The primary outcomes for these studies were the incidence of nausea, vomiting, or both at 0–6 h (early efficacy) or 0–48 h (late efficacy) after surgery. The non-pharmacological techniques employed in the selected clinical trials included acupuncture, EA, TENS, acupoint stimulation and acupressure. The meta-analysis indicated that generally acupuncture techniques were beneficial for PONV in adults, but ineffective in preventing PONV in children. Non-pharmacological techniques had the same efficacy as anti-emetics in the prevention of early and late PONV and also showed that they were better than placebo at preventing early PONV, although similar to placebo in preventing late PONV. They concluded that non-pharmacological techniques were similar to anti-emetics in preventing early and late vomiting in adults. Also, the number needed to treat (NNT) was between 4 and 5, i.e. between 25% and 20% of adults will not have early PONV compared with a placebo (Bandolier 2000). The lower the NNT, the better the anti-emetic. This compares favourably with anti-emetics such as 10 mg metoclopramide with a NNT of 9.1–10 (Henzi *et al.* 1999) and 8 mg ondansetron intravenously or 16 mg orally with a NNT of 5–6 (Tramer *et al.* 1997). They concluded that early nausea and vomiting was helped more than late nausea and vomiting, but that no benefit was found in children.

Subsequent to these reviews there have been numerous further studies in both adults and children. One recent study, in 191 patients undergoing upper and lower abdominal surgery, used short paravertebral semi-permanent indwelling needles in segments appropriate to the surgical incisions (Kotani *et al.* 2001). They also used epidural opioids post-operatively and showed reduction in pain, as well as nausea and vomiting, in the immediate post-operative follow-up period, prior to use of the epidural. They also showed reduced 'top-up' analgesic consumption in the acupuncture group and reduced nausea and vomiting. One abstract, on the use of acupuncture in 40 breast cancer patients, showed both a reduction in nausea and vomiting, and acute pain, following acupuncture versus standard anti-emetics and a control group without anti-emetics (Aldridge 2001).

Stener-Victorin *et al.* (1999) showed no difference in PONV after electro-acupuncture for women undergoing oocyte retrieval, compared with standard sedation. Windle *et al.* (2001), in an underpowered retrospective study, showed no added benefit when unilateral or bilateral acupuncture was applied at PC6, versus control, after surgical operations. TENS in combination with ondansetron was superior to either acupuncture or ondansetron alone in reduction of PONV and improved recovery in patients undergoing plastic surgery (White *et al.* 2002). A capsaicin impregnated plaster, placed on the skin either at PC6 or a Korean hand acupuncture point, reduced nausea and vomiting post-operatively and the requirements for rescue anti-emetics, compared with inactive tape in patients undergoing hysterectomy (Kim *et al.* 2002).

Several subsequent studies in paediatric patients were positive, using a variety of methods peri-operatively, compared with control groups (Schlager *et al.* 1998; Somri *et al.* 2001; Wang & Kain 2002). Schlager *et al.* (2000) subsequently showed an advantage of Korean hand acupressure, at point K-K9, versus a no-treatment control.

However, the study by Shenkman *et al.* (1999) was negative for children undergoing tonsillectomy, and that by Rusy *et al.* (2002) was somewhat equivocal.

One advantage of a single-point treatment, such as PC6, is that trial design is easier, with recruitment, relatively short-term follow-up and a placebo control intervention possible. However, challenges remain to prolong the effects of acupuncture for PONV beyond the early post-operative period. It would also be helpful if a more standardised way of measuring and reporting post-operative nausea and vomiting was in general use!

Acupuncture for chemotherapy-induced nausea and vomiting

Sixty per cent of all patients receiving cancer chemotherapy treatment experience nausea and vomiting (King 1997). Cisplastin, actinomycin D and methotrexate are highly emetogenic chemotherapy agents (Cunningham 1990). More than 90% of patients on cisplastin treatment would experience nausea and vomiting if untreated (Kris *et al.* 1985).

Sickness during chemotherapy occurs through multiple mechanisms (Hogan & Grant 1997). It is mediated through one or more locations, for example the chemoreceptor trigger zone, visceral irritation and release of 5-HT. Stimulation of the central nervous system can also occur, with an increase in intracranial pressure after intrathecal chemotherapy. Anxiety can lead to cortisol stimulation and activation of the vomiting centre and vestibular apparatus by acetylcholine and histamine. Anxiety states can contribute to anticipatory nausea and vomiting. This represents a form of conditioning that is largely mediated by the hypothalamic and limbic areas of the brain (Goodman 1997).

The serotonin (5 hydroxytryptamine$_3$: 5-HT$_3$) antagonists are now the most commonly used anti-emetics in the prevention and treatment of chemotherapy-induced nausea and vomiting (Campora *et al.* 1994). They are usually effective for early sickness (Cunningham 1997), but nausea and vomiting are occasionally refractory to anti-emetic treatment (Tonato *et al.* 1994).

Anticipatory nausea is more likely if the first treatment was complicated by nausea and vomiting (King 1997; Peters *et al.* 1994). This can lead to non-compliance with chemotherapy in extreme cases.

Acupuncture techniques have been largely used as adjuvants to anti-emetic treatment. Dundee *et al.* (1987) and Dundee & Yang (1990) conducted preliminary investigations of the anti-emetic activity of PC-6 stimulation in patients receiving chemotherapy while on anti-emetic treatment. These studies took place before the widespread use of 5-HT$_3$ antagonists. They showed that invasive acupuncture was more efficacious than non-invasive acupuncture, benefiting more than 90% of patients. However, the beneficial effects lasted less than 8 h. The efficacy of acupuncture was reduced in patients receiving highly emetogenic regimens (Dundee *et al.* 1987). Indirect TENS, especially applied in regular short intervals, benefited more than 85%

of patients (McMillan & Dundee 1990, 1991*b*). This was helped by the fact that TENS could be self-administered and 'topped up' at intervals of 2 h by further bursts of stimulation.

The findings from Dundee *et al.* (1987) were corroborated by evidence from work done by Aglietti *et al.* (1990). Liu *et al.* (1991) studied the magnetic stimulation of PC6 in patients in whom treatment of nausea and vomiting during chemotherapy with standard anti-emetics had been ineffective. The findings from their study indicated that magnetic discs at PC6 were also efficacious in preventing nausea and vomiting during chemotherapy.

Vickers' systematic review (Vickers 1996) included the efficacy of acupuncture, acupressure and TENS during chemotherapy. Five clinical trials met the inclusion criteria of this review and, although their quality was variable, all were positive.

Table 14.2 outlines some of the trials of acupuncture on chemotherapy-induced nausea and vomiting. One methodologically high-quality trial by Shen *et al.* (2000) was on 104 patients with breast cancer, receiving high-dose chemotherapy. The highly emetogenic treatment comprised cisplatin, cyclophosphamide and carmustine. Daily EA for 5 days at PC6 and ST36, a point with proven action on gastric function (Tougas *et al.* 1992), was compared with minimal needling at non-classical points, and conventional anti-emetics alone. The EA group was statistically significantly superior to both the minimal needling group and the conventional anti-emetic group. The minimal needling group was also statistically superior to the anti-emetic group, i.e. there were physiological effects at the non-specific site. It was therefore not an inactive control. The relief was maintained for 5 days when the patients had daily EA but not for the full 9-day study period. However, neither 5-HT_3 antagonists nor steroids were included in the conventional anti-emetic regimen, so future studies will need to compare acupuncture with current best anti-emetic medication. It is interesting to note that the negative study by Roscoe *et al.* (2002) used an electrical stimulus at PC6. It had promising aspects, but did not stipulate which electrical parameters were used, and may have been different from those found to give optimal effect by the late Professor John Dundee and Christine McMillan (Dundee & McMillan 1991).

On a practical note, it seems clear that PC6 stimulation is necessary before the emetogenic stimulus; that invasive treatment is more effective than non-invasive treatment; and that PC6 acupuncture is effective for approximately 8 h. TENS can help, but needs two-hourly stimulation at, ideally, low frequency. Future challenges remain to prolong the effects of PC6 acupuncture for patients undergoing emetogenic chemotherapy. Non-invasive transcutaneous forms of stimulation naturally seem safer and need developing and refining. Additionally, semi-permanent needles can be an attractive option and useful in the short-term, for example for 2–3 days post-emetogenic chemotherapy (J. Filshie, personal communication 2003). Patients can massage them two-hourly to maintain the anti-emetic effects. However, they can stay in for only a limited period of time as the needles might be a potential focus for infection if left *in situ* beyond a critical level of neutropenia.

Table 14.2 Summary of trials of acupuncture in the management of nausea and vomiting during chemotherapy

Study population	Number of patients	Acupuncture technique ± anti-emetic	Efficacy of acupuncture stimulation	Reference
Cisplatin treatment of testicular cancer	10	EA at PC6 vs EA at dummy point	Positive	Dundee et al. 1987
Patients receiving cisplatin treatment	77	Acupuncture vs historical control	Positive	Aglietti et al. 1990
General oncology	38	Seabands at PC6 vs Seabands at dummy point	Positive	Price et al. 1991
General oncology	18	Seabands at PC6 vs no intervention	Positive	Stannard 1989
Patients receiving highly emetogenic agents	8	TENS at PC6 + ondansetron vs ondansetron	Positive	McMillan et al. 1991
Mostly chemotherapy for breast cancer	27	Acupressure at PC6 vs acupressure at dummy site vs control	Negative	Roscoe et al. 2002
Chemotherapy for breast cancer	17	Acupressure at PC6 & ST6 + usual care	Positive	Dibble et al. 2000
High-dose chemotherapy for breast cancer	104	Daily EA 5 days SP6 + ST36 vs minimal needling vs standard anti-emetics	Positive 5 days	Shen et al. 2000

Acupuncture in nausea and vomiting in palliative care

Nausea and vomiting in advanced terminal care is considerably more complex (Filshie & Thompson 2003; Twycross & Back 1998). It may be due to one or more of the following causes: gastrointestinal problems, including varying degrees of intestinal obstruction; drugs, for example strong opioids such as morphine or some antibiotics; metabolic causes, including hypercalcaemia; renal failure; dehydration, and other electrolyte imbalances; brain metastases; pain and anxiety. The cause of the nausea and vomiting needs identifying by orthodox medical diagnosis and clinical investigation as appropriate, and acupuncture may or may not be indicated. If acupuncture is found to be of potential value, having excluded serious causes, points with known gastrointestinal physiological effects, for example ST36 (Tougas et al. 1992), or the segmental points CV12 or ST25, BL20 and BL21, may need to be added, if reversible gastrointestinal dysfunction is contributing to the nausea and vomiting.

Literature on the use of acupuncture for patients receiving palliative care is sparse. One study on only six patients in a hospice using an 'n of one design' had acupressure, a placebo wrist band or no band. No significant difference was found between them, though the sample size was too small to make any judgement (Brown et al. 1992).

Contraindications and cautions

The safety of acupuncture in palliative care has been reviewed (Filshie 2001). Direct needling with acupuncture will need to be avoided in a lymphoedematous limb, and may be contraindicated in a limb after axillary dissection. Non-invasive stimulation would be preferable if severe neutropenia complicates the clinical picture, or if a patient has extreme clotting dysfunction. One must note that the point PC6 lies above and relatively close to the median nerve, and so paraesthesia may occur if needles are inserted too deeply.

Mechanisms underlying the anti-emetic activity of acupuncture

Animal and human studies have revealed that acupuncture results in numerous neurophysiological responses (see Table 14.1). These responses occur both locally, at the site of application, and within the central nervous system, by complex ascending pathways, intracranial connections and descending pathways (Bowsher 1998; Lundeberg 1999; White 1999). Acupuncture releases β-endorphin and enkephalins, which act on μ and δ receptors, which can cause anti-emetic and pro-emetic actions, respectively. So far, the 'dose' of acupuncture must be in favour of the anti-emetic actions in the positive trials of acupuncture for anti-emesis. Acupuncture releases 5-HT and endogenous steroids, both of which may contribute to anti-emesis. Local anaesthetic injected at PC6, before acupuncture, blocks anti-emetic action (Dundee & Ghaly 1991). However, the precise underlying mechanisms for acupuncture anti-emetic activity are as yet unknown and likely to be complex. Furthermore, there are likely to be non-specific psychological effects. Nevertheless, the body of evidence for PC6 acupuncture so far demonstrates a specific effect of treatment over control groups (Lee & Done 1999; Vickers 1996). Acupuncture releases oxytocin, which is both analgesic and anxiolytic (Uvnas-Moberg *et al.* 1993) and this may contribute to relief of anxiety, which may be of particular help in cases of anticipatory nausea and vomiting. For post-operative nausea, it is possible that effective management of pain helps prevent it (Andersen & Krohg 1976). However, Lenhard and Waite (1983) showed that a decreased incidence in sickness after acupuncture in patients with migraine was not necessarily associated with pain relief, thus suggesting different mechanisms for acupuncture analgesia and acupuncture anti-emetic effects. Until further research is performed specifically to identify the contributions of these different effects, most theories remain speculative.

Conclusion

In conclusion, acupuncture has developed an established role in the treatment of PONV and also for chemotherapy-induced nausea and vomiting. Logical combinations of anti-emetics may eventually be found to be more effective when used in conjunction with acupuncture, than when used as direct alternatives. It may be particularly helpful for patients at high risk for PONV or with the more emetogenic chemotherapy regimens.

The types of stimulation, manual or electrical, and parameters of electrical stimulation, if used, need to be systematically investigated – as has been studied for pain (Chesterton *et al.* 2002, 2003) – to find the optimal relief, as well as the methods by which the anti-emetic action of acupuncture can be effectively prolonged.

Hypnosis

Trance experiences have been described since the time of the ancient Greeks, and 'animal magnetism' was popularised by Anton Mesmer in the 18th century, who used it for a range of psychosomatic conditions. James Braid coined the term 'hypnosis' in the 1840s. Hypnosis is an altered state of consciousness in a trusting relationship with a therapist. It involves a curious distortion of time awareness, thoughts and memories and greater access to the unconscious mind.

Spiegal & Moore (1997) have defined it as 'a natural state of aroused, attentive local concentration coupled with a relative suspension of peripheral awareness'. There are three principal components: absorption in the process, dissociation and suggestibility. Most of the normal critical faculties are suspended, and suggestions implanted in this state continue to affect the patient once aroused – the phenomenon of 'post-hypnotic suggestion'.

The methods rely more on the individual subject than on the skill of the hypnotist (Orne 1980). Hypnotisability is a stable, measurable state (Hilgard & Hilgard 1975; Spiegel & Spiegel 1978), with up to two-thirds of patients being hypnotisable, and approximately 10% highly responsive. There are direct and indirect methods. Indirect methods are gentle and less power-implicit approaches, and have been used successfully in cancer patients with low susceptibility (Barber 1982; Barber & Gitelson 1980).

Though more often used for relaxation, psychological support and 'ego strengthening', hypnosis has also been found to have a strong role in alleviation of pain associated with cancer (National Institutes of Health Technology Assessment Panel on Integration of Behavioral and Relaxation Approaches into the Treatment of Chronic Pain and Insomnia 1996). Furthermore, a meta-analysis of 20 studies of adjuvant hypnosis for surgery revealed significant benefits for 89% of surgical patients undergoing hypnosis, compared with a control (Montgomery *et al.* 2002). While in the UK general anaesthesia is almost exclusively used for painful procedures such as bone marrow aspiration and lumbar puncture, in children, hypnosis is often added to sedation techniques in other parts of the world to reduce the distress of these procedures. These have been reviewed by Steggles *et al.* (1986, 1997), Sutters & Miaskowski (1992), Ellis & Spanos (1994) and Genuis (1995).

Hypnosis for procedural, anticipatory and chemotherapy-related nausea and vomiting

The principal aim of hypnosis treatment is anxiety reduction, often employing guided imagery and progressive relaxation. The unpleasant sensations of nausea and vomiting are often displaced by the substitution of pleasant feelings. Multiple sessions of treatment may be required to gain effective symptom control. 'Auto-hypnosis' is frequently taught, so that patients can, at will, re-enter the pleasant frame of mind attained during hypnosis, when confronted with a challenging episode. Patients often have their imagery individually tailored to reflect their interests. Audio tapes can be made to back-up instructions given at consultation. Hilgard & LeBaron (1982) developed an imagination-focused form of clinical hypnosis for problems with paediatric cancer patients. Imagination is at its height in childhood, when imaginative play is of paramount importance to a child's development. To implement imagination-focused hypnosis, the child is interviewed about his/her favourite interests and activities, games, television characters, family and pets. The child is then guided through a tailor-made profoundly distracting fantasy sequence into the hypnotic state, when post-hypnotic suggestions can be successfully implanted.

Zeltzer and colleagues performed a series of studies of children. Initially these were observational. In 1983 they showed a reduction in nausea and vomiting, using patients as their own control (Zeltzer *et al.* 1983). In 1984 they showed a reduction in symptoms of both frequency and intensity of chemotherapy-related vomiting, compared with no intervention (Zeltzer *et al.* 1984). In 1991 they showed a reduction in symptoms when comparing hypnosis with a relaxation/distraction technique, using a standard treatment control group (Zelter *et al.* 1991). They demonstrated that distraction alone also reduced symptoms. Cotanch *et al.* (1985), Jacknow *et al.* (1994) and Hawkins *et al.* (1995) demonstrated in randomised controlled trials (RCTs) a reduction of symptoms of anticipatory nausea and vomiting or use of rescue medication, in children, compared with control groups. However, the effect was found to tail off in the four- to six-months follow-up period (Jacknow *et al.* 1994). Liossi (2000) has recently reviewed the use of hypnosis in paediatric oncology for both nausea and vomiting and procedure-related pain. She concluded that the use of hypnosis is extremely promising. However, she highlighted the need for further studies using hypnosis *in addition* to standard approaches, as did Montgomery *et al.* (2002), and also further refinement to trial methodology. Kuttner *et al.* (1988) have highlighted the fact that different approaches to hypnosis for pain and anxiety have different effects, based partly on the age of the child. Hypnosis may be better for age group 3–6 years, whereas both hypnosis and behavioural distraction may help 7–10 year-olds, though more than one session may be required.

Numerous studies have been performed on adults with anticipatory nausea and vomiting around chemotherapy. Marchioro *et al.* (2000) demonstrated a beneficial effect in 16 patients who had failed to be controlled by a $5-HT_3$ antagonist after previous highly emetogenic chemotherapy. They used a combination of relaxation and then hypnotherapy immediately before chemotherapy, with beneficial effects. Syrjala *et al.* (1992), though they demonstrated a reduction in mucositis pain visual analogue scale (VAS) scores in patients having hypnosis and undergoing bone marrow transplantation, failed to show a reduction in nausea, emesis and opioid use in the same group. Pre-treatment psychological distress strongly predicted nausea in this group during marrow transplantation, whereas pre-treatment physical dysfunction was a better predictor of emesis.

Hendler & Redd (1986) randomised patients to have identical interventions, different only in name. They were labelled hypnosis, relaxation or passive relaxation with guided imagery. The patients who had the intervention labelled hypnosis were significantly less likely to believe the procedure would effectively control nausea and vomiting, and less keen to try the intervention. On account of the fear or resistance towards the term 'hypnosis' an identical intervention may have different outcomes.

Hypnotherapy in palliative care

Although hypnosis has been found to be beneficial for relaxation, symptom control and coping skills in the care of terminally ill adults (Finlay & Jones 1996; Liossi & White 2001; O'Connell 1985) and children (Gardner 1988), there are only sporadic references to alleviation of nausea and vomiting.

There is no clear explanation for the effectiveness of hypnosis in symptom control of nausea and vomiting, based on the mechanisms of action understood at present. Table 14.3 shows some of the known effects of hypnosis as we currently understand them.

Table 14.3 Some of the known effects of hypnosis

Hypnosis is an altered state of consciousness with EEG patterns of alert wakefulness.	Alman & Lambrou 1993
Initially thought to be largely a right hemisphere orientated activity.	Pedersen 1995 Gruzelier 1996
Though much more complex than this in different circumstances depending on hypnotisable susceptibility, though frontal inhibition is also important.	Rainville *et al.* 1997
Hypnosis can affect the immune response.	Kiecolt-Glaser *et al.* 1986
The sensory and affective dimensions of pain are dissociated and PET scanning has shown changes in the anterior cingulate gyrus.	Rainville *et al.* 1997
However, the responses depend on the quality of the instructions given.	Rainville *et al.* 1999
There can be voluntary control of auditory evoked responses.	Hogan *et al.* 1984

Behavioural interventions including relaxation

Following early reports of reduced anticipatory nausea and vomiting after desensitisation (Morrow & Morrell 1982), a variety of approaches have been used (Carey & Burish 1988; King 1997). Virtual reality (VR) is an innovative form of distraction therapy for symptom control including nausea and vomiting in older children having chemotherapy (Schneider & Workman 2000) and adults with breast cancer (Schneider 2001). Most recently, Redd *et al.* (2001) have reviewed behavioural approaches, including hypnosis and relaxation, and have tabulated their efficacy for the treatment of nausea and vomiting.

Herbal medicine

Herbs are an integral part of traditional medicine in many cultures throughout the world, and numerous conventional drugs came into production by this route. The interface between drug and non-drug methods becomes somewhat blurred at this point! Aspirin from willow bark is one such example, and some herbs have been shown to have anti-tumour activity *in vitro* (Spaulding-Albright 1997). Cannabinoids have been used for a variety of symptoms in cancer patients (Kalant 2001). Several cannabinoids, derived from the plant/herb cannabis have been widely tested for control of chemotherapy-induced nausea and vomiting (Tramer *et al.* 2001). This systematic review did not include smoked cannabis. Although slightly superior to some conventional anti-emetics, such as metoclopramide, they had widespread effects on mood, some of which caused treatment withdrawal.

The powdered rhizomes of ginger have long been used in traditional medicine for alleviation of gastrointestinal illnesses. An anti-emetic effect was found, which reversed cisplatin-induced delay in gastric emptying, and the ginger juice preparation was found to be superior to ondansetron in dogs (Sharma *et al.* 1997) and rats (Sharma & Gupta 1998).

There is increasing evidence about herb–drug interactions (for example, Fugh-Berman 2000). Some commonly used herbal preparations adversely affect clotting function and antiviral and chemotherapy bioavailability (National Medicines Database, www.naturaldatabase.com). Quality assurance is also often variable. Clinicians need to be alert to this and should question their patients about any routine intake of herbal preparations.

Healing and therapeutic touch

Spiritual healing or 'therapeutic touch' is a systematic purposeful intervention by one or more persons aiming to help another living being by means of focused intention or hand contact to improve their condition (Abbot 2000; Benor 2001; The Prince of Wales's Foundation for Integrated Health 2003). Though there are many anecdotal reports of improvement in numerous symptoms, there is so far a lack of high-quality RCTs. Neil Abbot performed a systematic review of healing as a therapy for a variety of illnesses (Abbot 2000). He included one abstract of a dissertation by Sodergren (1994) on 80 patients who had 'therapeutic touch' versus an information group and a no-treatment group. Based on symptom scores, he showed a non-significant difference between the groups. Only a limited report on this study is available at present, so no further comment can be made.

Massage, aromatherapy and reflexology

Massage, aromatherapy and reflexology are widely available in hospices. These therapies and interventions have been reviewed by Wilkes (Wilkes 1992), Field (1998) and The Prince of Wales's Foundation for Integrated Health (2003). Ahles *et al.* (1999) have shown a reduction in distress, fatigue, nausea and anxiety immediately after three out of five massage sessions versus a control group with standard care. Foot massage was also helpful in reducing nausea and vomiting versus control (Grealish *et al.* 2000).

Music therapy

Music therapy has been shown to reduce anxiety and pain in a paediatric population around lumbar puncture (Rasco 1992). Music therapy has been used during a 48-h period as a diversional intervention during high-dose chemotherapy in patients receiving cyclophosphamide. It was found to reduce both nausea and vomiting as an adjunct to standard anti-emetic treatment (Ezzone *et al.* 1998). The intervention was simple to organise and deliver by nurses. It was individualised for each patient and seems worthy of further research, possibly including different chemotherapeutic regimens. Standley (1992) has also shown the benefit of music therapy for these symptoms.

Conclusion

Non-pharmacological interventions such as acupuncture and hypnosis have a strong evidence base to support their efficacy for nausea and vomiting in cancer patients. Additionally, behavioural treatment, herbal medicine, massage and music therapy have a lesser but accumulating evidence base. Many of these treatments have a low side-effect profile compared with drug treatment. Further work is recommended in these areas alongside conventional anti-emetic use, to try to reduce these symptoms even further in a group of patients already supremely challenged by a testing diagnosis and distressing symptom. More work is required to understand the basic neurophysiological mechanisms behind non-drug anti-emesis.

Acknowledgements

We acknowledge Professor J. W. Thompson for his considerable input to Table 14.1 and comments throughout the text; also Dr A. Vickers for his expertise and comments; Mrs J. Brooks for her invaluable secretarial support; and Mrs S. Cummings for help with the final editing.

References

Abbot, N. C. (2000). Healing as a therapy for human disease: a systematic review. *Journal of Alternative and Complementary Medicine* **6**, 159–169.

Abramowitz, M. D., Oh, T. H., Epstein, B. S., Ruttimann, U. E. & Friendly, D. S. (1983). The antiemetic effect of droperidol following outpatient strabismus surgery in children. *Anesthesiology* **59**, 579–583.

Aglietti, L., Roila, F., Tonato, M., Basurto, C., Bracarda, S., Picciafuoco, M., Ballatori, E. & Del Favero, A. (1990). A pilot study of metoclopramide, dexamethasone, diphenhydramine and acupuncture in women treated with cisplatin. *Cancer Chemotherapy and Pharmacology* **26**, 239–240.

Ahles, T. A., Tope, D. M., Pinkson, B., Walch, S., Hann, D., Whedon, M., Dain, B., Weiss, J. E., Mills, L. & Silberfarb, P. M. (1999). Massage therapy for patients undergoing autologous bone marrow transplantation. *Journal of Pain and Symptom Management* **18**, 157–163.

Aldridge, S. (2001). Acupuncture helps breast cancer patients (abstract), *American Society of Anaesthesiologists Annual Scientific Session*.

Alman, M. & Lambrou, P. (1993). *Self hypnosis*. London: Souvenir Press.

Andersen, R. & Krohg, K. (1976). Pain as a major cause of postoperative nausea. *Canadian Anaesthetists' Society Journal* **23**, 366–369.

Bandolier (2000). Non-pharmacological techniques prevent postoperative nausea and vomiting. http://www.jr2.ox.ac.uk/bandolier/band71/b71-9.html

Apfel, C. C., Laara, E., Koivuranta, M., Greim, C. A. & Roewer, N. (1999). A simplified risk score for predicting postoperative nausea and vomiting: conclusions from cross-validations between two centers. *Anesthesiology* **91**, 693–700.

Barber, J. (1982). Incorporating hypnosis in the management of chronic pain. In *Psychological approaches to the management of pain* (ed. J. Barber & C. Adrian), pp. 40–59. New York: Bunner/Mazel.

Barber, J. & Gitelson, J. (1980). Cancer pain: psychological management using hypnosis. *CA: A Cancer Journal for Clinicians* **30**, 130–136.

Bateman, N. (1991). Metoclopramide and acute movement disorders. *Prescribers' Journal* **31**, 212–215.

Belville, J. W. & Bross, I. D. J. (1960). Postoperative nausea and vomiting IV: factors related to postoperative nausea and vomiting. *Anesthesiology* **21**, 186–193.

Bender, C. M., McDaniel, R. W., Murphy-Ende, K., Pickett, M., Rittenberg, C. N., Rogers, M. P., Schneider, S. M. & Schwartz, R. N. (2002). Chemotherapy-induced nausea and vomiting. *Clinical Journal of Oncology Nursing* **6**, 94–102.

Benor, D. J. (2001). *Spiritual healing: scientific validation of a healing revolution*. Vision Publications, Southfield, MI.

Berman, B., Ezzo, J., Hadhazy, V. & Swyers, J. P. (1999). Is acupuncture effective in the treatment of fibromyalgia? *Journal of Family Practice* **48**, 213–218.

Bowsher, D. (1998). Mechanisms of acupuncture. In *Medical acupuncture: a western scientific approach* (ed. J. Filshie & A. White), pp. 69–82., Edinburgh: Churchill Livingstone.

Brown, S., North, D., Marvel, M. K. & Fons, R. (1992). Acupressure wrist bands to relieve nausea and vomiting in hospice patients: do they work? *American Journal of Hospital Palliative Care* **9**, 26–29.

Campora, E., Giudici, S., Merlini, L., Rubagotti, A. & Rosso, R. (1994). Ondansetron and dexamethasone versus standard combination antiemetic therapy. A randomized trial for the prevention of acute and delayed emesis induced by cyclophosphamide–doxorubicin chemotherapy and maintenance of antiemetic effect at subsequent courses. *American Journal of Clinical Oncology* **17**, 522–526.

Carey, M. P. & Burish, T. G. (1988). Etiology and treatment of the psychological side effects associated with cancer chemotherapy: a critical review and discussion. *Psychological Bulletin* **104**, 307–325.

Chesterton, L. S., Barlas, P., Foster, N. E., Lundeberg, T., Wright, C. C. & Baxter, G. D. (2002). Sensory stimulation (TENS): effects of parameter manipulation on mechanical pain thresholds in healthy human subjects. *Pain* **99**, 253–262.

Chesterton, L. S., Foster, N. E., Wright, C. C., Baxter, G. D. & Barlas, P. (2003). Effects of TENS frequency, intensity and stimulation site parameter manipulation on pressure pain thresholds in healthy human subjects. *Pain* **106**, 73–80.

Chiang, C.-Y., Chang, C.-T., Chu, H.-L. & Yang, L.-F. (1973). Peripheral afferent pathway for acupuncture analgesia. *Scientia Sinica* **16**, 210–217.

Cohen, M. M., Duncan, P. G., DeBoer, D. P. & Tweed, W. A. (1994). The postoperative interview: assessing risk factors for nausea and vomiting. *Anesthesia and Analgesia* **78**, 7–16.

Cohen, M. M., Duncan, P. G., Pope, W. D. B. & Wolkenstein, C. (1986). A survey of 112,000 anaesthetics at one teaching hospital (1975–83). *Canadian Anaesthetists' Society Journal* **33**, 22–31.

Cookson, R. F. (1986). Mechanisms and treatment of postoperative nausea and vomiting. In *Nausea and vomiting: mechanisms and treatment* (ed. C. J. Davis, G. V. Lake-Bakaar & D. G. Grahame-Smith), pp. 130–150. Berlin: Springer.

Cotanch, P., Hockenberry, M. & Herman, S. (1985). Self-hypnosis as antiemetic therapy in children receiving chemotherapy. *Oncology Nursing Forum* **12**, 41–46.

Cummings, M. (2000). Teasing apart the quality and validity in systematic reviews of acupuncture. *Acupuncture in Medicine* **18**(2), 104–107.

Cunningham, D. (1990). Treatment of emesis induced by cytotoxic drugs. *Hospital Update* **16**, 104.

Cunningham, R. S. (1997). 5-HT3-receptor antagonists: a review of pharmacology and clinical efficacy. *Oncology Nursing Forum* **24**(7) (Suppl.), 33–40.

Dibble, S. L., Chapman, J., Mack, K. A. & Shih, A. S. (2000). Acupressure for nausea: results of a pilot study. *Oncology Nursing Forum* **27**, 41–47.

Dickenson, A. H. (1996). Pain mechanisms and pain syndromes. In *Pain 1996 – an updated review* (ed. J. N. Campbell), pp. 113–121. Seattle: International Association for the Study of Pain.

Dorfer, L., Moser, M., Bahr, F., Spindler, K., Egarter-Vigl, E., Giullen, S., Dohr, G. & Kenner, T. (1999). A medical report from the stone age? *The Lancet* **354**, 1023–1025.

Dundee, J. W. (1990). Electro-acupuncture and postoperative emesis. *Anaesthesia* **45**, 789–790.

Dundee, J. W. & Ghaly, G. (1991). Local anesthesia blocks the antiemetic action of P6 acupuncture. *Clinical Pharmacology and Therapeutics* **50**, 78–80.

Dundee, J. W., Ghaly, R. G., Fitzpatrick, K. T. J., Lynch, G. A. & Abram, W. P. (1987). Acupuncture to prevent cisplatin-associated vomiting. *The Lancet* **i**, 1083.

Dundee, J. W. & McMillan, C. (1991). Positive evidence for P6 acupuncture antiemesis. *Postgraduate Medical Journal* **67**, 417–422.

Dundee, J. W. & Yang, J. (1990). Acupressure prolongs the antiemetic action of P6 acupuncture. *British Journal of Clinical Pharmacology* **29**, 644–645.

Dupeyron, J. P., Conseiller, C., Levarlet, M., Hemmingsen, C., Schoeffler, P., Pedersen, F. M., Gribomont, B. & Kaplan, L. A. (1993). The effect of oral ondansetron in the prevention of postoperative nausea and vomiting after major gynaecological surgery performed under general anaesthesia. *Anaesthesia* **48**, 214–218.

Ellis, J. A. & Spanos, N. P. (1994). Cognitive-behavioural interventions for children's distress during bone marrow aspirations and lumber punctures: a critical review. *Journal of Pain and Symptom Management* **9**, 96–108.

Ernst, E. & Pittler, M. H. (1998). The effectiveness of acupuncture in treating acute dental pain: a systematic review. *British Dental Journal* **184**, 443–447.

Ernst, E. & White, A. (1998). Acupuncture for back pain: a meta-analysis of randomized controlled trials. *Archives of Internal Medicine* **158**, 2235–2241.

Ezzo, J., Hadhazy, V., Birch, S., Lao, L., Kaplan, G., Hochberg, M. & Berman, B. (2001). Acupuncture for osteoarthritis of the knee: a systematic review. *Arthritis and Rheumatism* **44**, 819–825.

Ezzone, S., Baker, C., Rosselet, R. & Terepka, E. (1998). Music as an adjunct to antiemetic therapy. *Oncology Nursing Forum* **25**, 1551–1556.

Field, T. M. (1998). Massage therapy effects. *American Psychologist* **53**, 1270–1281.

Filshie, J. (2001). Safety aspects of acupuncture in palliative care. *Acupuncture in Medicine* **19**, 117–122.

Filshie, J. & Cummings, M. (1999). Western medical acupuncture. In *Acupuncture: a scientific appraisal* (ed. E. Ernst & A. White), pp. 31–59. Oxford: Butterworth-Heinemann.

Filshie, J. & Thompson, J. W. (2003). Acupuncture. In *Oxford textbook of palliative medicine*, 3rd edn (ed. D. Doyle *et al.*), pp. 410–423. Oxford: Oxford University Press.

Finlay, I. G. & Jones, O. L. (1996). Hypnotherapy in palliative care. *Journal of the Royal Society of Medicine* **89**, 493–496.

Fugh-Berman, A. (2000). Herb–drug interactions. *Lancet* **355**, 134–138.

Gardner, G. G. (1988). Hypnotherapy with the terminally ill child. In *Hypnosis and hypnotherapy with children* (ed G. G. Gardner and K. Olness), pp. 260–284. New York: Grune and Stratton.

Genuis, M. L. (1995). The use of hypnosis in helping cancer patients control anxiety, pain, and emesis: a review of recent empirical studies. *American Journal of Clinical Hypnosis* **37**, 316–325.

Goodman, M. (1997). Risk factors and antiemetic management of chemotherapy-induced nausea and vomiting. *Oncology Nursing Forum* **24**(7) (Suppl.), 20–32.

Grealish, L., Lomasney, A. & Whiteman, B. (2000). Foot massage. A nursing intervention to modify the distressing symptoms of pain and nausea in patients hospitalized with cancer. *Cancer Nursing* **23**, 237–243.

Gruzelier, J. (1996). The state of hypnosis: evidence and applications. *Quarterly Journal of Medicine* **89**, 313–317.

Grunwald, Z., Torjman, M., Schieren, H., & Bartkowski, R. R. (1993). The pharmacokinetics of droperidol in anesthetized children. *Anesthesia and Analgesia* **76**, 1238–1242.

Guo, H. F., Tian, J., Wang, X., Fang, Y., Hou, Y., & Han, J. (1996). Brain substrates activated by electroacupuncture of different frequencies (I): Comparative study on the expression of oncogene *c-fos* and genes coding for three opioid peptides, *Brain Research. Molecular Brain Research* **43**, 157–166.

Han, J. S. & Sun, S. (1990). Differential release of enkephalin and dynorphin by low and high frequencies electroacupuncture in the central nervous system. *Acupuncture: The Scientific International Journal (New York)* **1**, 19–27.

Han, J. S. & Terenius, L. 1982, Neurochemical basis of acupuncture analgesia. *Annual Review of Pharmacology and Toxicology* **22**, 193–220.

Han, J. S., Chen, X. H., Sun, S. L., Xu, X. J., Yuan, Y., Yan, S. C., Hao, J. X. & Terenius, L. (1991). Effect of low- and high-frequency TENS on Met-enkephalin-Arg-Phe and dynorphin A immunoreactivity in human lumbar CSF. *Pain* **47**, 295–298.

Hannallah, R. S., Britton, J. T., Schafer, P. G., Patel, R. I. & Norden, J. M. (1994). Propofol anaesthesia in paediatric ambulatory patients: a comparison with thiopentone and halothane. *Canadian Journal of Anaesthesia* **41**, 12–18.

Hawkins, P. J., Liossi, C., Ewart, B., Hatira, P., Kosmidis, H., Varvulsi, M. (1995). Hypnotherapy for control of anticipatory nausea and vomiting in children with cancer: preliminary findings. *Psycho-Oncology* **4**, 101–106.

Hendler, C. S. & Redd, W. H. (1986). Fear of hypnosis: the role of labeling in patients' acceptance of behavioral intervention. *Behavior Therapy* **17**, 2–13.

Henzi, I., Walder, B. & Tramer, M. R. (1999). Metoclopramide in the prevention of postoperative nausea and vomiting: a quantitative systematic review of randomized, placebo-controlled studies. *British Journal of Anaesthesia* **83**, 761–771.

Hilgard, E. R. & Hilgard, J. R. (1975). *Hypnosis in the relief of pain.* California: William Kaufmann.

Hilgard, J. R. & LeBaron, S. (1982). Relief of anxiety and pain in children and adolescents with cancer: quantitative measures and clinical observations. *International Journal of Clinical and Exprimental Hypnosis* **30**, 417–442.

Hogan, C. M. & Grant, M. (1997). Physiologic mechanisms of nausea and vomiting in patients with cancer. *Oncology Nursing Forum* **24**(7) (Suppl.), 8–12.

Hogan, M., MacDonald, J. & Olness, K. (1984). Voluntary control of auditory evoked responses by children with and without hypnosis. *American Journal of Clinical Hypnosis* **27**, 91–94.

Hovorka, J., Korttila, K. & Erkola, O. (1989). Nitrous oxide does not increase nausea and vomiting following gynaecological laparoscopy. *Canadian Journal of Anaesthesia* **36**, 145–148.

Jacknow, D. S., Tschann, J. M., Link, M. P. & Boyce, W. T. (1994). Hypnosis in the prevention of chemotherapy-related nausea and vomiting in children: a prospective study. *Developmental and Behavioral Pediatrics* **15**, 258–264.

Kalant, H. (2001). Medicinal use of cannabis: history and current status. *Pain Research and Management* **6**, 80–91.

Kenny, G. N. C. (1994). Risk factors for postoperative nausea and vomiting. *Anaesthesia* **49** (Suppl.), 6–10.

Kiecolt-Glaser, J. K., Glaser, R., Strain, E. C., Stout, J. C., Tarr, K. L., Holliday, J. E. & Speicher, C. E. (1986). Modulation of cellular immunity in medical students. *Journal of Behavioral Medicine* **9**, 5–21.

Kim, K. S., Koo, M. S., Jeon, J. W., Park, H. S. & Seung, I. S. (2002). Capsicum plaster at the Korean hand acupuncture point reduces postoperative nausea and vomiting after abdominal hysterectomy. *Anesthesia and Analgesia* **95**, 1103–1107.

King, C. R. (1997). Nonpharmacologic management of chemotherapy-induced nausea and vomiting. *Oncology Nursing Forum* **24**(7) (Suppl.), 41–48.

Korttila, K. (1992). The study of postoperative nausea and vomiting. *British Journal of Anaesthesia* **69**(7) (Suppl. 1), 20S–23S.

Korttila, K., Kauste, A. & Auvinen, J. (1979). Comparison of domperidone, droperidol, and metoclopramide in the prevention and treatment of nausea and vomiting after balanced general anesthesia. *Anesthesia and Analgesia* **58**, 396–400.

Kotani, N., Hashimoto, H., Sato, Y., Sessler, D. I., Yoshioka, H., Kitayama, M., Yasuda, T. & Matsuki, A. (2001). Preoperative intradermal acupuncture reduces postoperative pain, nausea and vomiting, analgesic requirement, and sympathoadrenal responses. *Anesthesiology* **95**, 349–356.

Kris, M. G., Gralla, R. J., Tyson, L. B., Clark, R. A., Kelsen, D. P., Reilly, L. K., Groshen, S., Bosl, G. J. & Kalman, L. A. (1985). Improved control of cisplatin-induced emesis with high-dose metoclopramide and with combinations of metoclopramide, dexamethasone, and diphenhydramine. Results of consecutive trials in 255 patients. *Cancer* **55**, 527–534.

Kuttner, L., Bowman, M. & Teasdale, M. (1988). Psychological treatment of distress, pain and anxiety for young children with cancer. *Developmental and Behavioral Pediatrics* **9**, 374–381.

Lee, A. & Done, M. L. (1999). The use of nonpharmacologic techniques to prevent postoperative nausea and vomiting: a meta-analysis. *Anesthesia and Analgesia* **88**, 1362–1369.

Lenhard, L. & Waite, P. M. (1983). Acupuncture in the prophylactic treatment of migraine headaches: pilot study. *New Zealand Medical Journal* **96**, 663–666.

Linde, K., Jobst, K. & Panton, J. (2000). Acupuncture for chronic asthma. *Cochrane Database Systematic Reviews* no. 2. CD000008.

Liossi, C. (2000). Clinical hypnosis in paediatric oncology: a critical review of the literature. *Sleep and Hypnosis* **2**, 125–131.

Liossi, C. & White, P. (2001). Efficacy of clinical hypnosis in the enhancement of quality of life of terminally ill cancer patients. *Contemporary Hypnosis* **18**, 145–160.

Liu, S., Chen, Z., Hou, J., Wang, J., Wang, J. & Zhang, X. (1991). Magnetic disk applied on Neiguan point for prevention and treatment of cisplatin-induced nausea and vomiting, *Journal of Traditional Chinese Medicine* **11**, 181–183.

Lundeberg, T. (1999). Effects of sensory stimulation (acupuncture) on circulatory and immune systems. In *Acupuncture: a scientific appraisal* (ed. E. Ernst & A. White), pp. 93–106. Oxford: Butterworth-Heinemann.

Ma, K. W. (1992). The roots and development of Chinese Acupuncture: from prehistory to early 20th century. *Acupuncture in Medicine* **10** (Suppl.), 92–99.

Madej, T. H. & Simpson, K. H. (1986). Comparison of the use of domperidone, droperidol and metoclopramide in the prevention of nausea and vomiting following gynaecological surgery in day cases. *British Journal of Anaesthesia* **58**, 879–883.

Marchioro, G., Azzarello, G., Viviani, F., Barbato, F., Pavanetto, M., Rosetti, F., Pappagallo, G. L. & Vinante, O. (2000). Hypnosis in the treatment of anticipatory nausea and vomiting in patients receiving cancer chemotherapy. *Oncology* **59**, 100–104.

McMillan, C. M. (1998). Acupuncture for nausea and vomiting. In *Medical acupuncture: a Western scientific approach* (ed. J. Filshie & A. White), pp. 295–317. Edinburgh: Churchill Livingstone.

McMillan, C. & Dundee, J. W. (1990). Problems of self-administration of P6 (Neiguan) antiemesis. *British Journal of Clinical Pharmacology* **31**, 236.

McMillan, C. & Dundee, J. W. (1991*a*). The role of transcutaneous electrical stimulation of Neiguan antiemetic acupuncture point in controlling sickness after cancer chemotherapy. *Physiotherapy* **77**, 499–502.

McMillan, C. & Dundee, J. W. (1991*b*). Is self-stimulation of P6 feasible as an antiemetic in cancer chemotherapy? *British Journal of Anaesthesia* **66**, 394–414.

McMillan, C. M., Dundee, J. W. & Abram, W. P. (1991). Enhancement of the antiemetic action of ondansetron by transcutaneous electrical stimulation of P6 antiemetic points in patients having highly emetic cytotoxic drugs. *British Journal of Cancer* **64**, 971–972.

Melchart, D., Linde, K., Fischer, P., Berman, B., White, A., Vickers, A. & Allais, G. (2001). Acupuncture for idiopathic headache. *Cochrane Database Systematic Reviews* no. 1, CD001218.

Montgomery, G. H., David, D., Winkel, G., Silverstein, J. H. & Bovbjerg, D. H. (2002). The effectiveness of adjunctive hypnosis with surgical patients: a meta-analysis. *Anesthesia and Analgesia* **94**, 1639–1645.

Morrow, G. R. & Morrell, C. (1982). Behavioral treatment for the anticipatory nausea and vomiting induced by cancer chemotherapy. *New England Journal of Medicine* **307**, 1476–1480.

National Institutes of Health Technology Assessment Panel on Integration of Behavioral and Relaxation Approaches into the Treatment of Chronic Pain and Insomnia. (1996). Integration of behavioral and relaxation approaches into the treatment of chronic pain and insomnia. *Journal of the American Medical Association* **276**, 313–318.

O'Connell, S. (1985). Hypnosis in terminal care: discussion paper. *Journal of the Royal Society of Medicine* **78**, 122–125.

Orne, M. T. (1980). Hypnotic control of pain: toward a clarification of the different psychological processes involved. *Research Publications – Association for Research in Nervous and Mental Disease* **58**, 155–172.

Palazzo, M. G. & Strunin, L. (1984). Anaesthesia and emesis. I. Etiology. *Canadian Anaesthetists' Society Journal* **31**, 178–187.

Park, J., Hopwood, V., White, A. R. & Ernst, E. (2001). Effectiveness of acupuncture for stroke: a systematic review. *Journal of Neurology* **248**, 558–563.

Pedersen, D. L. (1995). Hypnosis and the right hemisphere. *Proceedings of the British Society of Medical and Dental Hypnosis* **5**, 2–14.

Peters, D., Smith, J., Horrigan, C. & Mills, S. (1994). Chemotherapy-induced nausea. *Complementary Therapies in Medicine* **2**, 193–199.

Price, H., Lewith, G. & Williams, C. (1991). Acupressure as an antiemetic in cancer chemotherapy. *Complementary Medical Research* **5**, 93–94.

Rainville, P., Carrier, B., Hofbauer, R. K., Bushnell, M. C. & Duncan, G. H. (1999). Dissociation of sensory and affective dimensions of pain using hypnotic modulation. *Pain* **82**, 159–171.

Rainville, P., Duncan, G. H., Price, D. D., Carrier, B. & Bushnell, M. C. (1997). Pain affect encoded in human anterior cingulate but not somatosensory cortex. *Science* **277**, 968–971.

Rasco, C. (1992). Using music therapy as distraction during lumbar punctures. *Journal of Pediatric Oncology Nursing* **9**, 33–34.

Redd, W. H., Montgomery, G. H. & DuHamel, K. N. (2001). Behavioral intervention for cancer treatment side effects. *Journal of the National Cancer Institute* **93**, 810–823.

Roscoe, J. A., Morrow, G. R., Bushunow, P., Tian, L. & Matteson, S. (2002). Acustimulation wristbands for the relief of chemotherapy-induced nausea. *Alternative Therapies* **8**, 56–63.

Roth, L. U., Maret-Maric, A., Adler, R. H. & Neuenschwander, B. E. (1997). Acupuncture points have subjective (needling sensation) and objective (serum cortisol increase) specificity. *Acupuncture in Medicine* **15**, 2–5.

Rusy, L. M., Hoffman, G. M. & Weisman, S. J. (2002). Electroacupuncture prophylaxis of postoperative nausea and vomiting following pediatric tonsillectomy with or without adenoidectomy. *Anesthesiology* **96**, 300–305.

Schlager, A., Boehler, M. & Puhringer, F. (2000). Korean hand acupressure reduces postoperative vomiting in children after strabismus surgery. *British Journal of Anaesthesia* **85**, 267–270.

Schlager, A., Offer, T. & Baldissera, I. (1998). Laser stimulation of acupuncture point P6 reduces postoperative vomiting in children undergoing strabismus surgery. *British Journal of Anaesthesia* **81**, 529–532.

Schneider, S. M. (2001). Effect of virtual reality on symptom distress in breast cancer patients. *Oncology Nursing Forum* **28**, 341.

Schneider, S. M. & Workman, M. L. (2000). Virtual reality as a distraction intervention for older children receiving chemotherapy. *Pediatric Nursing* **26**, 593–597.

Sharma, S. S. & Gupta, Y. K. (1998). Reversal of cisplatin-induced delay in gastric emptying in rats by ginger (*Zingiber officinale*). *Journal of Ethnopharmacology* **62**, 49–55.

Sharma, S. S., Kochupillai, V., Gupta, S. K., Seth, S. D. & Gupta, Y. K. (1997). Antiemetic efficacy of ginger (*Zingiber officinale*) against cisplatin-induced emesis in dogs. *Journal of Ethnopharmacology* **57**, 93–96.

Shen, J., Wenger, N., Glaspy, J., Hays, R. D., Albert, P. S., Choi, C. & Shekelle, P. G. (2000). Electroacupuncture for control of myeloablative chemotherapy-induced emesis: a randomized controlled trial. *Journal of the American Medical Association* **284**, 2755–2761.

Shenkman, Z., Holzman, R. S., Kim, C., Ferrari, L. R., DiCanzio, J., Highfield, E. S., Van Keuren, K., Kaptchuk, T., Kenna, M. A., Berde, C. B. & Rockoff, M. A. (1999). Acupressure–acupuncture antiemetic prophylaxis in children undergoing tonsillectomy. *Anesthesiology* **90**, 1311–1316.

Smith, G. (1996). Inhalational anaesthetic agents. In *Textbook of anaesthesia*, 3rd edn (ed. A. R. Aitkenhead & G. Smith), pp. 121–138. Edinburgh: Churchill Livingstone.

Smith, L. A., Oldman, A. D., McQuay, H. J. & Moore, R. A. (2000). Teasing apart quality and validity in systematic reviews: an example from acupuncture trials in chronic neck and back pain. *Pain* **86**, 119–132.

Sodergren, K. A. (1994). The effect of absorption and social closeness on responses to educational and relaxation therapies in patients with anticipatory nausea and vomiting during cancer chemotherapy. *Dissertation Abstracts International* **54**, 6137.

Somri, M., Vaida, S. J., Sabo, E., Yassain, G., Gankin, I. & Gaitini, L. A. (2001). Acupuncture versus ondansetron in the prevention of postoperative vomiting. A study of children undergoing dental surgery. *Anaesthesia* **56**, 927–932.

Spaulding-Albright, N. (1997). A review of some herbal and related products commonly used in cancer patients. *Journal of the American Dietetic Association* **97**(10) (Suppl. 2), S208–S215.

Spiegel, D. & Moore, R. (1997). Imagery and hypnosis in the treatment of cancer patients. *Oncology* **11**, 1179–1189.

Spiegel, H. & Spiegel, D. (1978). *Trance and treatment.* Washington: American Psychiatric Press.

Standley, J. M. (1992). Clinical applications of music and chemotherapy: the effects on nausea and emesis. *Music Therapy Perspectives* **10**, 27–35.

Stannard, D. (1989). Pressure prevents nausea. *Nursing Times* **85**, 33–34.

Steggles, S., Damore-Petingola, S., Maxwell, J. & Lightfoot, N. (1997). Hypnosis for children and adolescents with cancer: an annotated bibliography, 1985–1995. *Journal of Pediatric Oncology Nursing* **14**, 27–32.

Steggles, S., Fehr, R. & Aucoin, P. (1986). Hypnosis for children and adolescents with cancer: an annotated bibliography 1960–1985. *Journal of the Association of Pediatric Oncology Nurses* **3**, 23–25.

Stener-Victorin, E., Waldenstrom, U., Nilsson, L., Wikland, M. & Janson, P. O. (1999). A prospective randomized study of electro-acupuncture versus alfentanil as anaesthesia during oocyte aspiration in in-vitro fertilization. *Human Reproduction* **14**, 2480–2484.

Sutters, K. A. & Miaskowski, C. (1992). The problem of pain in children with cancer: a research review. *Oncology Nursing Forum* **19**, 465–471.

Syrjala, K. L., Cummings, C. & Donaldson, G. W. (1992). Hypnosis or cognitive behavioral training for the reduction of pain and nausea during cancer treatment: a controlled clinical trial. *Pain* **48**, 137–146.

The Prince of Wales's Foundation for Integrated Health and National Council for Hospice and Specialist Palliative Care Services (2003). *National guidelines for the use of complementary therapies in palliative care.* London: The Prince of Wales's Foundation for Integrated Health.

Tian, J. *et al.* (1997). Involvement of endogenous orphanin FQ in electroacupuncture-induced analgesia. *Neuroreport* **8**, 497–500.

Tonato, M., Roila, F., Del Favero, A. & Ballatori, E. (1994). Antiemetics in cancer chemotherapy: historical perspective and current state of the art. *Support.Care Cancer* **2**, 150–160.

Tougas, G., Yuan, L. Y., Radamaker, J. W., Chiverton, S. G. & Hunt, R. H. (1992). Effect of acupuncture on gastric acid secretion in healthy male volunteers. *Digestive Diseases and Sciences* **37**, 1576–1582.

Tramer, M. R., Carroll, D., Campbell, F. A., Reynolds, D. J., Moore, R. A. & McQuay, H. J. (2001). Cannabinoids for control of chemotherapy induced nausea and vomiting: quantitative systematic review. *British Medical Journal* **323**, 16–21.

Tramer, M. R., Reynolds, D. J., Moore, R. A. & McQuay, H. J. (1997). Efficacy, dose–response, and safety of ondansetron in prevention of postoperative nausea and vomiting: a quantitative systematic review of randomized placebo-controlled trials. *Anesthesiology* **87**, 1277–1289.

Twycross, R. & Back, I. (1998). Nausea and vomiting in advanced cancer. *European Journal of Palliative Care* **5**, 39–45.

Uvnas-Moberg, K., Bruzelius, G., Alster, P. & Lundeberg, T. (1993). The antinociceptive effect of non-noxious sensory stimulation is mediated partly through oxytocinergic mechanisms. *Acta Physiologica Scandinavica* **149**, 199–204.

van Tulder, M. W., Cherkin, D. C., Berman, B., Lao, L. & Koes, B. W. (1999). The effectiveness of acupuncture in the management of acute and chronic low back pain: a systematic review within the framework of the Cochrane Collaboration Back Review Group. *Spine* **24**, 1113–1123.

Vickers, A. & Zollman, C. (1999). ABC of complementary medicine. Hypnosis and relaxation therapies. *British Medical Journal* **319**, 1346–1349.

Vickers, A. J. (1996). Can acupuncture have specific effects on health? A systematic review of acupuncture antiemesis trials. *Journal of the Royal Society of Medicine* **89**, 303–311.

Wang, S. M. & Kain, Z. N. (2002). P6 acupoint injections are as effective as droperidol in controlling early postoperative nausea and vomiting in children. *Anesthesiology* **97**, 359–366.

White, A. (1999). Neurophysiology of acupuncture analgesia. In *Acupuncture: a scientific appraisal* (ed. E. Ernst & A. White), pp. 60–92. Oxford: Butterworth-Heinemann.

White, P. F., Issioui, T., Hu, J., Jones, S. B., Coleman, J. E., Waddle, J. P., Markowitz, S. D., Coloma, M., Macaluso, A. R. & Ing, C. H. (2002). Comparative efficacy of acustimulation (ReliefBand) versus ondansetron (Zofran) in combination with droperidol for preventing nausea and vomiting. *Anesthesiology* **97**, 1075–1081.

Wilkes, E. (1992). Complementary therapy in hospice and palliative care. Report for Trent Palliative Care Centre.

Windle, P. E., Borromeo, A., Robles, H. & Ilacio-Uy, V. (2001). The effects of acupressure on the incidence of postoperative nausea and vomiting in postsurgical patients. *Journal of Perianesthetic Nursing* **16**, 158–162.

Zelter, L. K., Dolgin, M. J., LeBaron, S. & LeBaron, C. (1991). A randomized, controlled study of behavioural intervention for chemotherapy distress in children with cancer. *Pediatrics* **88**, 34–42.

Zeltzer, L., Kellerman J., Ellenberg, L. & Dash, J. (1983). Hypnosis for reduction of vomiting associated with chemotherapy and disease in adolescents with cancer. *Journal of Adolescent Health Care* **4**, 77–84.

Zeltzer, L., LeBaron, S. & Zeltzer, P. M. (1984). The effectiveness of behavioral intervention for reduction of nausea and vomiting in children and adolescents receiving chemotherapy. *Journal of Clinical Oncology* **2**, 683–690.

Zhou, Y., Sun, Y. H., Shen, J. M. & Han, J. S. (1993). Increased release of immunoreactive CCK-8 by electroacupuncture and enhancement of electroacupuncture analgesia by CCK-B antagonist in rat spinal cord. *Neuropeptides* **24**, 139–144.

PART 4

The prevention and control of depression, anorexia

Chapter 15

Assessment and management of depression in palliative care

Mari Lloyd-Williams, Fiona Taylor and Iain Lawrie

Introduction

Despite recent advances in health promotion, cancer screening, and the development of new chemotherapeutic agents, many patients will develop metastases and die of their advanced cancer. Much work has been done to evaluate the physical sequelae of advanced cancer, but relatively little research has been carried out into the psychological and psychiatric sequelae. Depression is a significant symptom for many palliative care patients but is under-recognised and frequently not treated (Lloyd-Williams 2000, 2002; Lloyd-Williams & Friedman 2001).

The prevalence of depression

The prevalence of depression in the general population is 6% (Bergevin & Bergevin 1995); therefore several patients diagnosed with advanced cancer may have a pre-existing psychiatric disorder. The exact prevalence of depression in palliative care patients is difficult to establish from the current literature. Reported rates, from studies using structured diagnostic interviews or well-defined criteria, vary from 5% to 26% solely for major depression and to 32% for all depressive disorders (Hoptopf *et al.* 2002). It is expected that approximately one in four patients admitted to a palliative care unit will have significant depressive symptoms (Buckberg *et al.* 1984; Lynch 1995).

What causes depression in palliative care patients?

It is not known why some patients with advanced cancer develop depression whereas others do not, but patients with advanced cancer face many stresses during the course of their illness. Such stresses include fears of dying, disability, disfigurement and dependence (Breitbart 1995), all of which are enhanced by the disease process (see Figure 15.1). Goldberg & Cullen (1985) described the role of key relationships, as an additional psychosocial factor in determining the onset of depression. Although, such concerns are universal, the level of psychological distress experienced differs between individuals depending on personality, coping ability, social support and medical factors (Breitbart 1995). The realisation that certain factors predispose to the development of depression can improve the ability to prevent patient suffering and therefore deserves further consideration (Martin *et al.* 1999).

Increased physical debility contributes to the development of psychiatric morbidity. Kurtz *et al.* (2001) found that a greater physical functioning deficit predicted higher levels of depressive symptomatology in newly diagnosed patients over the age of 65 years. Physical symptoms are more likely to correlate with depressive symptoms when they remain uncontrolled, have high severity and are numerous, thus adding to patient burden (Martin *et al.* 1999). Patients with pancreatic cancer have a higher prevalence of depression, possibly through the activity of paraneoplastic mechanisms (Holland *et al.* 1986). Factors, for example pain or knowledge of poor prognosis, are also thought to contribute to depression (Shakin *et al.* 1988). Evidence shows patients' awareness of their illness (for example, prognosis) and expectations about treatment outcomes are also important (Alexander *et al.* 1993).

Damage to the central nervous system or metabolic alterations, such as hypercalcaemia and hypercortisolism (Cushings syndrome), may also cause depressive symptoms. There are numerous explanatory mechanisms including secretion of toxins by the tumour, autoimmune reactions, viral infections, nutritional deficits and neuroendocrine dysfunction and as a side effect of treatment with corticosteroids (Breitbart *et al.* 1989). Chemotherapeutic agents (Weddington 1982) and whole-brain radiation (DeAngelis *et al.* 1989) have also been associated with the development of depression.

Personality factors

Personality factors, such as traits and attitudes, have been considered to determine the patient's perception of their environment and feelings associated with this (Lichter 1991). When symptom severity demands adaptation, the resulting loss of normal roles and independence contributes to the patient's emotional distress. A positive or negative outlook, the desire to maintain control, and traits such as pessimism, neuroticism and low self esteem all affect the patient's ability to cope and hinder adjustment.

Cancer imposes stress on a previously healthy individual. Such stresses are heightened at times of diagnosis, treatment, recurrence and when an individual is faced with a short prognosis. An overhanging threat of death elicits different coping strategies from different individuals, ranging from stoic acceptance to complete denial. However, when such defence mechanisms fail, the physical, psychological and spiritual burden upon the patient may take its toll and lead to an adjustment or psychiatric disorder.

Social factors

The ability of the patient to cope effectively is also influenced by the presence of social support, a mechanism whereby interpersonal relationships offer a source of comfort, confidence and protection. Isolation may occur through stigmatisation, a reluctance to voice problems to family or relatives or simply by living alone. Other social factors causing increased distress include, concurrent life stresses such as

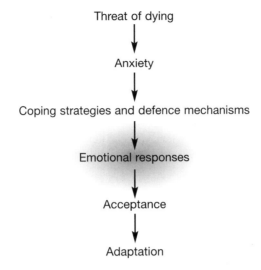

Figure 15.1 Processes occurring when facing death (Hodgson 1993)

financial or family problems. Lichter (1991) described how resolution of personal concerns expressed by patients alleviated psychological distress and led to peaceful deaths.

It is also important to recognise past episodes of depression and substance/alcohol abuse in a patient's history as these place them at greater risk (Massie *et al.* 1990).

The role of gender is less obvious. In the general population, females have twice the rate of major depression than men, but in a review, looking specifically at gender differences in cancer patients, depression was found to be equally prevalent in men and women (DeFlorio *et al.* 1995).

Age may also play a role, although this is harder to establish because cancer mainly develops in later life. In a retrospective study involving 1,046 patients who had been admitted to palliative care units, patients prescribed antidepressants were significantly younger than those that were not (Lloyd-Williams *et al.* 1999).

The exact aetiology of depression is unknown but it is important to recognise predisposing factors to improve the physicians' ability to detect those patients at greater risk.

The diagnosis of depression

Depression is characterised by persistent low mood (dysphoria) and loss of interest in activities (anhedonia). The clinical diagnosis of depression is made according to criteria, e.g. DSM-IV criteria (Figure 15.2). These criteria have been developed largely in psychiatric settings and recommend that to diagnose depression at least five of the listed symptoms must be present. Each symptom must also meet standards of severity (most of the day, nearly every day) and duration (longer than 2 weeks).

Depressed mood most of the day, nearly every day (dysphoria).

Markedly diminished interest or pleasure in all, or almost all, activities most of the day (anhedonia).

Significant weight loss or gain or decrease or increase in appetite.

Psychomotor agitation or retardation (mental and physical slowing).

Fatigue or loss of energy.

Feelings of worthlessness or excessive or inappropriate guilt.

Diminished ability to think or concentrate, or indecisiveness.

Recurrent thoughts of death (not just fear of dying), or suicidal thoughts/actions.

Figure 15.2 DSM-IV criteria to identify major depression (American Psychiatric Association 1996).

Much of the work on examining diagnostic criteria for depression in patients with cancer has been done with those at an early stage of the illness.

Endicott (1984) had discussed the complex problem of deciding which symptoms may be attributable to the cancer and which may be due to depression. She proposed that the somatic symptoms listed should be substituted in the patient with cancer, i.e.:

- Poor appetite or weight gain; substituted for fearfulness or depressed appearance in body or face.
- Insomnia/hypersomnia; substituted for social withdrawal or decreased talkativeness.
- Loss of energy, fatigue; substituted for brooding, self pity, pessimism.
- Diminished concentration or slowed thinking; substituted for; cannot be cheered up, does not smile, no response to good news or funny situations.

Endicott also stressed the importance of asking patients with cancer about suicidal ideation.

Detecting depression

Depression is an illness with no distinct biological markers or effective diagnostic test. The physician must rely upon skill and knowledge in differentiating depression from 'appropriate sadness' or grief reactions as the end of life approaches (Casey 1994). Low mood can be seen as a continuous variable in cancer patients. Physicians need to seek symptoms actively and not expect the patient to report them spontaneously. Non-disclosure by the patient may occur for several reasons. Patients may emphasise physical symptoms, as they believe that the physician is most helpful in this area, and perceive emotional problems as wasting the doctor's time. It must be noted that patient's attitudes may be reinforced by familial or cultural beliefs. The cancer patient may already feel stigmatised and the physician may believe that the added label of depression may enhance stigmatisation and therefore mental suffering; however, most patients are accepting of treatment (Maguire 2000).

There is uncertainty as to how to address such psychological issues with the terminally ill. Staff may perceive enquiries as adding to the patient's distress and are afraid of the consequences of asking direct questions about feelings. Razavi *et al.* (1994) stated that patients do not feel such questions are stressful as long as they are asked in an empathetic way. Thus staff confidence may be an issue or simply a lack of time (Barraclough 1997). Many professionals are involved in the care of the patient with advanced cancer and therefore it is possible that psychological issues may be perceived as someone else's responsibility and therefore overlooked.

Physicians may attribute somatic symptoms of depression to the cancer illness, highlighting their tendency to separate mental from physical health as described by Tucker (1999).

Block (2000) suggested hopelessness, helplessness, worthlessness, guilt and suicidal ideation as better indicators of depression. However, Chochinov (1994) found that a high threshold approach did not increase diagnostic accuracy if somatic symptoms were excluded and that the prevalence rate of major depression is only increased when somatic symptoms are assessed less stringently. It can be argued that a high threshold approach leads to a high number of false negatives and therefore untreated patients, an argument also valid against the total exclusion of somatic symptoms.

Chochinov *et al.* (1994) also looked at the application of diagnostic criteria and small differences in interpreting the severity of symptoms were found to confer with large differences in depressive rates. The diagnosis of depression relies on clinical judgment. The recognition of predisposing factors and the role of non-somatic symptoms in assessing cancer patients are important. However, poor detection remains a significant problem; Maguire (1985) stated that up to 80% of developed psychological morbidity remains unrecognised and untreated. Methods of improving detection of depression are clearly needed.

Structured clinical interviews are the best way to identify depression (McDaniel *et al.* 1995), but time, training, skill and expense limit large-scale usage. Validated screening instruments must not be viewed as substituting a clinical interview but have a role in contributing towards the assessment of probable cases. Self-administered tools would allow many patients to be surveyed with relatively little cost.

Screening for depression in palliative care

Screening tools for depression were originally designed for the physically well population. Hence their validity in palliative care patients is questionable and the debate over the inclusion of somatic or non-somatic symptoms resurfaces. Validity refers to whether or not the intended outcome variable is measured by the tool in the specified population. Reliability measurements are also important to calculate when establishing scales to determine the degree whereby results are consistent and reproducible.

Several tools have been validated in the palliative care population against 'gold standard' criteria, and cut-off points have been established to direct the physician towards possible depressive cases. The best cut-off point is decided upon by evaluating corresponding sensitivity and specificity values.

The Hospital Anxiety and Depression Scale

The Hospital Anxiety and Depression Scale (HADS) is the most frequently used tool in palliative care settings (Hoptopf *et al.* 2002). The scale (devised by Zigmond and Snaith (1983)) excludes confounding somatic symptoms, which could have a physical or emotional aetiology. The HADS consists of fourteen items, seven relate to anxiety and seven relate to depression. The patient has a choice of four responses for each item, scored on a likert scale of 0–3. The depression subscale is based on the concept of anhedonia, with five out of seven items reflecting loss of pleasure. This incites criticism because it excludes other non-somatic aspects of depression and it reduces its discriminatory power among palliative care patients, where suicide and feelings such as worthlessness, guilt and hopelessness are deemed important. Le Fevre *et al.* (1999) found the anxiety subscale performed better than the depressive subscale. Although this result was not statistically significant, it implies the co-existence of symptoms, and recommended a cut off of 20 when the total HAD score is evaluated. A further paper by Lloyd-Williams *et al.* (2001) found that using a combined cut-off threshold of 19 gave the optimum sensitivity and specificity but these were both below 70%.

Are you depressed?

The single item 'Are you depressed? 'Yes' or 'No' is orally administered and requires an oral answer from the patient. In a study by Chochinov *et al.* (1997) the single item regarding depressed mood, from the Schedule of Affective Disorders and Schizophrenia (SADS) diagnostic criteria, correctly predicted the diagnostic outcome for all the 197 advanced cancer patients assessed with a sensitivity and specificity 100%. These values suggest that the single item could work as a diagnostic rather than as a screening tool. The addition of another item regarding loss of pleasure reduced sensitivity to 98% but specificity remained at 100%.

A similar question, 'Do you often feel sad or miserable?' 'Yes' or 'No', was compared with the Montgomery Asberg depression rating scale (MADRS) in stroke patients (Watkins *et al.* 2001) and to a semi-structured interview in geriatric patients (Mahoney *et al.* 1994). In both studies, patients' responses to the single item, 'Yes' or 'No', correctly classified them as depressed or non-depressed respectively, in over 80% of the sample.

The Edinburgh Postnatal Depression Scale

The Edinburgh Postnatal Depression Scale (Edinburgh scale) is a self-assessment scale consisting of ten items corresponding to the non-somatic symptoms of depression, including subjective sadness, hopelessness, guilt and thoughts of self-harm. For every item there are four possible responses, each response is rated on a 4-point scale ranging from 0 to 3 in severity. The patient selects the statement in each item that seems to fit best with their mood over the past 7 days. The total is calculated from a maximum score of 30. The Edinburgh scale was originally designed to screen females for depression in the postnatal period and to be administered by healthcare workers with no background in psychiatry (Cox *et al.* 1987, 1996). The Edinburgh scale has been validated in a group of 100 metastatic advanced cancer patients (Lloyd-Williams *et al.* 2000). A cut-off score of 13, was found to have a sensitivity of 0.81 and specificity of 0.79 for detecting cases of depression and a positive and negative predictive value of 0.53 and 0.94, respectively.

Difficulties associated with screening tools in palliative care patients

Problems exist with the use of screening tools in the terminally ill population. In a study where the Hospital Anxiety and Depression Scale was administered to 52 hospice inpatients, only 33% completed the initial form (Urch *et al.* 1998). This highlights the relevance of short, simple assessment tools in this population. Visual Analogue Scales (VAS) may be useful (Lees & Lloyd-Williams 1999) but they have yet to be validated against a clinical interview for terminally ill patients.

The ethos behind screening is to detect patients who would benefit from further interventions. The identification of high-risk groups improves the odds of identifying patients with a mental illness (Hoeper *et al.* 1984). The relief of unnecessary suffering justifies the costs and implementation of a screening programme. Screening also allows many patients to be assessed without the involvement of psychiatric staff. Numerous tools have been described, yet the best time to screen for depression in palliative care patients is still subject to debate. Two issues are paramount: when to screen and how frequently to screen. Screening must initially occur at a point that will allow time for subsequent interventions to be effective. How frequently one should screen is more difficult to establish and depends upon the stability of depression over time. Lloyd-Williams & Riddleston (2002), in a study of palliative day-care patients, concluded that screening at initial referral is beneficial; having found that patient-rated depressive scores remained largely constant over a period of three months.

Antidepressant drugs

Antidepressants elevate mood, concurrently enhancing interest and drive, thus restoring normal social behaviour and preventing further depressive episodes. Evidence has shown that depression involves the under-activity of central neuronal pathways where the monoamines, norepinephrine and serotonin, act as neurotransmitters (Hollister 1995). Antidepressants are effective in blocking the re-uptake or breakdown of these neurotransmitters thus increasing their concentration within the synaptic cleft and enhancing neuronal activity. In a study of cancer patients referred to liaison psychiatry services, 67% were prescribed antidepressants, and 80% of these patients showed good clinical response (Chaturvedi *et al.* 1994).

Antidepressants take at least two to three weeks for a therapeutic response; hence prognosis is the most important factor when deciding upon an appropriate drug. Tricyclic antidepressants and selective serotonin reuptake inhibitors (SSRIs) are commonly used. SSRIs are specific to blocking the reuptake of serotonin and hence are better tolerated by terminally ill patients because the autonomic and sedating side effects, found with tricyclic antidepressants, are absent. Tricyclic antidepressants also have greater toxicity in overdose and cannot be used in patients with cardiac complications.

Psychostimulants are worth considering in patients with a short lifespan, because a therapeutic response can take days rather than weeks (Martin *et al.* 2000). Fatigue is reduced, appetite stimulated and overall sense of well-being improved (Homsi *et al.* 2001). They are widely prescribed in the USA yet their use within the UK remains limited. The treatment of depression in the terminally ill should be the same as for other patients with depression. All patients require good psychological support, together with antidepressant medication at an appropriate dosage and for an adequate length of time. Few patients with advanced metastatic cancer are prescribed antidepressant medication (Lloyd-Williams *et al.* 1999), there is a reluctance to prescribe antidepressant medication by some medical staff who have the mistaken belief that patients with cancer do not warrant or need treatment as their depression is in some way 'understandable'. There is also the misconception of antidepressant drugs being addictive (Maguire 2000; Martin & Jackson 2000). These misconceptions are unfounded and there are many effective antidepressants available with good side-effect profiles.

Counselling

There is considerable interest in the role of counselling for depression in palliative care patients. Counselling is defined as giving the client an opportunity to explore, discover and clarify ways of living more resourcefully and towards greater well-being. Many patients find the opportunity to talk about their concerns and fears to be helpful and may find this opportunity from their clinical nurse specialist and other nurse, doctor, paramedical staff and clergy. A recent study in primary care suggested that although counselling can be considered an appropriate treatment in some cases (Chilvers *et al* 2001), antidepressants have a faster onset of action and are therefore more appropriate for patients with a short life expectancy. For palliative care patients, the need is for psychological support from empathic professionals, but the energy and effort required to engage in a therapeutic relationship with a counsellor may be too great. Additionally, these patients are already in contact with many professionals and attend many hospital and clinic appointments; suggesting they see a counsellor weekly may be yet another burden and there is no evidence to suggest that designated counsellors are more effective than medical, nursing or allied staff who have built a caring relationship and are able to listen effectively. Indeed, one of the crucial aspects of providing good, effective psychosocial support is the giving of information (Fallowfield *et al.* 1995). Patients have frequent concerns about treatment options, prognosis and what will happen to them as they deteriorate; such questions can only be answered by medical and nursing staff with clinical knowledge.

Difficulties in managing the depressed patient

The presence of depression can make the general management and treatment of the patient difficult for the physician, especially as it is difficult to detect. Depression can lead to increased perception of pain and other physical symptoms. Such difficulties lead to earlier inpatient or hospice admission, longer periods of hospitalisation and therefore increased costs over non-depressed physically ill patients (Levenson *et al.* 1990). Intervention could also prevent co-morbidity in family members (Hopwood *et al.* 2000), another factor that may lead to early patient admission. Depression may cause the patient to be non-compliant with treatment and staff requests, and to withdraw from family and friends.

The patient's quality of life is affected not only through the amplification of physical symptoms but also through emotional suffering. Such distress impairs the patient's capacity for pleasure and reduces the ability to do the emotional work of separating and saying goodbye before death (Block 2000).

Depression is a factor in requests to hasten death (Chochinov *et al.* 1995). Depression has been found to correlate with suicidal ideation in advanced cancer patients, but as the feeling of hopelessness correlated higher in a study by Chochinov *et al.* (1998) this association cannot be explained by depression alone. The identification and treatment of depression may evoke a will to live and hence enable patients to make the most of their remaining time rather than wishing it all to end quickly.

Conclusions

Depression is a distressing and disabling symptom for many patients with advanced cancer. Prompt identification and treatment can do much to improved the quality of life for patients. Screening may be an aid to better recognition of depressive symptoms. The newer antidepressants with good side-effect profiles should be used for patients with advanced cancer and although supportive care is paramount, there is no evidence to suggest that interventions such as counselling confer any benefit in this population.

References

Alexander, P., Dinesh, N. & Vidyasagar, M. (1993). Psychiatric morbidity among cancer patients and its relationship with awareness of illness and expectation about treatment outcome. *Acta Oncologia* **46**, 623–626.

Barraclough, J. (1997). ABC of palliative care: depression, anxiety and confusion. *British Medical Journal* **315**, 1365–1368.

Bergevin, P. & Bergevin, R. (1995). Recognising depression. *American Journal of Hospice and Palliative Care* **12**, 22–23.

Block, S. (2000). Assessing and managing depression in the terminally ill patient. *Annals of Internal Medicine* **132**, 209–218.

Breitbart, W. (1995). Identifying patients at risk for, and treatment of major psychiatric complications of cancer. *Supportive Care in Cancer* **3**, 45–60.

Breitbart, W., Holland, J. & Stiefel F. (1989). Corticosteroids in cancer: neuropsychiatric complications. *Cancer Investigation* **7**, 479–491.

Buckberg, J., Penman, D. & Holland, J. (1984). Depression in hospitalised cancer patients. *Psychosomatic medicine* **46**, 199–211.

Casey, P. (1994). Depression in the dying disorder or distress. *Progress in Palliaitve Care* **2**, 1–3.

Chaturvedi, S., Maguire, P. & Hopwood, P. (1994). Antidepressant medications in cancer patients. *Psycho-Oncology* **3**, 57–60.

Chilvers, C., Dewey, M., Fielding, K., Gretton, V., Miller, P., Palmer, B., Weller, D., Churchill, R., Williams, I., Bedi, N. *et al.* (2001). Antidepressant drugs and generic counselling for treatment of major depression in primary care: randomised trial with patient preference arms. *British Medical Journal* **322**, 772–775.

Chochinov, H., Wilson, K., Enns, M. & Lander, S. (1994). Prevalence of depression in the terminally ill: effects of diagnostic criteria and symptom threshold judgements. *American Journal of Psychiatry* **151**, 537–540.

Chochinov, H., Wilson, K., Enns, M., Mowchun, N., Lander, S., Levitt, M. & Clinch, J. J. (1995). Desire for death in the terminally ill. *American Journal of Psychiatry* **152**, 1185–1191.

Chochinov, H., Wilson, K., Enns, M. & Lander, S. (1997). 'Are you depressed?' Screening for depression in the terminally ill. *American Journal of Psychiatry* **154**, 674–676.

Chochinov, H., Keith, G., Wilson, K., Enns, M. & Lander, R. (1998). Depression, hopelessness and suicidal ideation in the terminally ill. *Psychosomatics* **39**, 366–370.

Cox, J., Holden, J. & Sagovsky, R. (1987). Detection of postnatal depression: Development of 10 item Edinburgh Postnatal Depression Scale. *British Journal of Psychiatry* **150**, 782–786.

Cox, J., Chapman, G., Murray, D. & Jones, P. (1996). Validation of the Edinburgh Postnatal Scale (EPDS) in postnatal women. *Journal of Affective Disorders* **39**, 185–189.

DeAngelis, L., Delattre, J. & Posner, J. (1989). Radiation induced dementia in patients cured of brain metastasis. *Neurology* **39**, 789–796.

DeFlorio, M. & Massie, M. (1995). Review of depression in cancer: gender differences. *Depression* **3**, 66–80.

American Psychiatric Association (1996). *Diagnostic and Statistical Manual of Mental Disorder*, 4th edn. American Psychiatric Association.

Endicott, J. (1984). Measurement of depression in patients with cancer. *Cancer* **10** (Suppl.), 2243–2249.

Fallowfield, L., Ford, S. & Lewis, S. (1995). No news is not good news: information preferences of patients with cancer. *Psycho-Oncology* **4**, 197–202

Goldberg, R. & Cullen, L. (1985). Factors important to psychosocial adjustment to cancer; a review of the evidence. *Social Science of Medicine* **20**, 803–807.

Hodgson, G. (1993). Depression, sadness and anxiety. In *The management of terminal malignant disease* (ed. C. Saunders & N. Sykes), 3rd edn. London: Edward Arnold.

Hoeper, E., Nycz, G., Kessler, L., Burke, J. & Pierce, W. (1984). The usefulness of screening for mental illness. *The Lancet* **i**, 33–35.

Holland, J., Hughes, A., Tross, S., Perry, M., Oster, M. & Cormis, R. (1986). Comparative disturbance in patients with pancreatic and gastric cancers. *American Journal of Psychiatry* **143**, 982–986.

Hollister, L. (1995). Antidepressant agents. In *Basic and clinical pharmacology*, 6th edition (ed. B. Katzung). USA: Appleton & Lange.

Homsi, J., Nelson, K., Sarhill, N., Rybicki, L., LeGrand, S., Davis, M. & Walsh, D. (2001). A phase II study of methylphenidate for depression in advanced cancer. *American Journal of Hospice and Palliative Care* **18**, 403–407.

Hotopf, M., Chidgey, J., Addington-Hall, J., Lan Ly, K. (2002). Depression in advanced disease: a systematic review. Part 1: prevalence and case finding. *Palliative Medicine* **16**, 81–97.

Hopwood, P. & Stephens, J. (2000). Depression in patients with lung cancer: prevalence and risk factors derived from quality of life data. *Journal of Clinical Oncology* **18**, 893–903.

Kurtz, M., Kurtz, J., Stommel, M., Given, C. & Given, B. (2001). Physical functioning and depression among older persons with cancer. *Cancer Practice* **9**, 11–18.

Le Fevre, P., Devereux, J., Smith, S., Lawrie, S. & Cornbleet, M. (1999). Screening for psychiatric illness in the palliative care inpatient setting: a comparison between the Hospital Anxiety and Depression Scale and the General Health Questionnaire-12. *Palliative Medicine* **13**, 399–407.

Lees, N. & Lloyd-Williams, M. (1999). Assessing depression in palliative care patients using the visual analogue scale: a pilot study. *European Journal of Cancer Care* **8**, 220–223.

Levenson, J., Hamer, R. & Rossite, R. (1990). Relationship of psychopathology in general medical inpatients to use and cost of service. *American Journal of Psychiatry* **147**, 1491–1503.

Lichter, I. (1991). Some psychological causes of distress in the terminally ill. *Palliative Medicine* **5**, 138–146.

Lloyd-Williams, M. (2000).The assessment and treatment of depression in palliative care patients. *Postgraduate Medical Journal* **76**, 555–558.

Lloyd-Williams, M., Friedman, T. & Rudd, N. (2001). The validation of the Hospital Anxiety and Depression scale in terminally ill patients. *Journal of Pain and Symptom Management* **22**, 990–996.

Lloyd-Williams, M. & Friedman, T. (2001). The prevalence of depression in terminally ill patients. *European Journal of Cancer Care* **10**, 270–274.

Lloyd-Williams, M. (2002). Should we screen for depression in palliative care patients? *American Journal of Hospice and Palliative Care* **19**, 112–114.

Lloyd-Williams, M., Friedman T. & Rudd, N. (1999). A survey of antidepressant prescribing in the terminally ill. *Palliative Medicine* **13**, 243–248.

Lloyd-Williams, M., Freidman, T. & Rudd, N. (2000). Criterion validation of the Edinburgh Postnatal Depression Scale as a screening tool for depression in patients with advanced metastatic cancer. *Journal of Pain and Symptom Management* **20**, 259–265.

Lloyd-Williams, M. & Riddleston, H. (2002). The stability of depression scores in patients who are receiving palliative care. *Journal of Pain and Symptom Management* **24**, 593–597.

Lynch, M. (1995). The assessment and prevalence of affective disorders in advanced cancer. *Journal of Palliative Care* **11**, 10–18.

Maguire, P. (1985). Improving the detection of psychiatric problems in cancer patients. *Social Science of Medicine* **20**, 819–823.

Maguire, P. (2000). The use of antidepressants in patients with advanced cancer. *Supportive Care in Cancer* **8**, 265–267.

Mahoney, J., Drinka, T., Abler, R., Gunter-Hunt, G., Matthews, C., Gravenstein, S. & Carnes, M. (1994). Screening for depression: Single Question versus GSD. *Journal of American Geriatric Society* **42**, 1006–1008.

Martin, A. & Jackson, K. (1999). Depression in palliative care patients. *Journal of Pharmaceutical Care in Pain and Symptom Control* **7**, 71–89.

Martin, A. & Jackson, K. (2000). Depression in palliative care patients. *Hospice Journal* **7**, 71–78.

Massie, M. & Holland, J. (1990). Depression and the cancer patient. *Journal of Clinical Psychiatry* **51**, 12–17.

McDaniel, J., Musselman, D., Porter Redd, D. & Nemeroff, C. (1995). Depression in patients with cancer. *Archives of General Psychiatry* **52**, 90–99.

Razavi, D. & Stiefel, F. (1994). Common psychiatric disorders in cancer patients: adjustment disorders and depressive disorders. Review article. *Support Cancer Care* **2**, 223–232.

Shakin, E. & Holland, J. (1988). Depression and pancreatic cancer. *Journal of Pain and Symptom Management* **3**, 194–198.

Tucker, J. (1999). Modification of attitudes to influence survival from breast cancer. *The Lancet* **354**, 1320.

Urch, C., Chamberlain, J. & Field, G. (1998). The drawback of the hospital anxiety and depression scale in the assessment of depression in hospice inpatients. *Palliative Medicine* **12**, 395–396.

Watkins, C., Daniels, L., Jack, C., Dickinson, H. & van den Broek, M. (2001). Accuracy of a single question in screening for depression in a cohort of patients after stroke: comparative study. *British Medical Journal* **323**, 1159.

Weddington, W. (1982). Delirium and depression associated with amphotericin B. *Psychosomatics* **23**, 1076–1078.

Zigmond, A. & Snaith, R. (1983). The Hospital Anxiety and Depression Scale. *Acta Psychiatrica Scandinavica* **67**, 361–70.

Chapter 16

The management of anorexia

Samantha Jayasekera and Patrick Stone

> '*My father holds a trembling spoon and sucks at it, the liquid only, not the little*
> *vegetables floating around, which he avoids as if they were the equivalent size and*
> *hardness of a chop…Ah, chicken. But it might as well be stone. My father chews away*
> *for a minute or two, then spits it out. There are two little mounds of mashed potatoes,*
> *too, but he ignores these completely. "It tastes like paraffin," he says, not whingeing,*
> *merely reporting. "And it's so dry. It's like swallowing sawdust, or twigs."* '
>
> Blake Morrison (1993)

Introduction

Patients with cancer commonly complain of profound involuntary weight loss and absence or loss of appetite. These are the clinical signs that form the hallmarks of cachexia. Cachexia is also characterised by abnormalities in carbohydrate, fat, protein and energy metabolism, which manifest as weakness, fatigue, malaise and loss of skeletal muscle and adipose tissue (Doyle *et al.* 1998). Anorexia is defined as a loss of appetite and may occur in the absence of other features of cachexia. The focus of this chapter is the management of the *symptom* of anorexia rather than the *syndrome* of cancer cachexia. Where possible, recommendations will be evidence-based.

The causes of anorexia

Anorexia often develops in the context of cancer cachexia. Current evidence suggests that cachexia arises as a result of the interplay between host factors (e.g. cytokines) and tumour-derived products (e.g. lipid-mobilising factor). An in-depth review of the pathophysiology of this syndrome is beyond the scope of this article. Anorexia may also develop independently of the cachexia syndrome. Common causes for anorexia include:

1. Anorexia developing as part of the syndrome of cancer cachexia.
2. Poor oral hygiene, oral candida, ill-fitting dentures and dysphagia.
3. Poorly controlled pain, dyspnoea, nausea and constipation leading to reduced food intake and anorexia.
4. Chemotherapy and radiotherapy resulting in gastric dysfunction and/or mucositis. Treatment-related nausea and/or fatigue may also contribute to anorexia.
5. Tumour or surgery affecting the gastrointestinal tract leading to obstruction or absorption problems.

6. Many drugs can cause gastro-intestinal upset and/or nausea and may thus contribute to anorexia, e.g. selective serotonin re-uptake inhibitors (SSRIs), non-steroidal anti-inflammatory drugs (NSAIDs) and antibiotics (e.g. metronidazole).

Aim of management

For patients with advanced cancer it may not be appropriate to manage weight loss and anorexia aggressively. Often it is relatives rather than patients themselves who are more concerned about anorexia and weight loss. For this reason a careful exploration of the meaning that this symptom holds for patients and their carers is a useful starting point before embarking on active interventions. Some patients may simply wish that they had a slightly better appetite so that they can join in family meals. Other patients may be more concerned about actually putting on some weight because of the distress that can be caused by altered body image.

In this review we will consider both non-pharmacological and pharmacological treatment strategies.

Non-pharmacological management of anorexia

Several non-pharmacological methods have been used in the management of anorexia.

1. Treating the underlying cause. If a treatable underlying cause for the anorexia is identified then this should be managed appropriately. Thus patients with oral thrush will benefit from anti-fungal treatment and patients with chronic nausea secondary to delayed gastric emptying may benefit from a pro-kinetic anti-emetic (e.g. metoclopramide). Attention should also be paid to the presence of co-existing symptoms such as pain, anxiety or depression which may indirectly lead to anorexia.
2. General dietary advice. Cancer patients are often provided with non-specific or 'common sense' advice. Many cancer charities and organisations provide leaflets containing such advice (see Figure 16.1). The effectiveness of this type of advice on improving nutritional outcomes and/or anorexia has not been adequately evaluated.
3. Specific nutritional advice. More in-depth advice is usually provided by a dietician. A recent systematic review (Brown 2002) reviewed the evidence for the effectiveness of such an approach. The authors reviewed seven randomised controlled trials and reported that although dietetic advice resulted in increased calorie and protein intake there was no difference in survival, tumour response, nutritional status or quality of life.
4. Enteral/parenteral nutrition (EPN). The use of enteral/parenteral nutrition is controversial and initial attempts to combat cancer cachexia with enteral or parenteral nutrition have not been very successful (Nixon 1996). In one study (Jatoi et al. 2002) it was reported that patients retained water and fat but did not

---

General dietary advice

1. Eat frequent, small meals.
2. Remember that many people have a better appetite in the morning.
3. Increase calories and protein in diet.
4. Drink small amounts of liquids with meals.
5. Avoid noxious odours.
6. Find a nutritional supplement that is appealing.
7. Exercise as tolerated with your doctor's permission.
8. Make mealtimes relaxing by adding music, candles, etc.
9. Soft, cool, frozen foods may be more appealing.
10. Keep healthy snacks handy.

Figure 16.1 Adapted from *Eating hints for cancer patients* (http://www.nci.nih.gov/cancerinfo/eatinghints)

build up lean body mass. No systematic review of EPN was identified; however, most authors seem to agree with the sentiments expressed by Inui (2002) who stated that 'the place of aggressive nutritional treatment in malignant disease remains ill-defined…most systematic studies…have been disappointing'. If there is any role for EPN it is probably confined to patients with decreased food intake due to mechanical obstruction of their gastro-intestinal tract. Sikora *et al.* (1998) showed that parenteral nutrition facilitated the complete administration of chemo-radiation doses in patients with oesophageal cancer. Whereas the benefits of EPN remain unclear, there is good evidence of morbidity associated with this approach (e.g. infection). There is even a theoretical risk that EPN may lead to an increase in tumour growth.

5. Physical exercise. Courneya *et al.* (1999) have systematically reviewed the evidence for the benefits of exercise in cancer patients. They found that patients who took regular physical exercise showed improved functional capacity, muscle strength, body composition, haematological indicators, and less nausea, fatigue, anxiety and depression. There were no studies in the systematic review that specifically addressed the effect of physical exercise on appetite. One of the studies in the review (Winningham *et al.* 1989) reported that supervised exercise resulted in a decrease in percentage body fat and an increase in lean body mass in a cohort of patients with stage II breast cancer in contrast with the control group. Another study (Winningham *et al.* 1988), also done with patients with a diagnosis of stage II breast cancer, showed that supervised exercise led to a larger decrease in symptoms of nausea when compared with the control group. Although neither study had anorexia as a specific endpoint, the results may still be relevant because of the expected close relation between nausea and loss of appetite.

Pharmacological management of anorexia

Although many pharmacological approaches have been suggested as treatments for anorexia, very few of them have been adequately evaluated or have been found to be of benefit. The best evidence seems to be for the use of progestagens and corticosteroids.

1. Progestagens. There is good evidence that progestagens are an effective treatment in cancer anorexia. A recent systematic review and meta-analysis (Maltoni *et al.* 2001) found that there was a statistically significant improvement in appetite in patients taking high-dose progestagens (odds ratio 4.23, 95% confidence interval: 2.53–7.04). However, the benefits of progestagens seem to be restricted to increased appetite and increased weight. Most studies have failed to find any other quality-of-life benefits with this group of drugs (Bruera *et al.* 1998; Feliu *et al.* 1992). The optimal time at which to start treatment with progestagens is yet to be determined. Some studies have suggested that the effects of progestagens are greater in patients with earlier stage disease (Simons *et al.* 1996; Beller *et al.* 1997). Progestagens can take many weeks to have their full effect and this may limit their usefulness in patients with advanced disease.

2. Corticosteroids. In patients with advanced cancer it is probably more common for patients to be prescribed corticosteroids than progestational steroids. Mantovani *et al.* (2001) have recently reviewed five randomised controlled trials which showed that glucocorticoids had significant effects on appetite, food intake, sensation of well-being and performance status although a beneficial effect on body weight was not shown. In these studies the beneficial effects were limited to about four weeks. There is no evidence that one glucocorticoid is superior to any other in its appetite stimulating ability (Nelson 2000). Because of the well-documented side-effects of corticosteroids, it is important that these drugs are not prescribed without a proper assessment of their effectiveness in individual patients. It is the authors' own clinical practice to prescribe 4 mg dexamethasone once a day for a one-week trial period and then to review. If there is no evidence of benefit then the steroids are stopped immediately; if there is an improvement in appetite then the steroids are reduced to the lowest maintenance dose compatible with continued symptom control.

3. Fish-oil extracts. Early studies of fish-oil-based interventions in cancer cachexia have yielded promising results. The benefits of fish-oil, especially eicosapentaenoic acid (EPA), were initially demonstrated in the field of cardiology, where it was shown that consumption was associated with a reduced tendency to platelet aggregation, reduced blood viscosity, and an improvement in lipid profile (Leaf *et al.* 1988). Individuals who consume fish at least twice a week have been shown to have a reduction in mortality after myocardial infarct (Burr *et al.* 1989). More recently, there is some evidence that fish-oil extracts may also have beneficial

effects in cancer patients. In an uncontrolled, open-label study, Barber *et al.* (1999) reported that patients gained a median of 2.5 kg of body weight after seven weeks of consuming a fish-oil-enriched nutritional supplement. Body-composition analysis suggested no change in fat mass but a significant gain in lean body mass. The functional ability of patients was seen to improve significantly in these patients, as measured by the Karnofsky performance score. Appetite was also seen to improve significantly. A preliminary report of a study by Fearon *et al.* (2001) has suggested that patients who consume one and a half to two cans per day of a fish-oil-enriched nutritional supplement experience a net gain in body weight. A definitive report of this study has not yet been published. Until such time, it is difficult to draw firm conclusions about the role of these supplements in managing anorexia.

4. Other approaches. There are many other potential agents that have been suggested or tried for cancer cachexia. These include cannabinoids, melatonin, branched-chain amino acids, thalidomide, clenbuterol, anabolic steroids and NSAIDS. Although some of these drugs have shown promising early results or have good theoretical grounds for suggesting that they may be effective treatments for anorexia, none of them has yet been adequately evaluated.

Conclusion

The management of anorexia is an important aspect of the care of patients with cancer, with the potential to improve both quality of life and survival. Progestational drugs are the treatment with the best evidence for effectiveness. Treatment strategies should be tailored to the individual patient, with attention paid to the management of reversible causes of anorexia (e.g. poor oral hygiene). However, because anorexia is a multi-factorial problem, it is unlikely that any single treatment will prove to be effective. A combination of approaches may be more successful.

References

Barber, M. D., Ross, J. A., Voss, A. C., Tisdale, M. J. & Fearon, K. C. (1999). The effect of an oral nutritional supplement enriched with fish-oil on weight loss in patients with pancreatic cancer. *British Journal of Cancer* **81**, 80.

Beller, E., Tattersall, M., Lumley, T., Levi, J., Dalley, D., Olver, I., Page, J., Abdi, E., Wynne, C., Friedlander, M. *et al.* (1997). Improved quality of life with megestrol acetate in patients with endocrine-insensitive advanced cancer: a randomised placebo-controlled trial. Australasian megestrol acetate cooperative study group. *Annals of Oncology* **8**, 277–283.

Brown, J. K. (2002). A systematic review of the evidence on symptom management of cancer related anorexia and cachexia. *Oncology Nursing Forum* **29**, 517–530

Bruera, E., Ernst, S., Hagen, N., Spachynski, K., Belzile, M., Hanson, J., Summers, N., Brown, B., Dulude, H. & Gallant, G. (1998). Effectiveness of megestrol acetate in patients with advanced cancer: a randomised double-blind crossover study. *Cancer Prevention and Control* **2**, 74–78.

Burr, M. L., Fehily, A. M., Gilbert, J. F., Rogers, S., Holliday, R. M., Sweetnam, P. M., Elwood, P. C. & Deadman, N. M. (1989). Effects of changes in fat, fish and fibre intakes on death and myocardial reinfarction: Diet and Re-infarction Trial (DART). *The Lancet* ii, 757.

Courneya, K. & Friedenreich, C. M. (1999). Physical exercise and Quality of life following cancer diagnosis: a literature review. *Annals of Behavioral Medicine* **21**, 171–179.

Doyle, D., Hanks, G. & MacDonald, N. (eds) (1998). *Oxford textbook of palliative medicine*, 2nd edn, pp. 548–556. Oxford: Oxford University Press.

Fearon, K. C. H., von Meyenfeldt, M., Moses, A., Geenen, R. V., Roy, A., Gouma, D., Giacosa, A., Gossum, A. V. & Tisdale, M. (2001). An energy and protein dense, high n-3 fatty acid oral supplement promotes weight gain in cancer cachexia. *European Journal of Cancer* **37**(6) (Suppl.), p. 90 (abstract).

Feliu, J., Gonzalez-Baron, M., Berrocal. A,, Artal, A., Ordonez, A., Garrido, P., Zamora, P., Garcia de Paredes, M. L. & Montero, J. M. (1992). Usefulness of megestrol acetate in cancer cachexia and anorexia. *American Journal of Clinical Oncology* (CCT) **15**, 436–440.

Inui, A. (2002). Cancer anorexia–cachexia syndrome. *CA: A Cancer Journal for Clinicians* **52**, 72–91.

Jatoi, A. & Loprinzi, C. L. (2002). Adenosine triphosphate: does it help cancer patients get bigger and strong? *Journal of Clinical Oncology* **20**, 362–363.

Leaf, A. & Weber, P. C. (1988). Cardiovascular effects of n-3 fatty acids. *New England Journal of Medicine* **318**, 549.

Mantovani, G., Maccio, A., Massa, E. & Madeddu, C. (2001). Managing cancer related anorexia/cachexia. *Drugs* **61**, 499–514.

Morrison, B. (1993). *And when did you last see your father?* London: Granta Books.

Nelson, K. A. (2000). The cancer anorexia-cachexia syndrome. *Seminars in Oncology* **27**, 64–68.

Nixon, D. W. (1996). Cancer, cancer cachexia and diet: lessons from clinical research. *Nutrition* **12**, 525–565.

Simons, J. P. F. H. A., Aaronson, N. K., Vansteenkiste, J. F., ten Velde, G. P., Muller, M. J., Drenth, B. M., Erdkamp, F. L., Cobben, E. G., Schoon, E. J., Smeets, J. B. *et al.* (1996). Effects of medroxyprogesterone acetate on appetite, weight and quality of life in advanced stage non-hormone-sensitive cancer: a placebo controlled multicentric study. *Journal of Clinical Oncology* **14**, 1077–1084.

Sikora, S. S., Ribeiro, U., Kane, J. M., 3rd, Landreneau, R. J., Lembersky, B. & Posner, M. C. (1998). Role of nutrition support during induction chemo-radiation treatment in esophageal cancer. *Journal of Parenteral and Enteral Nutrition* **22**, 18–21.

Winningham, M. L. & MacVicar, M. G. (1988). The effect of aerobic exercise on patient reports of nausea. *Oncology Nursing Forum* **15**, 447–450.

Winningham, M. L, MacVicar, M.G., Bondoc, M., Anderson, J. & Minton, J. (1989). Effect of aerobic exercise on body weight and composition in patients with breast cancer on adjuvant chemotherapy. *Oncology Nursing Forum* **16**, 683–689.

PART 5

Perspectives in clinical management at the end of life

Withholding versus withdrawing treatment, 'Do Not Attempt Resuscitation' orders and advance directives: perspectives in medical law and professional ethics

John Keown

Introduction

When is it lawful and ethical to withhold or withdraw a life-prolonging treatment? Recent years have witnessed a burgeoning interest in this question, not least because of the increasing technological ability of modern medicine to prolong life. The growing significance of the issue has been reflected by important judgments handed down by the courts and guidance issued by the British Medical Association (BMA).

These judicial decisions and professional guidelines have generated animated ethical debate. One major criticism has been that the law and guidance are ethically inconsistent. Although they prohibit acts which have as their intention (aim) the shortening of a patient's life, they permit intentionally shortening patients' lives by omission. In other words, they are Hippocratic in prohibiting 'active euthanasia' but hypocritical in allowing 'passive euthanasia'. This paper considers whether this charge of ethical inconsistency is justified. The paper falls into three parts which address, respectively, the law; the BMA guidance; and ethics.

Part I. The law

Competence

In law, a patient is competent to consent to treatment, or to refuse consent, if they have the capacity to understand and retain information and weigh it in the balance to arrive at a decision. All adult patients are presumed to be competent, though the presumption is rebuttable. If a competent refuses a treatment, a doctor who overrides their refusal is liable for battery. This could result in the doctor being sued for damages in the civil courts or even prosecuted in the criminal courts.

The courts appear to have granted competent (adult) patients an *absolute* right to refuse treatment, even if non-treatment spells death. For example, in the case of Ms B, a paralysed patient was being kept alive by a ventilator. She asked her doctors to withdraw the ventilator; they refused. The court held that as Ms B was competent she had a right to refuse even life-saving treatment and that her doctors were, therefore, acting unlawfully in maintaining her ventilation. The right to refuse treatment established by such cases appears to be unqualified and to extend even to refusals of treatment which are clearly suicidal.

Whereas the right to refuse medical interventions appears to be absolute, the right to consent to such interventions is not. If a doctor were to inject a patient with a lethal dose of potassium chloride, it would be no defence to a charge of murder for the doctor to plead that the patient had requested it. Dr Nigel Cox, a consultant, was convicted of the attempted murder of one of his elderly patients by administering potassium chloride to her, even though she had repeatedly requested that he end her life.

Similarly, it would not be a defence to a charge of assisted suicide that the patient, to whom the doctor had handed the lethal substance for self-administration, had asked for it. As the case of Diane Pretty confirmed, a patient has no right to assisted suicide and the law against assisted suicide is consistent with the European Convention on Human Rights.

Incompetence: advance directive or 'living will'

If the patient is not competent, the next question is whether the patient was previously competent and made an anticipatory refusal of the treatment. Such anticipatory refusals are often described as 'advance directives' or 'living wills'. Unlike wills, however, there are no formalities provided for the making of advance refusals, which may be either written or oral. The courts have held that provided the advance refusal is 'clearly established and applicable to the circumstances' which have materalised, it is legally binding. As with a contemporaneous refusal of treatment, a doctor who overrides a binding advance directive incurs liability for battery even if, it appears, the advance refusal is clearly suicidal.

No advance directive

If the incompetent patient has made no advance directive, then the legal duty of the doctor is to act in the patient's 'best interests'. This vague concept lacks legal definition. However, it is widely agreed that it is not in a patient's best interests to be subjected to treatment that is futile, that is, has no reasonable hope of therapeutic benefit. For example, if a dying patient were beyond resuscitation, cardiopulmonary resuscitation (CPR) would clearly be futile. (So too would CPR which would succeed only in resuscitating a patient who is close to death. It would serve only to prolong the dying process, which is not a proper goal of medicine.)

It is also widely agreed that it is not in a patient's best interests to be subjected to a treatment which offers a reasonable hope of therapeutic benefit but which would inflict excessive burdens on the patient. For example, the possible benefits of courses of chemotherapy might be outweighed by their burdensome side-effects.

So far, so uncontroversial. But does the law go further? Does it allow a doctor to withhold and withdraw treatment and tube-feeding not because the *treatment* is worthless (as being either futile or too burdensome) but because the doctor thinks that the patient's *life* is worthless? In 1993, that question was answered by the Law Lords in the Tony Bland case.

The Tony Bland case

Tony Bland was crushed into unconsciousness during the Hillsborough football stadium disaster. He was admitted to hospital and was later diagnosed as being in a 'persistent vegetative state' (PVS). He was fed by nasogastric tube. His parents and doctor wanted to withdraw his tube-feeding but because of doubts about the lawfulness of this action the hospital applied for a judicial declaration that withdrawal would be lawful.

The barrister representing Tony opposed withdrawal. He argued that removing Tony's tube-feeding would be murder: it would be just like severing the air-pipe of a deep-sea diver. The High Court disagreed, and granted the declaration. Its decision was affirmed by the Court of Appeal and by the Law Lords. Tony's tube-feeding was withdrawn and he died.

Why was it not murder? In summary, the Law Lords reasoned as follows.

1. Murder consists of the intentional termination of life by an act and may be committed *by omission* only where there is a *legal duty to act*. (If a father deliberately let his infant daughter starve to death he could not escape a murder conviction on the ground that he killed her by omission: parents are under a legal duty to feed their children.)
2. Withdrawal of Tony's tube-feeding was an *omission*.
3. And it was an omission not of *basic care* (which his doctor might be thought to be under a virtually absolute duty to provide) but of *medical treatment*.
4. His doctor was under *no duty to continue* this treatment because it was *not in Tony's best interests*.
5. It was not in his best interests because it was *futile*.
6. And it was futile because *life in persistent vegetative state was not a benefit, at least in the opinion of a responsible body of doctors.*
7. In short, the Law Lords held that Tony's tube-feeding was no longer worthwhile because his *life* was no longer worthwhile, at least in the opinion of a responsible body of doctors. Indeed, most of the Law Lords held withdrawal lawful *even though they thought that the doctor's intention was to kill Tony.*

Part II. Professional guidance

In 1999, the BMA published guidance concerning the withholding and withdrawal of medical treatment (which, like the Law Lords in *Bland*, it defines, not uncontroversially, to include tube-feeding). A second edition, lightly revised in the wake of the incorporation into English law of the European Convention on Human Rights, appeared in 2001.

The guidance endorses those court decisions which have granted competent patients a seemingly absolute right to refuse treatment, whether the refusal relates to a currently proposed treatment or treatment during a future period of incompetence.

In relation to incompetent patients, the guidance states that the primary goal of treatment is to benefit the patient by restoring or maintaining health, maximising benefit and minimising harm. Does it take the view that a patient may be better off dead?

On the one hand, the guidance holds that the criterion governing non-treatment decisions should be the worth of the treatment, not the worth of the patient. Moreover, the guidance opposes the active intentional killing of patients. On the other hand, however, the guidance endorses the law as laid down in the *Bland* case. It is difficult to see how the guidance can endorse that law without also embracing the notion that the lives of some patients are no longer worthwhile and that it is unacceptable to withhold or withdraw treatment (and tube-feeding) for that reason, and with intent to kill.

Part III. Three ethical questions

Parts I and II give rise to at least three major ethical questions.

1. Do the law and BMA guidance permit 'passive euthanasia'?

'Passive euthanasia' is not used here to mean the withholding or withdrawal of treatment which a doctor *foresees* will shorten the patient's life. A doctor whose intention (aim) is to withhold or withdraw a life-preserving treatment because it is futile or too burdensome, merely foreseeing that the patient will therefore die sooner, is not committing passive euthanasia. Rather, passive euthanasia means the *intentional* hastening of the patient's death by withholding or withdrawing treatment: where causing death is the doctor's aim. Passive euthanasia is not about stopping treatments the doctor thinks worthless, but stopping lives the doctor thinks worthless. The Law Lords in *Bland* explicitly condoned the intentional termination of the life of a patient which was judged by 'a responsible body of medical opinion' no longer to be a benefit to the patient. The law therefore permits passive euthanasia, at least of patients in PVS.

This leaves the law, as one of the Law Lords put it in *Bland*, in a 'morally and intellectually misshapen' state. The law prohibits, as murder, the intentional hastening of a patient's death by an act but permits the intentional hastening of a patient's death by withholding or withdrawing treatment. Yet there is surely no moral difference between giving a patient a lethal injection of potassium chloride, and intentionally starving a patient to death by withdrawing tube-feeding.

What about the BMA guidance? In short, it is difficult to read its endorsement of *Bland* as anything other than an endorsement of passive euthanasia.

2. Are the law and BMA guidance on a 'slippery slope'?

The Law Lords were careful to limit their judgments to PVS. For example, one commented that he expressed no opinion whether his decision would be the same if the patient had 'glimmerings of awareness'. The BMA guidance, however, exhibits no such reservations; it goes beyond PVS and applies to those with advanced dementia and serious stroke.

Nevertheless, it is likely that when a case comes to court in which a doctor wishes (say) to withdraw tube-feeding from a patient with advanced dementia in accordance with the BMA guidance, the court will declare withdrawal lawful, even if the doctor's intent is to kill. There are three reasons why the courts are likely to follow the BMA.

First, the court would be likely to hold that the BMA guidance reflects the views of a 'responsible body of medical opinion' and that a doctor who acts in accordance with it is therefore acting reasonably and lawfully.

Secondly, the ethical proposition informing *Bland* is that there are certain patients whose lives are no longer worth living. Once the courts have accepted that such a category of patients exists, it is difficult to see how they can sensibly limit it to patients in PVS. The category of 'worthless lives' is inherently arbitrary and liable to slippage.

Thirdly, courts in cases before and after *Bland*, cases that have not received as much attention, have held it lawful to withhold or withdraw treatment from patients who have some degree of awareness. For example, in one case the question was whether an infant who was physically and mentally disabled should be ventilated if it stopped breathing. The Court of Appeal held that ventilation could be withheld if the child's 'quality of life' after ventilation would be 'so afflicted as to be intolerable to that child'.

'Quality of life' is a chameleon phrase. In one sense it can refer to an assessment of the patient's condition as it is now, and as it would be after a proposed treatment, in order to determine whether the treatment would improve the patient's condition and whether the *treatment* would therefore be worthwhile. Its use in this manner is ethically uncontroversial; it implies no judgment about the worth of the patient's life.

But 'quality of life' can also be used in another, ethically controversial sense, as part of assessment whether, however successful the treatment, the *patient's life* would be worth living. It was clearly in this second sense that the phrase was used by the Court of Appeal. It was the baby's life, not the ventilation, which it regarded as 'intolerable'.

3. Do the law and BMA guidance permit passive assistance in suicide?

The right to refuse futile or excessively burdensome treatments is ethically uncontroversial. But a right to refuse treatment *in order to kill oneself* is not. The right to refuse treatment conceded by the law and the guidance, because it is unqualified, appears to extend to even suicidally motivated refusals. The law and guidance therefore appear to endorse a right to commit suicide. This inevitably undermines the opposition of the law and the BMA to active assistance in suicide. For, if there is a right to commit suicide why is it wrong intentionally to assist someone to exercise this right?

Indeed, the courts and guidelines appear to allow doctors intentionally to assist suicidal refusals. That is, they appear to allow doctors to withhold or withdraw treatment in accordance with a clearly suicidal refusal even if the doctor's intention is to assist the patient's suicidal enterprise. In other words, they appear to allow passive assistance in suicide.

Conclusion

By reasoning that to cause Tony Bland's death by withdrawing his tube-feeding with intent to kill was not murder, because it was an omission and not an act, the Law Lords were distracted from the sound moral distinction between *intending* and *foreseeing* death by the morally irrelevant distinction between killing a patient *by an act* and killing a patient *by omission*. Hence the 'morally and intellectually misshapen' state of the law, and of the BMA guidance which has embraced it.

The courts' and the BMA guidance's apparent endorsement of suicide and assisted suicide by omission tracks the same irrelevant moral distinction between acts and omissions.

The courts and the BMA would have avoided moral and intellectual misshapenness had they reasoned as follows:

1. that doctors are under an absolute duty not to try to kill their patients, whether by act or omission;
2. that it is proper to withdraw futile treatments, even if an earlier death is foreseen as certain;
3. and *either* that tube-feeding patients in PVS is futile (because it cannot serve the core purpose of medicine of restoring the patient to health), and may therefore be withdrawn;
4. *or* that tube-feeding a PVS patient is, at least once it has been instituted, basic care which must, in general, be continued;
5. and that competent patients have a right to refuse treatment, but no right to commit suicide or to be assisted in suicide, and that doctors should not intentionally assist suicidal refusals.

Further reading

Keown, J. (2002). Euthanasia, ethics and public policy. An argument against legalisation. Cambridge: Cambridge University Press.

Montgomery, J. (2003). Health Care Law. 2nd Edition. Oxford: Oxford University Press.

Chapter 18

The management of the last 48 hours of life: The Liverpool Integrated Care Pathway for the Dying Patient

John Ellershaw

What are integrated care pathways?

There is an increasing movement in healthcare towards continuous quality improvement and guideline based practice. The focus is to promote high quality, efficient, cost-effective care. An integrated care pathway provides a flowsheet that outlines the expected and realistic course of a patient's care. Each episode can be described, tracked and monitored to ensure that intermediate and final outcomes are within an accepted range of quality. A pathway specifies an agreed plan of care by contributing professionals—including members of the core professional team and those who are on the periphery (Kitchener *et al.* 1996; Berwick 1996; Zander *et al.* 1994). If a pathway is not followed at any point, the healthcare professional records a reason for the deviation as a 'variance'. Analysis of this variance provides a mechanism for analysing the reasons for not achieving the desired outcomes of care. It is an important part of implementing and using the care pathway that variances are analysed and acted on when appropriate, this includes education, training and resource issues.

Integrated care pathways promote an outcome-based culture; education therefore plays an important role in the introduction of a care pathway. For the integrated care pathway to be successful, all professionals must use this document in place of previous documentation. In this way, it becomes a central organising tool for clinical activity and is an ideal model for multiprofessional notes.

Integrated care pathways and palliative care

Care pathways are used to plan and document care for patients and can provide a method of co-ordinating and standardising care across geographical settings. They are potentially appropriate tools for developing, monitoring and improving the delivery of palliative care in hospice, hospital and community.

Palliative care has developed a model of excellence in the care of the dying patient (National Council of Hospice and Specialist Palliative Services 1997). However, there has been concern that this model of excellence is poorly understood and practised outside the specialist palliative care unit or hospice setting. Important steps in the care of the dying are often considered to be routine in a palliative care setting but may be partially or poorly performed in other health care environments. As only 12% of all deaths in the UK occur in a hospice setting (Office of National Statistics 2000), it is essential to capture this model of excellence in the care of the dying so it can be translated for use by all healthcare professionals. This is endorsed by the National Cancer Plan, which states 'the care of the dying must improved to the level of the best' (Department of Health 2000*a*). The issue of improved care of the dying has also been highlighted in other National Service Frameworks (see Figure 18.1).

National Service Framework for Coronary Heart Disease
'When the underlying aim of treatment is to control symptoms, a palliative approach with help from palliative care specialists can improve a patient's quality of life.' (Department of Health 2000*b*).

National Service Framework for Older People
'In stroke where recovery is not possible, this should be recognised by staff. The care of the patient should be discussed with them as far as possible and with their carers as appropriate. The principles of palliative care should inform the care plan, with priority being given to supporting the patient to die with dignity, without unnecessary suffering and in the place of their choice wherever possible'. (Department of Health 2001).

National Cancer Plan
'Too many patients will experience distressing symptoms, poor nursing care, poor psychological and social support and inadequate communication from healthcare professionals during the final stages of an illness. This can have a lasting effect on carers and those close to the patient, who often carry the burden of care. The care of all dying patients must improve to the level of the best' (Department of Health 2000a).

Figure 18.1 Quotes from National Service Frameworks relating to Care of the Dying

The Liverpool Integrated Care Pathway for the Dying Patient

In response to this need to transfer the hospice model of care of the dying patient to other settings, the Royal Liverpool University Hospitals and the Marie Curie Centre in Liverpool have developed the Liverpool Integrated Care Pathway for the Dying Patient (LCP). The LCP gives the clinical freedom to provide care within an evidence-based framework, and acts as a multiprofessional document which staff can use to co-ordinate and record the care of the dying patient (Ellershaw & Wilkinson 2003).

The LCP highlights the need to deliver holistic care during the dying phase and gives guidance on the different aspects of care required. It particularly recognises the areas of care which may present most difficulties such as recognising that a patient is entering the terminal phase of their illness. The multiprofessional emphasis ensures that all team members are involved in the decision making process.

The average length of time that a patient is cared for on the pathway is 48 h, although the range can vary from a few hours up to ten days. There is also a Care after Death Section which looks at the immediate support and bereavement needs of the patient's family.

The practical problems of implementing the LCP and delivering a high standard of care for the dying patient should not be underestimated. First, there needs to be an executive-level decision to implement the LCP within the organisation, followed by a comprehensive educational programme about the aims and use of the LCP. It may take 6–12 months to introduce the LCP into a new clinical area.

Components of the LCP

1. Initial assessment and care of the dying patient (see Figure 18.2)

Cancer patients in the final stages of their illness generally become weaker and spend a greater proportion of time in bed. They are more drowsy and less able to tolerate fluids, food or oral medication. A diagnosis of dying can be made using these criteria which will allow the team caring for the patient to deliver active and appropriate care. A team approach to the diagnosis of dying avoids giving conflicting messages to the family and/or carers. The pathway uses several criteria to facilitate this diagnosis of dying:

- a reduction in consciousness;
- an inability to take medication;
- becoming bed-bound;
- only able to take sips of fluid.

It is important to recognise that these criteria cannot always be extended to non-cancer patients, because the course of the terminal phase may vary in different disease processes.

The pathway identifies that the active care of a dying patient should include:

- reviewing the medication;
- discontinuing non-essential medication;
- the prescribing of p.r.n. (as required) medication for pain, agitation, nausea/vomiting and respiratory-tract secretions according to agreed guidelines.

It also highlights the need to discuss that the patient is dying with the family and ensure that the religious and spiritual needs of the patient are addressed.

Comfort measures

Goal 1: current medication assessed and non essentials discontinued.

Goal 2: as required subcutaneous medication written up as per protocol (pain, agitation, respiratory tract secretions, nausea and vomiting).

Goal 3: discontinue inappropriate interventions (blood tests, antibiotics, intravenous fluids/medications—not for cardiopulmonary resuscitation documented, turning regimes/vital signs).

Psychological/insight

Goal 4: ability to communicate in English assessed as adequate (translator not needed).

Goal 5: insight into condition assessed.

Religious/spiritual support

Goal 6: religious/spiritual needs assessed with patient/family.

Communication with family/other

Goal 7: identify how family/other are to be informed of patients impending death.

Goal 8: family/other given relevant hospital information; communication with primary healthcare team.

Goal 9: general practitioner is aware of patient's condition.

Summary

Goal 10: plan of care explained and discussed with patient/family.

Goal 11: family/other express understanding of plan of care.

Figure 18.2 Initial assessment and care goals for patients in the dying phase (adapted from the LCP (Ellershaw *et al.* 2003))

2. Ongoing care of the dying patient

The pathway emphasises the importance of regular patient review with at least observations every 4 h of symptom control and the need to act appropriately if there are any problems. Particular attention is given to pain, agitation, respiratory secretions, nausea and vomiting, mouth care and micturition problems. It is of vital importance to consider psychological and spiritual support for the family and patient.

3. Care of family and carers after death of the patient

After the patient's death the pathway focuses on the care and support of the family and carers. It includes catering for the information needs of the family and any special requests about the care of the body.

Clinical effectiveness of the integrated care pathway for the dying patient

1. Education

Key educational objectives to overcoming the barriers in caring for the dying can be identified (see Figure 18.3).

---

1. To be able to communicate sensitively regarding issues related to death and dying.

2. To work as a member of a multiprofessional team.

3. To be able to prescribe appropriately for dying patients:
   (a) to discontinue inappropriate medication;
   (b) to convert oral to subcutaneous medication;
   (c) to prescribe as needed medication appropriately including for pain and agitation;
   (d) to prescribe subcutaneous drugs for delivery by a syringe driver.

4. To be competent in the use of a syringe driver.

5. To recognise the key signs and symptoms of the dying patient, i.e. being able to diagnose dying.

6. To describe an ethical framework which deals with issues related to the dying patient, including cardiopulmonary resuscitation, withholding and withdrawing treatment, foreshortening life and futility.

7. To appreciate cultural and religious traditions related to the dying phase.

8. To be aware of medico-legal issues.

9. To be able to refer appropriately to a specialist palliative care team.

Figure 18.3 Education objectives for care of the dying (Ellershaw & Ward (2003), with permission from the BMJ Publishing Group)

The LCP provides a framework to support these educational objectives. Medical education is increasingly recognising the importance of care for dying patients and it is a core objective identified in '*Tomorrow's doctors*' (General Medical Council 2002) directing the development of the undergraduate medical curriculum. Recently, the Royal College of Physicians has produced generic competencies for all physicians in training and care of the dying is identified as a core skill (Joint Committee on Higher

Medical Training 2003). The LCP can be incorporated into training to meet the educational objectives outlined in these documents. The fourth year medical students who are studying at the University of Liverpool are introduced to the use of the LCP while participating in a four-week placement within the specialist palliative care setting. As a result, they become familiar with the document and are therefore familiar with it when they begin work as house officers.

2. Improving care

The introduction of the LCP can have many benefits. It improves knowledge and helps staff caring for dying patients to acquire the necessary skills. It also empowers staff working outside specialist palliative care to deliver high quality, evidence based care to dying patients.

Variance

By analysis of individual variances, particular events and trends can be identified which may lead to resource issues or highlight educational needs. An example of this could be the need for additional specialised mattresses in the community or to provide a more favourable environment within a hospital setting for relatives. The analysis may also identify issues relating to symptom control; for example, accessibility to 'as required' drugs for pain and agitation in the dying phase. This analysis of variance is best done directly in the health care setting which then directly drives and influences change in clinical practice.

Promoting the palliative care approach

The LCP not only influences the care of the dying patient but also impacts on the care received by patients earlier in the course of their disease, particularly for improved symptom control and communication. It promotes specialist palliative care teams in hospital and community to be used more appropriately in their clinical and educational roles, by encouraging generic staff to become more skilled at dealing with the common problems experienced by palliative care patients.

3. Clinical governance: setting standards

The LCP identifies demonstrable outcomes of care which can be audited and used to set standards and encourage reflective practice. The outcome measures represent the multidimensional nature of care, which includes the physical, psychological, social and spiritual concerns. These outcome measures can be measured in several care settings including specialist palliative care units (hospice), hospital settings in the community and in nursing homes. By auditing the care of the dying it can inform the clinical governance agenda and as a result promote best practice. It is not uncommon for complaints based in the acute setting to be linked with care of the dying including poor symptom control and poor communication. The LCP can therefore act as a tool to help prevent such complaints and also the complex bereavement issues that may arise from them.

4. Research

Analysis of the LCP provides an evidence base for care of the dying, which has not previously not been described. The current evidence base about care of the dying is limited, partly because of the practicalities of researching within this difficult area of care and partly because of the ethical limitations of randomised trials in this patient cohort. However, the LCP provides an objective measurement about standard of care, and from this an evidence base is being developed. Analysis of symptoms of pain, respiratory tract secretions and agitation have been analysed in the last 48 h of life (Ellershaw *et al.* 2001). Pain control in patients who continue the transdermal fentanyl patch in the dying phase has also been investigated (Ellershaw *et al.* 2002). By providing an objective measurement for care of the dying, current development of practice can be influenced from a stronger research base than has previously been possible. Further work in this area is in progress.

Dissemination of the LCP

Over the past five years, study days have been established to describe and support the implementation of the LCP. Over 500 people have attended the foundation study day, and the advanced study day has been attended by those who wish to implement the pathway in their unit.

Currently, there are 121 services around the country at various stages of implementation of the LCP. It has been adopted locally within our cancer network for implementation in all care settings including the hospital, hospice, community and nursing home. An exciting advance is the development of a Dutch translation of the LCP, which is currently being piloted in the Rotterdam region. The Royal Liverpool University Hospital and The Marie Curie Centre Liverpool were awarded Beacon Status in September 2000. The Handbook was published in November 2001.

Conclusion

The LCP provides a template to enable healthcare professionals to deliver a model of excellence of care for dying patients. The pathway can be used to promote the educational role of specialist palliative care teams within generic care settings. It can also be used to help to set standards and assess quality assurance within a specialist palliative care unit. The LCP has a significant role to play in improving the care of the dying to the highest level.

References

Berwick, D. M. (1996). A primer on leading the improvement of systems. *British Medical Journal* **312**, 619–622.

Department of Health (2000*a*). *The NHS Cancer Plan – A Plan For Investment, A Plan For Reform*, chapter 7, p. 66.

Department of Health (2000*b*). *National Service Framework for Coronary Heart Disease*, chapter 6, p. 18, website www.doh.gov.uk/nsf

Department of Health (2001). *National Service Framework for Older People*, chapter 5, p. 23.

Ellershaw, J. E., Smith, C., Overill, S., Walker, S. E. & Aldridge, J. (2001). Care of the dying: setting standards for symptom control in the last 48 hours of life *Journal of Pain and Symptom Management* **21**, 12–17.

Ellershaw, J. E., Kinder, C., Aldridge, J., Allison, M. & Smith, J. (2002). Care of the dying: is pain control compromised or enhanced by continuation of the fentanyl transdermal patch in the dying phase? *Journal of Pain and Symptom Management* **24**, 398–403.

Ellershaw, J. E. & Ward, C. (2003). Care of the dying patient: the last hours or days of life. *British Medical Journal* **326**, 30–34.

Ellershaw, J. E. & Wilkinson, S. (eds) (2003). *Care for the dying: a pathway to excellence.* Oxford: Oxford University Press.

General Medical Council (2002). *Tomorrow's doctors – recommendations on undergraduate medical education.* London: General Medical Council.

Joint Committee on Higher Medical Training (2003). *Higher medical training – generic curriculum.* London: Joint Committee on Higher Medical Training.

Kitchiner, D., Davidson, C. & Bundred, P. (1996). Integrated care pathways: effective tools for continuous evaluation of clinical practice. *Journal of Evaluation in Clinical Practice* **2**, 650–669.

NHS Modernisation Agency (2001). *NHS beacon learning handbook – spreading good practice across the NHS*, volume 4, p. 128.

Office of National Statistics (2000). www.statisticss.gov.uk/downloads/theme_health/DHI_33/Table17.xls; http://www.statistics.gov.uk

Working Party of Clinical Guidelines in Palliative Care (1997). *Changing Gear. Guidelines for managing last days of life in adults.* National Council of Hospice and Specialist Palliative Care Services. Northamptonshire: Land and Unwin (Data Sciences) Ltd.

Zander, K. & McGill, R. (1994). Critical and anticipated recovery paths: only the beginning. *Nursing Management* **25**, 34–40.

Index